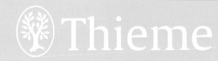
Before you begin,
you should read the
Some Practical Hints on the
facing infold. They will help you
make the most of all the practical aspects
of the book; for example, finding a particular
stucture, and will enable you to optimize your
learning efforts. The manual contains a system
of numbered legends to consult when you are
repeating a chapter or simply brushing up your
knowledge. Each chapter closes with several
Test Yourself! questions, the solutions to which
are at the back of the book. Most CT images
are accompanied by gray scale drawings
that indicate the type of tissue
or organ according to the
following examples:

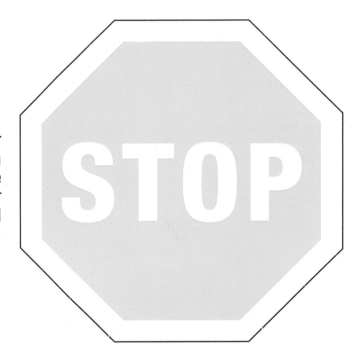

Schemata for CT Drawings

All the drawings have been done according to a gray scale. Air or gas, regardless of where they are found, are black; bone is white. Between these extremes, the shading varies for tissues, organs, and abnormalities independent of the image display settings. In addition, abnormalities such as metastases can be recognized by their specific patterns.

Air (black)

in the trachea

in the colon

Fat or CSF (charcoal)

Muscle (dark gray)

transverse section

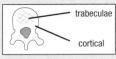
longitudinal section

Bone (white)

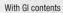
trabeculae

cortical

Blood vessels (light gray)

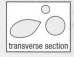
transverse section

longitudinal section

Pancreas, salivary glands

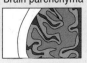

Parenchyma of larger organs (medium gray)

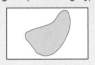

Small intestine (thin walls)

With GI contents

With some CM

With dense CM

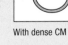

Colon with fecal residue and gas

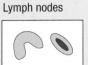

Lymph nodes

Brain parenchyma

Hemorrhage

Metastases

Library of Congress Cataloging-in-Publication Data
is available from the publisher.

Matthias Hofer, MD, MPH,
Master of Medical Education (MME)
Assistant Professor for Diagnostic Radiology,
Director of Education, Institute for Diagnostic,
Interventional and Pediatric Radiology (DIPR),
Head: Professor Johannes Heverhagen, MD
Inselspital Bern, Bern University, Switzerland

Contributor: Ingrid Boehm, MD, Assistant Professor
for Diagnostic Radiology, (DIPR)
Inselspital Bern, Bern University, Switzerland

PET/CT images from

Professor Gerald Antoch, MD
Director, Institute for Diagnostic,
Pediatric and Interventional Radiology
Heinrich Heine University, Düsseldorf, Germany

Till-Alexander Heusner, MD
Professor for Diagnostic Radiology
Head of Radiology Dept.
Sankt Elisabeth Hospital, Gütersloh, Germany

© 2021. Thieme. All rights reserved.
Georg Thieme Verlag KG
Rüdigerstrasse 14, D-70469 Stuttgart, Germany
www.thieme.de

New parts translated by
John Grossman, Schrepkow, Germany
www.john-grossman.com

Cover Design: Thieme Publishing Group
Cover Image source - the cover image was
composed by Thieme using the following images:
Siemens Healthineers CT SOMATOM Force:
© Siemens Healthcare GmbH, 2020
Cardiac Images: Deutsches Herzzentrum, München, Germany
Hepatic PET/CT Images: Professor Gerald Antoch,
Düsseldorf, Germany

Typesetting by Ramona Sprenger, Cologne, Germany
www.einraumapartment.de

Printed in Germany by
Druckerei Steinmeier, Deiningen

DOI 10.1055/b000000534

ISBN 978-3-13-244263-4   5 4 3 2 1

Also available as an ebook:
eISBN (PDF):   978-3-13-244264-1
eISBN (ePub):   978-3-13-244265-8

1st	German edition	1997	1st	Korean edition	2006
1st	English edition	1998	3rd	English edition	2007
2nd	German edition	1999	2nd	Italian edition	2007
1st	Spanish edition	2000	1st	Polish edition	2007
3rd	German edition	2000	1st	Greek edition	2008
2nd	Spanish edition	2003	2nd	Russian edition	2008
4th	German edition	2003	6th	German edition	2008
1st	Italian edition	2005	2nd	Brazilian edition	2010
1st	Portuguese edition	2005	7th	German edition	2010
3rd	Spanish edition	2005	4th	English edition	2010
2nd	English edition	2005	8th	German edition	2014
1st	Brazilian edition	2005	9th	German edition	2016
1st	Russian edition	2006	10th	German edition	2021
5th	German edition	2006	5th	English edition	2021

Computed tomography has become an integral and indispensable part of clinical diagnostics, with which special clinical questions can be answered with high accuracy in only a short time latency. The recent technical developments enable a spatial resolution in the submillimeter range for CT-supported angiographies, and with the help of dual source CT, also statements about the chemical composition of tissues or e.g. kidney stones. Above all, the development of PET/CT has made possible immense progress in oncology with regard to the diagnostic accuracy in the question of metastases or tumor recurrences. Modern imaging modalities are often not satisfactorily covered when teaching medical students in lectures and clinical courses. When leaving medical school, the knowledge gaps in this area can often be considerable.

All these aspects and recent developments have already been taken into account in this standard book on CT diagnostics, so that it offers the necessary basics for beginners, who are just familiarizing themselves with the subject, and is suitable for advanced users with a special radiological interest. The quiz cases, in particular, will hopefully arouse many readers` detective ambition to check their diagnostic skills themselves. The success story of 28 editions in 9 languages speaks for itself, and proves the broad acceptance of this book among German-speaking and international colleagues. I wish you a high learning benefit and lots of fun using this teaching manual!

Bern, January 2021

Professor Johannes Heverhagen, MD
Dept. Head of University Institute for Diagnostic,
Interventional and Pediatric Radiology (DIPR)
Inselspital Bern, Bern University, Switzerland

List of Abbreviations

3D	Three-dimensional	ESWL	Extracorporal shock wave lithotripsy	NHL	Non-Hodgkin Lymphoma
a, ant.	Anterior	FDG	Fluorodeoxyglucose: a form of sugar,	Nn.	Nerves
A.	Artery		marked with radioactive	NPP	Nucleus pulposus prolapse
Aa.	Arteries		short-living tracers	PET	Positron Emission Tomograhy
ADR	Adverse drug reaction	FET	Fluorethylthyrosin (radioactive tracer)	p.i.	Post injection
AG	Adrenal gland	FNH	Focal nodular hyperplasia of the liver	Pixel	Picture element (two-dimensional)
Amp.	Ampulla	FOV	Field of view	PNS	Paranasal sinuses
AO	Aorta	GB	Gallbladder	p.o.	Per oral
AP	Anteroposterior	GIT	Gastrointestinal tract	post.	Posterior
AR	Area = size of an ROI in cm^2	HCC	Hepatocellular carcinoma	PRIND	Prolonged reversible ischemic
BBB	Blood-brain barrier	HRCT	High resolution CT		neurologic deficit
BC	Bronchial carcinoma	HU	Hounsfield unit(s)	Proc.	Process
BE	Barium enema	i.m.	Intramuscular	PSMA	Prostate-specific membrane antigen
BT	Bolus tracking	IM	Intramuscular	ROI	Region of interest
BW	Body weight	i.v.	Intravenous	RT	Renal transplant
Ca	Carcinoma	IV	Intravenous	s.c.	Subcutaneous
CAD	Coronary artery disease	IUD	Intrauterine device	SC	Subcutaneous
CARE	Combined applications to reduce exposure	IVU	Intravenous urogram	SAC	Subarachnoid space
CCT	Cranial CT	kg	Kilogram	SAH	Subarachnoid hemorrhage
CCT	Craniocerebral trauma	LA	Lower abdomen	SD	Standard deviation
ChE	Cholecystectomy	lat.	Lateral	SMA	Superior mesenteric artery
CI	Cortical index	Lig.	Ligament	ST	Section or slice thickness
CKD-EPI	Chronic Kidney Disease	LL	Lower leg	SUV$_{max}$	Maximum standardized uptake value
	Epidemiologic Collaboration	LN	Lymph node	TACE	Transarterial chemoembolization
CM	Contrast medium	L-spine	Lumbar spine	Tg	Thyroid gland
CN	Cranial nerve	LV	Lumbar vertebra	TIA	Transient ischemic attack
CSF	Cerebrospinal fluid	mBq	millibequerel (unit for radiation)	T-spine	Thoracic spine
C-spine	Cervical spine	M.	Muscle	TV	Thoracic vertebra
CT	Computed tomography	MA	Mid abdomen	UA	Upper abdomen
CTA	CT angiography	ME	Mean	UB	Urinary bladder
CV	Cervical vertebra	med.	Medial	UGI	Upper GI series
d	Diameter or day	MIP	Maximum intensity projection	UL	Upper leg
DD	Differential diagnosis	Mm.	Muscles	V.	Vein
DOTATOC	Edotreotid (radioactive tracer)	MPR	Multiplanar reconstruction	Vol	Volume
DIC	Disseminated intravascular coagulopathy	MRI	Magnetic resonance imaging	Voxel	Voxel element (three-dimensional)
ECG	Electrocardiogram	MSCT	Multislice CT	Vv.	Veins
ERCP	Endoscopic retrograde	mSv	millisievert (unit for radiation)		
	cholangiopancreatography	N.	Nerve		

4   Table of Contents

Table of Contents

General Principles of CT

Computed tomography is a special type of x-ray procedure that involves the indirect measurement of the weakening, or attenua-tion, of x-rays at numerous positions located around the patient being investigated. Basically speaking, all we know is

- what leaves the x-ray tube,
- what arrives at the detector and
- the position of the x-ray tube and detector for each position.

Simply stated, everything else is deduced from this information. Most CT slices are oriented vertical to the body`s axis. They are usually called axial or transverse sections. For each section the x-ray tube rotates around the patient to obtain a preselected section thickness (Fig. 6.1). Most CT systems employ the continuous rotation and fan beam design: with this design, the x-ray tube and detector are rigidly coupled and rotate continuously around the scan field while x-rays are emitted and detected. Thus, the x-rays, which have passed through the patient, reach the detectors on the opposite side of the tube. The fan beam opening ranges from 40° to 60°, depending on the particular system design, and is defined by the angle originating at the focus of the x-ray tube and extending to the outer limits of the detector array.

Typically, images are produced for each 360° rotation, permitting a high number of measurement data to be acquired and sufficient dose to be applied. While the scan is being performed, attenuation profiles, also referred to as samples or projections, are obtained. Attenuation profiles are really nothing other than a collection of the signals obtained from all the detector channels at a given angular position of the tube-detector unit. Modern CT systems (Fig. 6.4) acquire approximately 1400 projections over 360°, or about four projections per degree. Each attenuation profile comprises the data obtained from about 1500 detector channels, about 30 channels per degree in case of a 50° fan beam. While the patient table is moving continuously through the gantry, a digital radiograph ("scanogramm" or "localizer", Fig. 6.2) is produced on which the desired sections can be planned. For a CT examination of the spine or the head, the gantry is angled to the optimal orientation (Fig. 6.3).

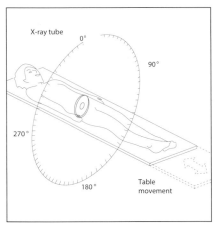

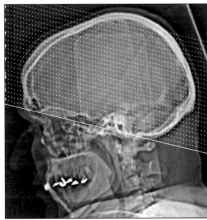

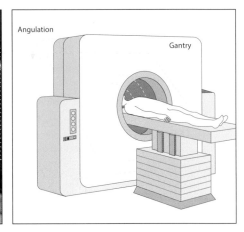

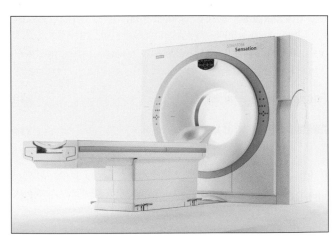

Multiple-Row Detector Spiral CT

Multiple-row detector CT (MDCT) is the latest scanner development. Rather than one detector row, multiple detector rows are placed opposite the x-ray tube. This shortens the examination time and improves the temporal resolution, allowing, for instance, the determination of the rate of vascular enhancement.

The detector rows along the z-axis opposite the x-ray tube are unequal in width, with the outer rows wider than the inner rows to provide better conditions for image reconstruction after data acquisition (see pages 9-11 and 206).

Dual Source CT

This newest technique features two detector units and two X-ray tubes in one gantry and is described in more detail on pages 198-201.

Comparison of Conventional CT with Spiral CT

In conventional CT, a series of equally spaced images is acquired sequentially through a specific region, e.g. the abdomen or the head (Fig. 7.1). There is a short pause after each section in order to advance the patient table to the next preset position. The section thickness and overlap/intersection gap are selected at the outset. The raw data for each image level is stored separately. The short pause between sections allows the conscious patient to breathe without causing major respiratory artifacts.

Both single-row detector CT (SDCT) and multiple-row detector CT (MDCT) continuously acquire data of the patient while the examination table moves through the gantry. The x-ray tube describes an apparent helical path around the patient (Fig. 7.2). If table advance is coordinated with the time required for a 360° rotation (pitch factor), data acquisition is complete and uninterrupted. This modern technique has greatly improved CT because respiratory artifacts and inconsistencies do not affect the single dataset as markedly as in conventional CT. The single dataset can be used to reconstruct slices of differing thickness or at differing intervals. Even overlapping slices can be reconstructed.

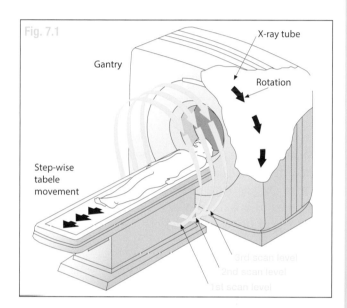

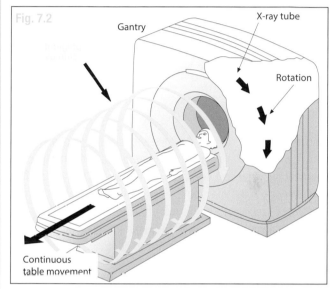

However, the examination may take several minutes, depending on the body region and the size of the patient. Proper timing of image acquisition after i.v. contrast media is particularly important for assessing perfusion effects. CT is the technique of choice for acquiring complete 2D axial images of the body without the disadvantages of superimposed bone and / or air as seen in conventional x-ray images.

In modern MDCT units with 16 up to 64 detector rows, data acquisition time for e.g. the thorax no longer exceeds the duration most patients can hold their breath: Even with narrow collimations, the entire thorax can be scanned within 7-10 seconds [47]. Even a CTA of the carotid arteries and circle of Willis with a pitch of 1.5 and rotation time of 0.37 seconds/rotation requires only 5 seconds for a scan range of 350 mm (64 x 0.6 mm collimation). Due to increased speed, most modern CT units would pass the renal excretion of CM, so that a longer delay time or a short break are required to document the patient`s renal excretion function. Therefore, the „neck of the bottle" in the workflow is no longer the data acquisition time, but sometimes the size of the corresponding data files in cases of complex MIP- / MPR-recontructions at the local workstation.

One of the advantages of the helical technique is that lesions smaller than the conventional thickness of a slice can be detected. Small liver metastases (**7**) will be missed if inconsistent depth

of respiration results in them not being included in the section (Fig. 7.3a). The metastases would appear in overlapping reconstructions from the dataset of the helical technique (Fig. 7.3b).

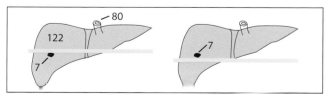

Fig. 7.3a Conventional CT

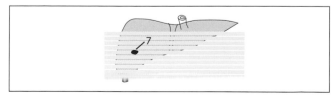

Fig. 7.3b Spiral-CT

Spatial Resolution

The reconstructed images should have a high temporal resolution to separate even small structures from each other. This generally creates no problem along the x- or y-axis of the image since the selected field of view (FOV) typically encompasses 1024 x 1024 or more picture elements (pixel). These pixels appear on the monitor as grey values proportionate to their attenuation (Fig. 8.1b). In reality, however, they are not squares but cubes (voxel = volume element) with their length along the body axis defined by the section thickness (Fig. 8.1a).

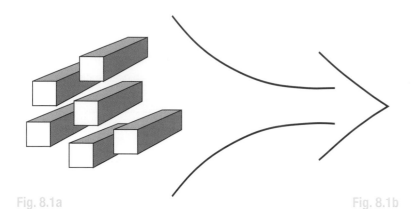

Fig. 8.1a

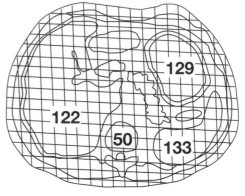

Fig. 8.1b

The image quality should improve with smaller voxels, but this only applies to the spatial resolution since a thinner section lowers the signal-to-noise ratio. Another disadvantage of thinner sections is the inevitable increase in the radiation dose to the patient (see page 175). Nonetheless, smaller voxels with identical measurements in all three dimensions (isotropic voxels) offer a crucial advantage: The multiplanar reconstruction (MPR) in coronal, sagittal or other planes displays the reconstructed images free of any step-like contour (Fig. 8.2). Using voxels of unequal dimension (anisotropic voxels) for MPR is burdened by a serrated appearance of the reconstructed images (Fig. 8.3), which, for instance, can make it difficult to exclude a fracture (Fig. 148.5b).

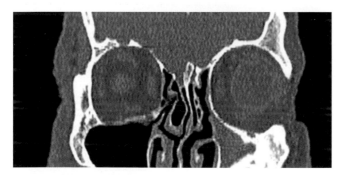

Fig. 8.2 MPR from isotropic voxels

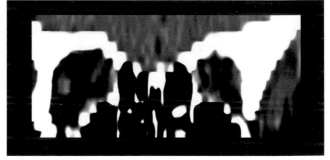

Fig. 8.3 MPR from anisotropic voxels

Pitch

By now, several definitions exist for the pitch, which describes the rate of table increment per rotation in millimeter and section thickness.

A slowly moving table per rotation generates a tight acquisition spiral (Fig. 8.4a). Increasing the table increment per rotation without changing section thickness or rotation speed creates interscan spaces of the acquisition spiral (Fig. 8.4b).

The mostly used definition of the pitch describes the table travel (feed) per gantry rotation, expressed in millimeters, and selected collimation, also expressed in millimeters.

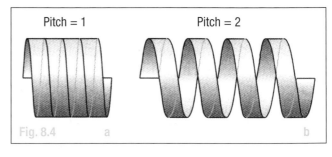

Pitch = 1   Pitch = 2

Fig. 8.4   a   b

$$\text{Pitch} = \frac{\text{Table travel / rotation}}{\text{Collimation}}$$

$$\text{Pitch} = \frac{\text{Feed / rotation}}{\text{Collimation}} \qquad \text{e.g.:} \quad \frac{24 \text{ mm / rotation}}{16 \times 1.5 \text{ mm}} = \frac{24 \text{ mm}}{24 \text{ mm}} = 1$$

Since the units (mm) in the numerator and denominator cancel out, the pitch is a dimensionless number. For a while, a so-called volume pitch was stated for multiple-row detector CT scanners, which relates the table feed to a single section rather than to the entire array of sections along the z-axis. For the example given above, this means a volume pitch of 24 mm / 1.5 mm = 16. However, there seems to be a trend to returning to the original definition of the pitch.

The new scanners give the examiner the option to select the craniocaudal extension (z-axis) of the region to be examined on the topogram as well as the rotation time, section collimation (thin or thick sections?) and examination time (breath-holding intervals?). The software, e.g., "SureView®," calculates the suitable pitch, usually providing values between 0.5 and 2.0.

Section Collimation: Resolution Along the Z-Axis

The resolution (along the body axis or z-axis) of the images can also be adapted to the particular clinical question by the choice of the collimation. Sections between 5 and 8 mm gen-erally are total-ly adequate for standard examinations of the abdomen. However, the exact localization of small fracture fragments or the evaluation of subtle pulmonary changes require thin slices between 0.5 and 2 mm. What determines the section thickness?

The term collimation describes how thin or thick the acquired slices can be preselected along the longitudinal axis of the patient (= z-axis). The examiner can limit the fan-like x-ray beam emitted from the x-ray tube by a collimator, whereby the collimator's aper-ture determines whether the fan passing through the collimator and collected by the detector units behind the patient is either wide (Fig. 9.1) or narrow (Fig. 9.2), with the narrow beam allow-ing a better spatial resolution along the z-axis of the patient. The collimator cannot only be placed next to the x-ray tube, but also in front of the detectors, i.e., "behind" the patient as seen from the x-ray source.

Depending on the width of collimator's aperture, the units

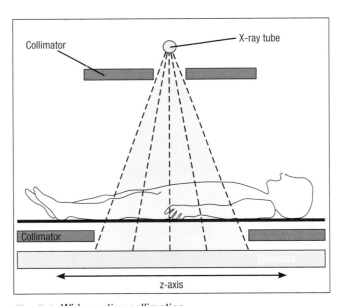

Fig. 9.1 Wide section collimation

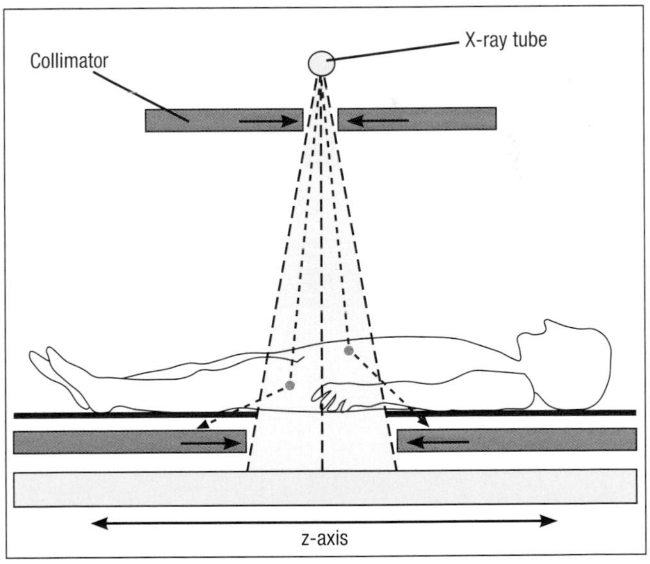

Fig. 9.2 Narrow section collimation

with only one detector row behind the patient (single section) can generate sections with a width of 10 mm, 8 mm, 5 mm or even 1 mm. A CT examination obtained with very thin sections is also called a high resolution CT (HRCT) and, if the sections are at the sub-millimeter level, ultra high reso-lution CT (UHRCT). The UHRCT is used for the petrous bone

with about 0.5 mm sections to detect delicate fracture lines through the cranial base or auditory ossicles in the tympanic cavity (see pages 46–49). For the liver, however, the exam-ination is dominated by the contrast resolution since the question here is the detectability of hepatic metastases (here somewhat thicker sections).

Adaptive Array Design

A further development of the single-slice spiral technology is the introduction of the multislice technique, which has not one detector rows but several detector rows stacked perpendicular to the z-axis opposite the x-ray source. This enables the simultaneous acquisition of several sections.

The detector rows are not inevitably equal in width. The adaptive array design consists of detectors that increase in width from the center to the edge of the detector ring and consequently allows various combinations of thickness and numbers of acquired sections.

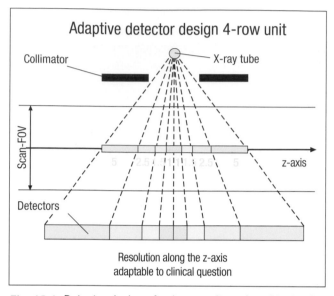

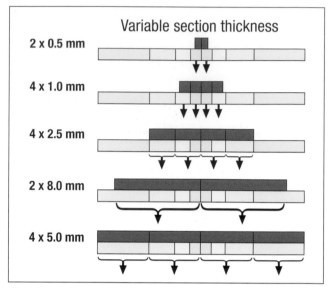

Fig. 10.1   Detector design of a 4-row unit, as found in the Siemens Sensation 4

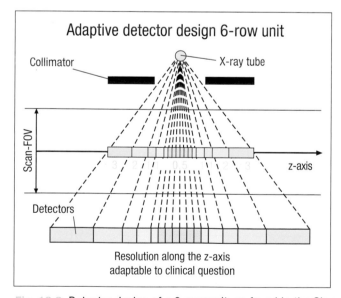

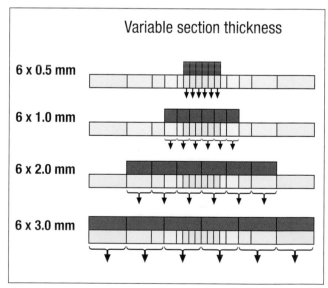

Fig. 10.2   Detector design of a 6-row unit, as found in the Siemens Emotion 6

For instance, a 16-slice examination can be performed with 16 thin sections of a higher resolution (for the Siemens Sensation 16, this means 16 x 0.75 mm) or with 16 sections of twice the thickness. For an iliofemoral CTA (see page 188), it is preferable to acquire a long volume along the z-axis in a single run, of course with a selected wide collimation of 16 x 1.5 mm.

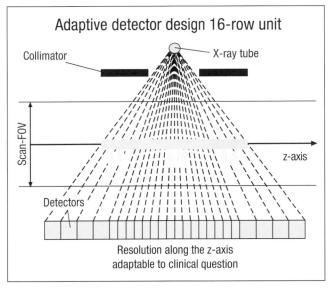

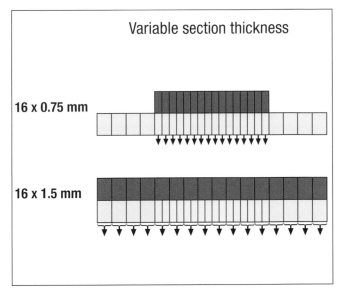

Fig. 11.1 Detector design of a 16-row unit, as found in the Siemens Sensation 16

The development of the CT hardware did not end with 16 slices and faster data acquisition can already be achieved with 32- and 64-row scanners. The trend to thinner slices is associated with higher patient exposure to radiation, requiring additional and already introduced measures for exposure reduction (see pages 174-177).

When both liver and pancreas are included, many users prefer a reduced slice thickness from 10 mm to 3 mm to improve image sharpness. This increases, however, the noise level by approxi-mately 80%. Therefore it would be necessary to employ 80% more mA or to lengthen the scan time (this increases the mAs product) to maintain image quality.

Reconstruction Algorithm

Spiral users have an additional advantage: In the spiral image reconstruction process, most of the data points were not actually measured in the particular slice being reconstructed (Fig. 11.2). Instead, data are acquired outside this slice (●) and interpolated with more importance, or "contribution", being attached to the data located closest to the slice (X). In other words: The data point closest to the slice receives more weight, or counts more, in the reconstruction of an image at the desired table position.

This results in an interesting phenomenon. The patient dose (actually given in mGy) is determined by the mAs per rotation divided by the pitch, and the image dose is equal to the mAs per rotation without considering the pitch. If for instance 150 mAs per rotation with a pitch of 1.5 are employed, the patient dose in mGy is linear related to 100 mAs, and the image dose is related to 150 mAs. Therefore spiral users can improve contrast detectability by selecting high mA values, increase

the spatial resolution (image sharpness) by reducing slice thickness, and employ pitch to adjust the length of the spiral range as desired, all while reducing the patient's dose! More slices can be acquired without increasing the dose or stressing the x-ray tube.

This technique is especially helpful when data are reformatted to create other 2D views, like sagittal, oblique, coronal, or 3D views (MIP, surface shaded imaging, see pp. 8 and 13).

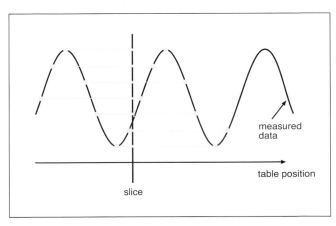

Fig. 11.2 Wide (360°) spiral reconstruction algorithm

The data obtained at the detector channel are passed on, profile for profile, to the detector electronics as electric signals corresponding to the actual x-ray attenuation. These electric signals are digitized and then transmitted to the image processor. At this stage, the images are reconstructed by means of the "pipeline principle", consisting of preprocessing, convolution, and back projection (Fig. 12.1).

Preprocessing includes all the corrections taken to prepare the measured scan data for reconstruction, e.g., correction for dark current, dose output, calibration, channel correction, beam hardening, and spacing errors. These corrections are performed to further minimize the slight variations inherently found in the tube and detector components of the imaging chain.

Convolution is basically the use of negative values to correct for smearing inherent to simple back projection. If, for instance, a cylindric water phantom is scanned and reconstructed without convolution, the edges of this phantom will be extremely blurry (Fig. 12.2a): What happens when just eight attenuation profiles of a small, highly absorbent cylindrical object are superimposed to create an image? Since the same part of the cylinder is measured by two overlapping projections, a star-shaped image is produced instead of what is in reality a cylinder. By introducing negative values just beyond the positive portion of the attenuation profiles, the edges of this cylinder can be sharply depicted (Fig. 12.2b).

Back projection involves the reassigning of the convolved scan data to a 2D image matrix representing the section of the patient that is scanned. This is performed profile for profile for the entire image reconstruction process. The image matrix can be thought of as analogous to a chessboard, consisting of typically 512 x 512 or 1024 x 1024 picture elements, usually called "pixels". Back projection results in an exact density being assigned to each of these pixels, which are then displayed as a lighter or darker shade of gray. The lighter the shade of gray, the higher the density of the tissue within the pixel (e.g., bone).

The Influence of kV

When examining anatomic regions with higher absorption (e.g., CT of the head, shoulders, thoracic or lumbar spine, pelvis, and larger patients), it is often advisable to use higher kV levels in addition to, or instead of, higher mA values: when you choose higher kV, you are hardening the x-ray beam. Thus x-rays can penetrate anatomic regions with higher absorption more easily. As a positive side effect, the lower energy components of the radiation are reduced, which is desirable since low energy x-rays are absorbed by the patient and do not contribute to the image. For imaging of infants or bolus tracking, it may be advisable to utilize kV lower than the standard setting.

Tube Current [mAs]

The tube current, stated in milliampere-seconds [mAs], also has a significant effect on the radiation dose delivered to the patient. A patient with more body width requires an increase in the tube current to achieve an adequate image quality. Thus, more corpulent patients receive a larger radiation dose than, for instance, children with a markedly smaller body width. Body regions with skeletal structures that absorb or scatter radiation, such as shoulder and pelvis, require a higher tube current than, for instance, the neck, a slender abdominal torso or the legs. This relationship has been actively applied to radiation protection for some time now (compare with page 177).

Scan Time

It is advantageous to select a scan time as short as possible, particularly in abdominal or chest studies where heart movement and peristalsis may degrade image quality. Other CT investigations can also benefit from fast scan times due to decreased probability of involuntary patient motion. On the other hand, it may be necessary to select a longer scan time to provide sufficient dose or to enable more samples for maximal spatial resolution. Some users may also consciously choose longer scan times to lower the mA setting and thus increase the likelihood of longer x-ray tube life.

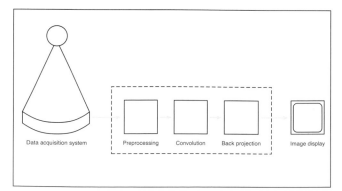

Fig. 12.1   The pipeline principle of image reconstruction

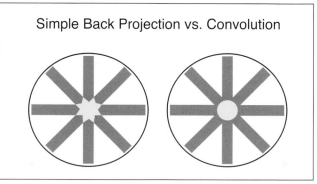

Fig. 12.2a   Back projection without convolution   Fig. 12.2b   Back projection with convolution

3D Reconstructions

Because the helical or spiral technique acquires a continuous, single volume dataset for an entire body region, imaging of fractures and blood vessels has improved markedly. Several different methods of 3D reconstruction have become established:

Maximal Intensity Projection

MIP is a mathematical method that extracts hyperintense voxels from 2D or 3D datasets [6, 7]. These voxels are selected from several different angles through the dataset and then projected as a 2D image (Fig. 13.1). A 3D impression is acquired by altering the projection angle in small steps and then viewing the reconstructed images in quick succession (i.e., in cine mode). This procedure is also used for examining contrast-enhanced blood vessels.

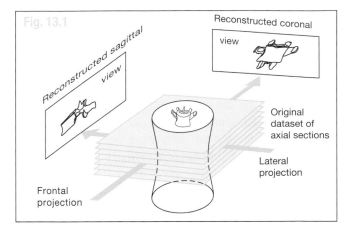

Fig. 13.1

Multiplanar Reconstruction

This technique makes it possible to reconstruct coronal and sagittal as well as oblique planes. MPR has become a valuable tool in the diagnosis of fractures and other orthopedic indications. For example, conventional axial sections do not always provide enough information about fractures. A good example is the undisplaced hairline fracture (*) without cortical discontinuity that can be more effectively demonstrated by MPR (Fig. 13.2a).

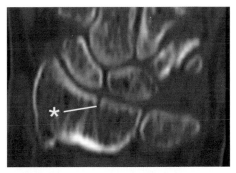

Fig. 13.2a

3D Surface Shaded Display

This method shows the surface of an organ or a bone that has been defined in Hounsfield units above a particular threshold value. The angle of view, as well as the location of a hypothetical source of light (from which the computer calculates shadowing) are crucial for obtaining optimal reconstructions. The fracture of the distal radius shown in the MPR in Figure 13.2a is seen clearly in the bone surface in Figure 13.2b.

(Figs. 13.2a and 13.2b supplied with the kind permission of J. Brackins Romero, M. D., Recklinghausen, Germany)

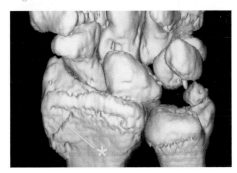

Fig. 13.2b

3D surface shaded displays are also valuable in planning surgery as in the case of the traumatic injury to the spinal column seen in Figures 13.3 a, b, and c. Since the angle of view can be freely determined, the thoracic compression fracture (*) and the state of the intervertebral foramina can be examined from several different angles (anterior in Fig. 13.3a and lateral in Fig. 13.3b). The sagittal MPR in Figure 13.3c determines whether any bone fragments have become dislocated into the spinal canal (compare with myelography CT on page 147).

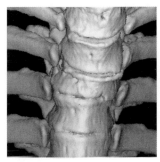

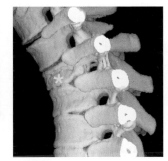

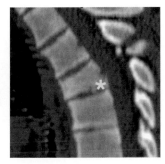

Fig. 13.3a

Fig. 13.3b

Fig. 13.3c

Anatomic Orientation

An image on the display is not only a 2D representation of anatomy, it contains information about the mean attenuation of tissue in a matrix consisting of about 1024 x 1024 elements (**pixels**). A section (Fig. 14.1) has a defined thickness (d_S) and is composed of a matrix of cubic or cuboid units (**voxels**) of identical size. This technical aspect is the reason for the partial volume effects explained below. An image is usually displayed as if the body were viewed from caudal. Thus the right side of the patient is on the left side of the image and vice versa (Fig. 14.1). For example, the liver (**122**) is located in the right half of the body, but appears in the left half of the image. Organs of the left side such as the stomach (**129**) and the spleen (**133**) appear on the right half of an image. Anterior aspects of the body, for example the abdominal wall, are represented in the upper parts of an image, posterior aspects such as the spine (**50**) are lower. With this system CT images are more easily compared with conventional x-ray-images.

Fig. 14.1

Partial Volume Effects

The radiologist determines the thickness of the image (d_S). 4–6 mm are usually chosen for thoracic or abdominal examinations, and 2–5 mm for the skull, spine, orbits, or petrosal bones. A structure may therefore be included in the entire thickness of a slice (Fig. 14.2a) or in only a part of it (Fig. 14.3a). The gray scale value of a voxel depends on the mean attenuation of all structures within it. If a structure has a regular shape within a section, it will appear well defined. This is the case for the abdominal aorta (**89**) and the inferior vena cava (**80**) shown in Figures 14.2a, b.

Partial volume effects occur when structures do not occupy the entire thickness of a slice, for example when a section includes part of a vertebral body (**50**) and part of a disk (**50e**) the anatomy will be poorly defined (Figs. 14.3a, b). This is also true if an organ tapers within a section as seen in Figures 14.4a, b. This is the reason for the poor definition of the renal poles or the borders of the gallbladder (**126**) or urinary bladder. Artifacts caused by breathing during image acquisition are discussed on page 19.

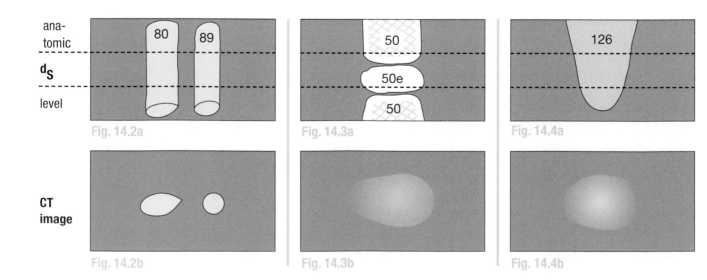

Fig. 14.2a

Fig. 14.3a

Fig. 14.4a

Fig. 14.2b

Fig. 14.3b

Fig. 14.4b

Distinguishing Between Nodular and Tubular Structures

It is essential to differentiate between possibly enlarged or affected LNs and vessels or muscles which have been cut in transverse section. This may be extremely difficult in a single image because these structures have similar density values (gray tones). One should therefore always analyze adjacent cranial and caudal images and compare the structures in question to determine whether they are nodular swellings or continue as more or less tubular structures (Fig. 15.1): A lymph node (**6**) will appear in only one or two slices and cannot be traced in adjacent images (compare Figs. 15.1a, b, and c). The aorta (**89**) or the inferior cava (**80**), or a muscle, for example the iliopsoas (**31**), can be traced through a cranio-caudal series of images.

If there is a suspicious nodular swelling in one image, it should become an automatic reaction to compare adjacent levels to clarify whether it is simply a vessel or muscle in cross-section. This procedure will also enable quick identification of the partial volume effects described on the previous page.

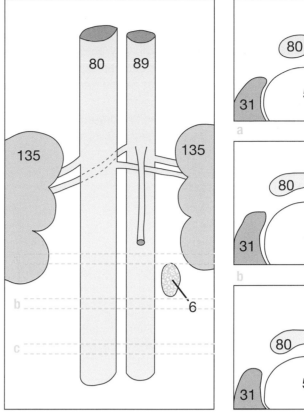

Fig. 15.1

Densitometry (Measurement of Density)

If it is uncertain, for example, whether fluid found in the pleural cavity is a pleural effusion or a hemothorax, a measurement of the liquid's density will clarify the differential diagnosis. The same applies to focal lesions in the parenchyma of the liver or the kidney. However, it is not advisable to carry out measurements of single voxels (=volume element, see Fig. 14.1) since such data are liable to statistical fluctuations which can make the attenuation unreliable. It is more accurate to position a larger "region of interest" (ROI) consisting of several voxels in a focal lesion, a structure, or an amount of fluid. The computer calculates the mean density levels of all voxels and also provides the standard deviation (SD).

One must be particularly careful not to overlook beam-hardening artifacts (Fig. 19.2) or partial volume effects. If a mass does not extend through the entire thickness of a slice, measurements of density will include the tissue next to it (Figs. 121.2 and 133.1–133.3). The density of a mass will be measured correctly only if it fills the entire thickness of the slice (d_S) (Fig. 15.2). It is then more likely that measurements will include only the mass (hatched area in Fig. 15.2a). If d_S is greater than the mass's diameter, for example a small lesion in an unfavorable position, it can only appear in partial volume at any scan level (Fig. 15.2b).

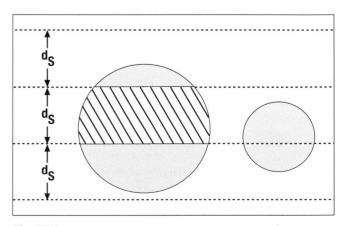

Fig. 15.2   a   b

Density Levels of Different Types of Tissues

Modern equipment has a capacity of 4096 gray tones, which represent different density levels in HUs. The density of water was arbitrarily set at 0 HU and that of air at −1000 HU (Table 16.1a). The monitor can display a maximum of 256 gray tones. However, the human eye is able to discriminate only approximately 20. Since the densities of human tissues extend over a fairly narrow range (a window) of the total spectrum (Table 16.1b), it is possible to select a window setting to represent the density of the tissue of interest. The mean density level of the window should be set as close as possible to the density level of the tissue to be examined. The lung, with its high air content, is best examined at a low HU window setting (Fig. 17.1c), whereas bones require an adjustment to high levels (Fig. 17.2c). The width of the window influences the contrast of the images: the narrower the window, the greater the contrast since the 20 gray tones cover only a small scale of densities.

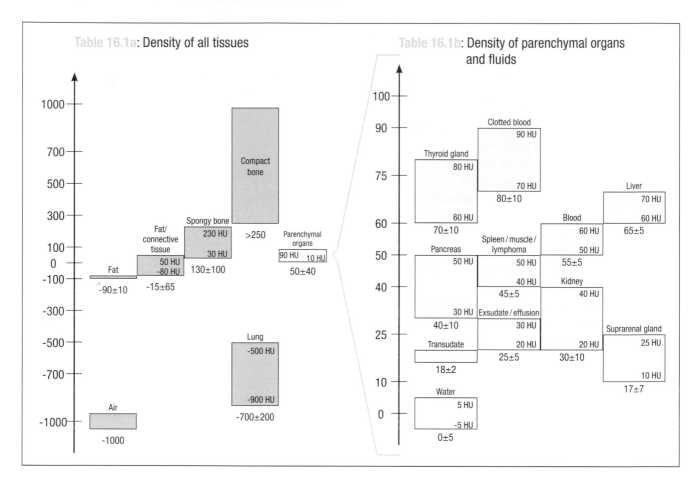

Table 16.1a: Density of all tissues

Table 16.1b: Density of parenchymal organs and fluids

It is noteworthy that the density levels of almost all soft-tissue organs lie within a narrow range between 10 and 90 HUs (Table 16.1b). The only exception is the lung and, as mentioned above, this requires a special window setting (Figs. 17.1a–c). With respect to hemorrhages, it should be taken into account that the density level of recently coagulated blood lies about 30 HU above that of fresh blood. This density drops again in older hemorrhages or liquefied thromboses. An exudate with a protein content above 30 g/l cannot be readily distinguished from a transudate (protein content below 30 g/l) at conventional window settings. In addition, the high degree of overlap between the densities of, for example, lymphomas, spleen, muscles, and pancreas makes it clear that it is not possible to deduce, from density levels alone, what substance or tissue is present.

Finally, standard density values also fluctuate between individuals, depending as well on the amount of CM in the circulating blood and in the organs. The latter aspect is of particular importance for the examination of the urogenital system, since i.v. CM is rapidly excreted by the kidney, resulting in rising density levels in the parenchyma during the scanning procedure. This effect can be put to use when judging kidney function (see Fig. 135.1).

Documentation of Different Windows

When the images have been acquired, a hard copy is printed for documentation. For example: in order to examine the mediastinum and the soft tissues of the thoracic wall, the window is set such that muscles (**13, 14, 20–26**), vessels (**89, 90, 92...**), and fat are clearly represented in shades of gray. The soft-tissue window (Fig. 17.1a) is centered at 50HU with a width of about 350HU. The result is a representation of density values from −125HU (50–350/2) up to +225HU (50+350/2). All tissues with a density lower than −125HU,

such as the lung, are represented in black. Those with density levels above +225 appear white and their internal structural features cannot be differentiated.

If lung parenchyma is to be examined, for example when scanning for nodules, the window center will be lower at about −200HU, and the window wider (2000HU). Low-density pulmonary structures (**96**) can be much more clearly differentiated in this so-called lung window (Fig. 17.1c).

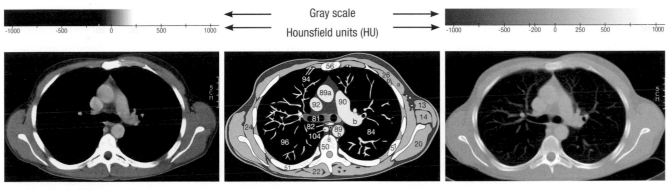

Gray scale
Hounsfield units (HU)

Fig. 17.1a Soft tissue window   Fig. 17.1b   Fig. 17.1c Lung window

In order to achieve maximal contrast between gray and white matter in the brain, it is necessary to select a special brain window because the density values of gray and white matter differ only slightly. The brain window must be very narrow (80 to 100HU => high contrast) and the center must lie close to the mean density of cerebral tissue (35HU) to demonstrate these slight differences (Fig. 17.2a). At this setting it is of course impossible to examine the skull since all structures hyperdense to 75–85HU appear white. The bone window should therefore have a much higher center, at about +300HU, and a sufficient width of about 1500HU.

The metastases (**7**) in the occipital bone (**55d**) would only be visible in the appropriate bone window (Fig. 17.2c), but not in the brain window (Fig. 17.2a). On the other hand, the brain is practically invisible in the bone window; small cerebral metastases would not be detected. One must always be aware of these technical aspects, especially since hard copies are not usually printed at each window setting. The examiner should review thoroughly the images on the screen in additional windows to avoid missing important pathologic features. Examination of the liver poses special problems and is dealt with separately on page 120.

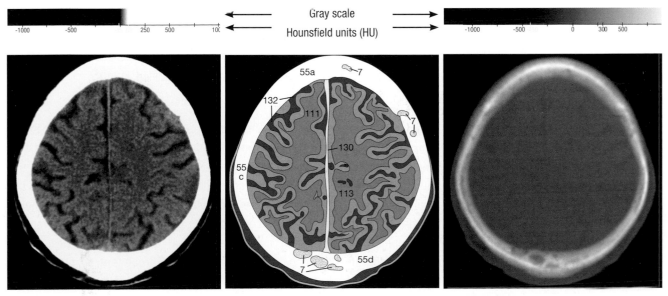

Gray scale
Hounsfield units (HU)

Fig. 17.2a Brain window   Fig. 17.2b   Fig. 17.2c Bone window

Medical History

Following a period of fasting (the day of the examination), and prior to any CT examination, a thorough medical history needs to be obtained which focuses on factors that may represent a contradiction to contrast media or indicate an increased likelihood of a reaction. In patients with suspected renal dysfunction baseline blood urea nitrogen and creatinine levels should be obtained (see below). It is important to note whether prior CT images are available for comparison. Information about prior surgery and radiation therapy in the anatomic region to be examined by CT is also important. Careful consideration of the pertinent radiologic findings on the current context with prior results and the patient's clinical history allow the radiologist to render a meaningful differential diagnosis.

Adverse CM-Induced Reactions and Their Prophylaxis

Contrast agents are drugs, and as such, have the ability to induce adverse reactions. CM-related adverse drug reactions (ADR) can be classified as type A (predictable, dose-dependent, related to the pharmacological properties), and type B reactions (unpredictable, uncommon, and usually not related to the pharmacological properties) [8].

Renal Toxicity (Type A Reactions)

All available and FDA-approved contrast agents are nephrotoxic. Iodinated contrast agents are renal excreted, and can disturb the renal hemodynamics, induce apoptosis, and have tubular toxicity [13a]. These pathological events may lead to contrast-induced acute kidney injury (CI-AKI). To avoid CI-AKI, serum creatinine should be measured (Table 18.1), and estimated glomerular filtration rate (eGFR) should be calculated (Table 18.2), before the patient receives the contrast medium [13c]. The body surface area can be calculated by the square root of (body weight [kg] x body height [cm], divided by the factor 3600), e.g.: 187 cm x 90 kg = 16830 / 3600 = 4.675; $\sqrt{4.675} = 2.16$ m^2 [13d]. Dependent on the eGFR value, different prophylactic actions (e.g., hydration, injection of low-dose contrast, omission of contrast, and performing a noncontrasted scan) are necessary.

Patients with dialysis-dependent renal insufficiency can be divided into two groups: with or without residual renal function. Preservation of the renal residual function is important because it is a predictor of higher survival. A recent meta-analysis showed that intravascular applied contrast might not result in a significant reduction of the residual renal function in such patients [13b]. Therefore, an immediate dialysis following the injection of an iodinated contrast agent is not necessary.

Male	Female
0.8–1.2 mg/dl	0.7–1.0 mg/dl
70–106 µmol/l	62–88 µmol/l

Ratio
1mg/dl = 88.42 µmol/l
1 µmol/l = 0.011 mg/dl

Table 18.1 Reference Values for Serum Creatinine Levels

Renal Insufficiency	GFR [ml/min/1.73m^2]	Clinical Correlation
I	> 90	Normal Findings
II	60–89	Mild Renal Insufficiency
III	30–59	Moderate Renal Insufficiency
IV	15–29	Severe Renal Insufficiency
V	< 15	Renal Failure

Table 18.2 Grading of Renal Insufficiency, according to CKD-EPI (Chronic Kidney Disease Epidemiology Collaboration, [13c])

Medication as Risk (Type A Reactions)

Diabetic patients on metformin therapy, an oral antihyperglycemic drug, seem to be at risk for the acquisition of a lactic acidosis, if they suffer from a renal complaint. A recent retrospective study shows that other factors, but not metformin use, are associated with metabolic acidosis in patients with reduced renal function [14a]. The authors conclude that there is no need to discontinue metformin before CT using contrast agents in patients with mild to moderate renal failure. Nephrotoxic drugs, such as cyclosporine A or nonsteroidal anti-inflammatory drugs, increase the risk for CI-AKI. Therefore, if contrast is necessary, a temporary stop of such medications could be useful. In contrast to previous assumptions, beta blockers do not increase the frequency of anaphylactic events, but do increase the risk for severe anaphylactic reactions and for treatment-refractory conditions [14b]. Although previous reports suggest an increased risk, a detailed analysis shows that patients on interleukin-2 treatment do not bear an increased risk for the acquisition of a hypersensitivity reaction following CM-application [14c].

Oral Administration of Contrast Agents

After a period of fasting, the patient should drink liquid contrast agents in small portions over a period of 30–60 minutes before the CT examination. As mentioned below (see also p. 20), the patient is given a water-soluble iodinated contrast agent.

Therefore, the patient should arrive at least 1 hour before an abdominal CT examination. Importantly, where possible, CT of the abdomen should be performed 3 days after a conventional barium examination has been carried out (for example: barium swallow, barium meal, small bowl enema, barium enema). Usually, the digital projection radiograph (scanogram Fig. 19.1a, scout view) would show that residual barium in the GIT would result in major artifacts (Fig. 19.1b), rendering CT valueless. The sequence of diagnostic procedures for patients with abdominal diseases should therefore be carefully planned.

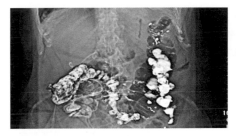

Fig. 19.1a

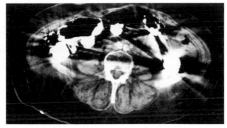

Fig. 19.1b

Informing the Patient

Possibly, patients fear the harmful effects of x-rays in CT-scanners. Concerns can usually be reduced if you relate diagnostic X-ray exposure to natural background radiation. Naturally, the patient must have the feeling that he or she is being taken seriously and his or her worries are understood, otherwise confidence and trust in the radiologist are threatened. Many patients are relieved to know that they can communicate with the radiographers in the control room via an intercom and that the examination can be interrupted or terminated at any time if there are unexpected problems. Patients with claustrophobia may feel more comfortable if they close their eyes during the examination; the close proximity of the gantry is then less of a problem. In very rare cases, a mild sedative may be helpful.

Controlling Respiration

Before starting the examination, the patient should be told of the need for controlled breathing. For conventional CT, the patient is instructed to breathe before each new image acquisition and then to hold his or her breath for a few seconds. In the helical technique, it is necessary to stop breathing for about 7–30 seconds. If the patient cannot comply, diaphragmatic movement will lead to image blur with a marked deterioration in image quality (Fig. 19.2). In the case of neck examinations, swallowing influences the quality of the images more than breathing.

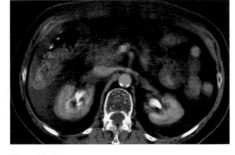

Fig. 19.2

Removal of All Metallic Objects

Naturally, jewelry of any kind and removable dental prostheses must be removed before the head or neck are examined in order to avoid artifacts. In Figs. 19.3a, b the effects of such artifacts (**3**) are obvious. Only the cervical vertebral body (**50**) and the adjacent vessels (**86**) are defined; the other structures are unrecognizable. For the same reason, all clothing with metallic hooks, buttons, or zippers should be removed before thoracic or abdominal CTs are performed.

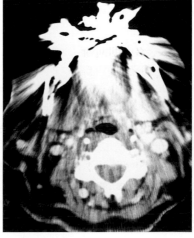

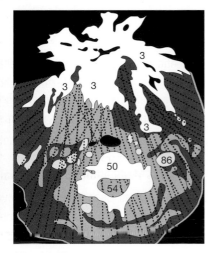

Fig. 19.3a

Fig. 19.3b

Contrast-Enhanced CT-Scans and Contrast Media

To achieve high-image quality for diagnostic approaches, radiologists perform most CT-examinations as contrast-enhanced scans. Only a minority of CT-exams (e.g., stone protocols, fracture assessments) are noncontrasted scans (i.e., without CM-application). In developed industrial countries, the preferred and most used contrast materials are iodinated and nonionic contrast media. These agents are water-soluble derivatives of the triiodobenzoic acid, and are of low osmolality.

Per Oral CM-application

In addition to intravenous contrast, the examination of the GI-tract needs per oral CM-application. Without such contrast, it is difficult or impossible to differentiate between the duodenum (**130**), and the head of the pancreas (**131** in Fig. 20.1).

Moreover, the differentiation between other GI parts (**140**) and neighboring structures could be also impossible. Following per oral contrasting, we can well delineate both the duodenum and the pancreas (Fig. 20.2a, b).

In contrast to the intravascular CM-application, we can use both low- and high-osmolar iodinated CM for the per oral application. Patients without any risk for an aspiration can receive a high-osmolar iodinated contrast medium (e.g., Gastrografin®), and patients at risk should receive a low-osmolar iodinated contrast medium (e.g., Ultravist®). One should be aware that the same precautions as mentioned below for intravenous contrast applications should also be used for the per oral application [18a].

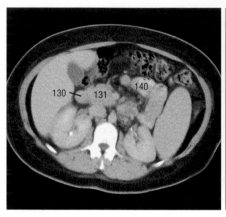 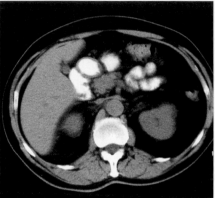 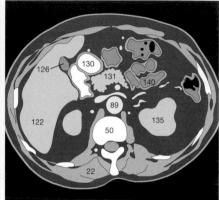

Fig. 20.1   Fig. 20.2a   Fig. 20.2b

The Procedure

Following a period of fasting (the day of the examination), the patient should drink an iodinated contrast medium in small portions over a period of 20–60 minutes before the CT examination starts. Therefore, the patient should arrive on time for an abdominal CT examination. To contrast the proximal GIT, the patient should drink the contrast agent 20–30 minutes before the CT scan starts. However, if the entire colon and the rectum will be scanned, it is recommended that the patient drinks the contrast medium approximately 45–60 minutes before the CT scan starts. In order to scan pelvic organs (e.g., bladder, cervix, or ovary), an additional rectal application of 100–200 ml iodinated contrast medium is necessary to differentiate tumors clearly from parts of the colon, sigmoid, or rectum, for example. To achieve complete contrast of the whole GIT, dilute Gastrografin® 1:3 up to 1:4 in water. If the upper part of the GIT should be examined only, use a reduced volume of diluted Gastrografin®.

If the urinary bladder has been removed and replaced by an ilial-conduit, initially the abdomen should be scanned by using an intravenous applied contrast agent only, which is excreted along with the urine in the conduit but not via the intestine. If necessary, a second scan with oral contrast may follow to delineate the intestine. Other protocols use mannitol and water, for example [18b].

Additional Medication for an Optimal Imaging Result

For an optimal assessment of the stomach walls, plain water is increasingly used as a hypodense contrast agent in combination with intravenous Buscopan® (scopolamine butylbromide), which relaxes muscles in gastric and bowel walls and thus reduces peristaltic movements [18c].

Intravenous CM-Application

Most commonly, we apply contrast materials as intravenous injection by using an automated power injector. We calculate the CM-dose on both the body weight, and the necessary diagnostic procedure: examinations of the neck or of an aortic aneurysm (to exclude a dissection flap), require higher concentrations than cranial CT-scans, for example. Usually, a CM-dose (e.g., iopromide) of 1.2 mL/kg body weight leads to excellent image results.

An increase in the density of blood vessels not only demarcates them better from muscles and organs but also provides information on the rate of blood perfusion (contrast agent uptake) in pathologically altered tissues: disturbances of the blood-brain barrier, the borders of abscesses, or the inhomogeneous uptake of contrast agents in tumorlike lesions are only some examples. We call this phenomenon contrast enhancement: the contrast agent increases, i.e., the density and thus the signal is intensified. Depending on the patient's health problem and an unenhanced (plain) scan should be obtained initially, followed by the intravenous injection of the contrast agent. We can more easily detect vascular grafts, inflammatory processes within bones, and abscess walls, if we compare unenhanced and contrast-enhanced images. The same holds true for focal liver lesions examined by using conventional CT techniques. Helical CT allows serial liver images in the early phase of arterial contrasting, followed by a series in the phasc of venous drainage [17]. This procedure even allows the detection of small focal lesions (see pp. 121–124).

Preparing the i.v. Line

The injected bolus of contrast is modified when passing through the pulmonary circulation. The injection should therefore ideally have a rapid flow rate of 2–6 mL/sec for achieving sufficient density enhancement of the blood vessels [29]. A Venflon® canula with a diameter of at least 1.0 mm (20G), or preferably 1.2–1.4 mm (18G–17G), is used. Checking that the canula is correctly in the vessel is essential. A trial injection of sterile saline into the vein at a high flow rate should be carried out before injecting contrast agents. The absence of subcutaneous swelling confirms proper positioning: Thus, the fact that the vein can accommodate the intended flow rate can also be confirmed.

Inflow Phenomena

The streaming artifact of enhanced and unenhanced blood results from a short time interval between the start of injection and the onset of data acquisition. Since inflow is usually from one side via the axillary, subclavian, and brachiocephalice veins (**91**) into the superior vena cava (**92**), there is an apparent filling defect within the vena cava (Figs. 21.1a–21.3b).

Knowing about such inflow phenomena avoids a false positive diagnosis of venous thrombosis. Using too high concentrations of contrast agents in this area could result in disturbing artifacts. More inflow phenomena are described on the next pages.

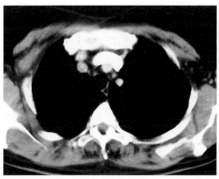

Fig. 21.1a

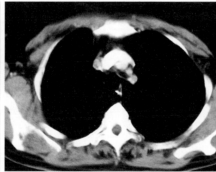

Fig. 21.2a

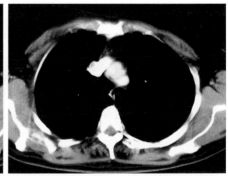

Fig. 21.3a

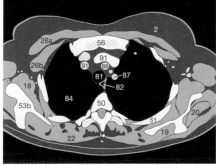

Fig. 21.1b

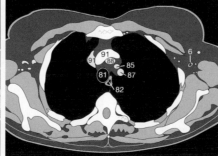

Fig. 21.2b

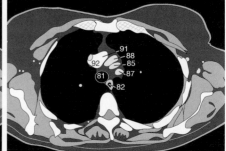

Fig. 21.3b

Abdominal Inflow Phenomena

Flow phenomena can also frequently be seen in the inferior vena cava (**80**) at the level of the renal veins (**111**). These veins may already contain blood which has a fairly high concentration of contrast agents, and this blood mixes with unenhanced blood flow returning from the lower extremities and pelvic organs. In the early postcontrast phase in the vena cava (**80**) caudal to the level of the renal veins, the density is hypodense relative to the adjacent aorta (**89**) as in Figs. 22.1a,b.

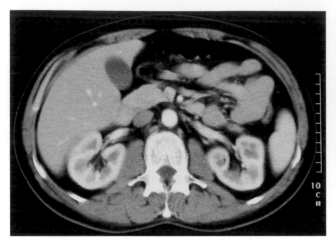

Fig. 22.1a

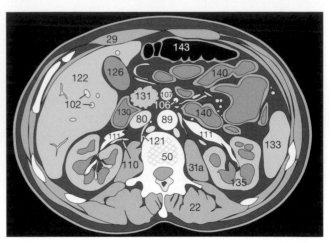

Fig. 22.1b

Immediately above the renal veins, the contents of the inferior vena cava may appear bilaterally enhanced by the blood from both kidneys, whereas the central part is still unenhanced (Fig. 22.2). If the renal veins do not empty into the cava at the same level or if a kidney has been removed, a unilateral enhancement may occur (Fig. 22.3). Such differences in density should not be mistaken for thrombosis of the inferior vena cava (see Figs. 23.1 and 144.1).

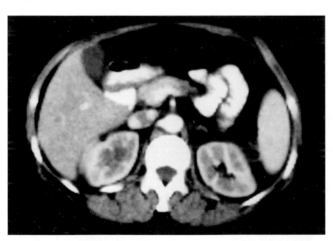

Fig. 22.2a

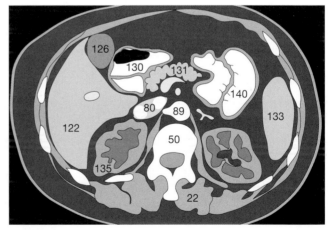

Fig. 22.2b

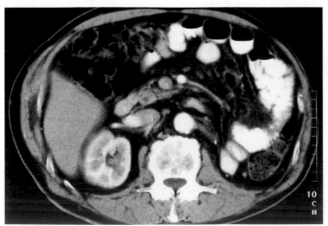

Fig. 22.3a

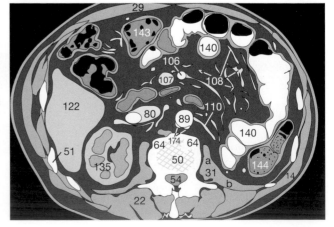

Fig. 22.3b

Flow Phenomena

If we trace the inferior vena cava (**80**) cranially toward the right atrium, additional flow phenomena become apparent as more veins empty into it. The cava has spiraling eddies of inhomogeneous density (⟹ in Fig. 23.1) caused by mixing of the blood as described on the previous page. Moments later such inhomogeneities are no longer evident in the

lumen (**80**) and density levels are identical to those in the aorta (**89**) in Fig. 23.2.

By the way, did you notice the artheroslerotic plaque in the posterior wall of the aorta (**174** in Fig. 23.2)? The patient has well-developed osteophytes (**64**) on the anterior border of the vertebral bodies (**50**).

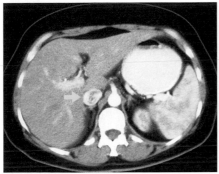 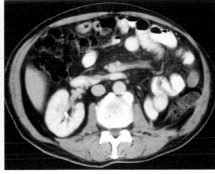 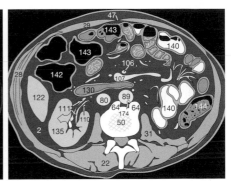

Fig. 23.1 Fig. 23.2a Fig. 23.2b

Hyperthyroidism (Type A Reactions)

Patients with thyroid disease can acquire delayed hyperthyroidism several weeks after the administration of iodinated contrast agents. In severe cases, preexisting hyperthyroidism can lead to a thyroid crisis [9a–9c]. Symptoms range from diarrhea, muscle weakness, fever, and excessive perspiration without any physical exercise, exsiccation, anxiety, and restlessness up to intense tachycardia or life-threatening tachyarrhythmia. Besides (very) late reactions, immediate adverse events are also possible [10a].

In order to identify patients with (latent) hyperthyroidism, the TSH value is determined by a screening test. Because of the negative feedback mechanism, the release of TSH-hormone in

the pituitary gland is reduced in cases with hyperactive thyroid gland, so that patients with **low** TSH levels are particularly sought out: TSH normal values range between 0.4 and 4.0 mU/L in adults, but vary significantly from laboratory to laboratory [10b] and are influenced by several drugs as well [10c]. Therefore, in order to prevent a hyperthyroidism/thyroid crisis in patients at risk (e.g., Graves' disease, thyroid adenoma), current thyroid hormone values should be mentioned on the CT request form. When we suspect hyperthyroidism, TSH and T3/T4 values should be analyzed before patients receive contrast injection. The ESUR Guidelines on Contrast Media (version 10.0) recommend (Table 23.3):

Recommendations on Contrast Media

- Iodine-based contrast media should not be given to patients with manifest hyperthyroidism.

- In selected high-risk patients, prophylactic treatment may be given by an endocrinologist.

- Patients at risk should be closely monitored by endocrinologists after iodine-based contrast medium injection.

- Intravenous cholangiographic contrast media should not be given to patients at risk.

Table 23.3 ESUR Guidelines on Contrast Media [11]

Patients with normal thyroid hormone values can receive iodinated CM. One should realize that even patients without thyroid disease have a significantly higher risk of thyroid dysfunction following iodinated CM exposure [12,12a].

If radioiodine therapy for hyperthyroidism or thyroid cancer is planned, the IV application of iodinated contrast agents could lead to a saturation of the iodine uptake system in the thyroid gland for several weeks. Therefore, radioiodine therapy is a contraindication for iodinated contrast media.

Hypersensitivity Reactions (Type B Reactions)

Hypersensitivity reactions to nonionic contrast media occur in approximately 2% of patients [15a] as mild, moderate, or severe. Most acquire mild reactions, a lesser number moderate ones, and only rarely we observe severe forms of hypersensitivity reactions (Table 24.1).

Usually, immediate adverse reactions manifest within the first 30 minutes, and 70% of adverse events occur within the first 5 minutes following the contrast injection [15a] with an individual or a combination of symptoms such as erythema, hives or urticaria, itching, nausea, vomiting, hypotension, tachycardia, circulatory shock, shortness of breath, for example [15b]. Moderate and severe immediate hypersensitivity reactions require an emergency treatment (see table on page 25). Serious events (such as pulmonary edema, severe circulatory disturbances, convulsions, and anaphylaxis) occur very rarely, and require immediate intensive care. Be sure to document carefully every adverse event in the record. We should document a minimum of three facts: date of the adverse reaction exact name of the culprit CM, and all clinical symptoms [15c]. It is important to document the date of an adverse reaction because CM-hypersensitivities have a limited duration [15d]. We should also be aware that so-called "iodine allergy" does not exist [15e–f] and, consequently, such a term should not be documented. Last but not least, hypersensitivities following the application of an contrast agent may be contrast-induced, but could be also induced by other drugs (e.g., Buscopen®) [15g].

who acquire immediate adverse reactions or have a history of adverse events should be monitored for a minimum of 30 minutes. at risk (with a history of an adverse event following contrast medium injection) should undergo an individual prophylactic management. A prerequisite is an exact documentation of such adverse reactions.

Adverse reactions to iodinated contrast agents do not show "cross-reactivity" to gadolinium-based MRI contrast agents. Patients with a history of a previous CM-induced hypersensitivity reaction, acute complaints of allergic asthma, and less frequently, other acute allergies requiring treatment are at increased risk. In these patients, the first decision is whether contrast should be given or not. This includes the following considerations: Is a noncontrasted scan possible? Should we use another imaging modality? Should we perform the scan later? If we decide to apply CM, the second consideration is, which CM should we apply?

Severity of immediate adverse reactions			Time points of manifestations of adverse CM reactions		
Mild	Moderate	Severe	Acute	Late	Very late
Erythema, mild urticaria	Generalized urticaria	Severe bronchial asthma, respiratory standstill	< 1 h following contrast	1h to 1 week after contrast	After several weeks
Itching	Facial or laryngeal edema (angioedema)	Severe drop of blood pressure, tachycardia up to cardiac arrest	Usually: < 30 minutes		
Nausea	Bronchospasm, difficulties breathing, mild bronchial asthma	Loss of consciousness and anaphylactic shock			
Vomiting	Vasovagal reaction, mild drop of blood pressure, mild tachycardia	Seizure		All immediate and delayed reactions (e.g., fixed drug eruption, DRESS, etc.)	Thyroid crisis

Table 24.1

Premedication

In the past, the usefulness of drug premedication has been questioned [16a]. Therefore, according to the ESUR Guidelines (version 10.0), premedication is no longer recommended [11]. Only in few selected cases, should premedication be applied. Recent prophylactic approaches omit the culprit CM [15e], and use a lower CM-dose and a lower injection speed, for example [16b].

Treatment of Adverse Reactions to Contrast Agents
Important: Read carefully and train such situations before a patient acquires an adverse reaction

▶ **Gastrointestinal reactions**
(nausea or vomiting)

- Mild forms ➡ wait and see, talk to the patient
- Severe forms H1 blockers, such as 1 ampule IV =
  2 mg in 5 mL clemastine (Tavegil®) IV slowly
- Very severe forms that do not respond to H1-blockers:
  antiemetics, such as 1 ampule IV =
  62 mg in 10 mL dimenhydrinate (Vomex AB)

▶ **Mild forms of skin or mucosal reactions / sensations**
(hot or cold feeling, erythema, pruritus, urticaria)

- Wait and see, talk to the patient

▶ **Moderate forms of skin or mucosal reactions**
(generalized urticaria, angioedema)

- H1 blockers, such as 1 ampule IV =
  2 mg in 5 mL clemastine (Tavegil®).
  If the reaction does not respond after 30–45 minutes,
  inject a second ampule clemastine IV.

▶ **Dyspnea or asthma attack**
(shortness of breathing, stridor, bronchospasm, laryngeal edema, pulmonary edema)

- Site the patient in an upright position, measure blood pressure
- Oxygen mask, 4–8 L O_2/min and pulse oximetry
- H1 blockers, such as 1 ampule IV =
  2 mg in 5 mL clemastine (Tavegil®).
- In severe forms: epinephrine as autoinjector (EPI-PEN®)
- Call the emergency team

▶ **Seizure**

- Protect patient from traumatic events
- Benzodiazepine such as clonazepam, 1 ampule IV =
  1 mg in 1 mL (Rivotril®)

▶ **Cardiovascular reactions**
(hypotension, tachycardia, arrhythmia, rarely bradycardia or hypertension)

- Elevate the patient's legs
- H1 blockers, such as 1 ampule IV =
  2 mg in 5 mL clemastine (Tavegil®) Oxygen mask, 4–8 L O_2/min
- Monitor blood pressure, pulse oximetry, ECG
- Volume replacement IV such as 500–1000 mL lactated Ringer solution
  or 0.9% sodium chloride solution
- In severe forms: epinephrine via autoinjector (EPI-PEN®)
- Call the emergency team

▶ **Anaphylactic shock**
(systolic pressure < 70 mm Hg, heart rate < 60/min, cardiac arrest, loss of consciousness)

- Immediately call the emergency team!
- Oxygen mask, 6–10 L O_2/min
- Position patient supine with the legs slightly elevated
- Epinephrine via autoinjector (EPI-PEN®)
- Volume replacement IV such as 500–1000 mL lactated Ringer solution or
  0.9% sodium chloride solution
- H1 blockers, such as 1 ampule IV =
  2 mg in 5 mL clemastine (Tavegil®)
- Monitor blood pressure, pulse oximetry, ECG
- In case of cardiac arrest: Resuscitate according to standard advanced cardiac
  life support (ACLS) procedure

Modified from the Guidelines of the European Society of Urogenital Radiology (ESUR) [11]
Also provided as a pocket-size card at the end of the book.

Many cranial CT (CCT) examinations can be performed without injection of contrast medium: For instance, the differential diagnosis (DD) of cerebral bleeding versus infarction in patient with sudden onset of neurologic deficits does not require the administration of contrast medium. However, intravenous injection of contrast medium is necessary to detect an impaired blood-brain barrier (BBB) as found in tumors, metastases or inflammations.

Selection of the Image Plane

The desired image planes parallel to the orbitomeatal line are selected on the sagittal localizer image (topogram) (Fig. 26.1). This is a readily reproducible line drawn from the supraorbital ridge to the external auditory meatus, allowing reliable comparison with follow-up CT examinations. The posterior fossa is scanned in thin sections (2-3 mm) to minimize beam hardening artifacts, and the supratentorial brain above the pyramids in thicker sections (5 mm).

The images are displayed as seen from below (caudal view) and consequently are laterally reversed, i.e., the left lateral ventricle is on the right and vice versa. Only CTs obtained for neurosurgical planning are often displayed as seen from above (right = right) since this cranial view corresponds to the neurosurgical approach for cranial trepanation.

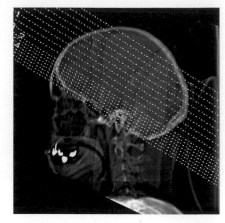

Fig. 26.1

Systematic Interpretation

Each examiner is free to find a preferred sequence for reviewing the images. This means that the examiner can choose between several acceptable approaches and is not restricted to a "one and only" strategy. However, staying with a consistent arrangement of the images to be interpreted has the advantage that fewer findings are overlooked, especially by the novice. The checklist below just contains recommendations that can serve as good guideline for the novice.

First, the size of the ventricles and extracerebral CSF spaces has to be evaluated to exclude a life threatening space-occupying process right away. Hereby, the patient's age has to be considered because of age-related widening of the CSF spaces. Any blurring of the grey-white matter junction as manifestation of cerebral edema should be looked for (see below). If a pathologic change is suspected, the adjacent sections should be inspected to avoid any misinterpretation due to a partial volume effect (see Fig. 29.1 and Fig. 52.2).

Always use the legends on the front cover flap for this chapter. The listed numbers apply to all head and neck images. The subsequent pages provide you with a survey of the normal anatomy, followed by normal variants and the most frequent pathologic findings.

Checklist for Reading Cranial CT

Age? (because of the age-related width of the CSF spaces / cerebral atrophy; see page 50)

Medical History: • Risk factors?   (Trauma ➡ Chance of intracranial bleeding)

                                       (Hypertension, diabetes, nicotine ➡ Vascular stenoses, infarcts)

Signs of space-occupying lesion:

- Normal configuration of the 4th ventricle? (posterior to the pons, see pages 28 / 29)
- Normal configuration of the 3rd ventricle? (interthalamic, narrow / slit-like, see page 30)
- Normal symmetry of the lateral ventricles?

  (concave lateral border of the anterior horn and central ventricular region?)

- Midline shift? (sign of large space-occupying process)
- Preserved basal cistern? (e.g., quadrigeminal cistern: smilie face / bat man figure, see Fig. 30.1)
- Cortex ◀▶ white matter demarcation OK? (blurred interface = sign of edema)
- Width of the extracerebral CSF OK for patient's age? (Sylvian fissure, refer to p.50)

Focal lesions: • Unenhanced: DD physiologic calcification (choroid plexus, pineal gland / partial volume;

                              refer to Figures 29.3 and 30.2) versus genuine hyperdense bleeding

                              (DD types of bleeding, see pages 54-57)

                     • Contrast enhanced: Sign of impaired BBB? (caused by tumors, metastases, inflammations, …)

Osseous lesions: • Check cranial vault and base in bone window for osteolytic lesions / osseous infiltration

                     • In trauma patient: Rule out fractures (especially cranial base, midfacial bones – DD sutures)

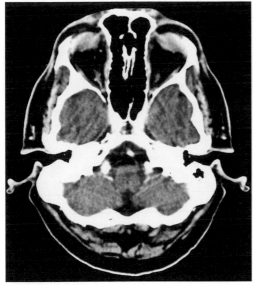

Fig. 27.1a

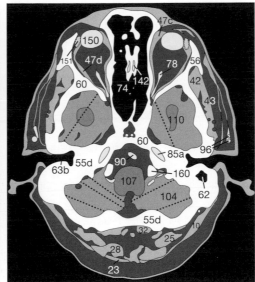

Fig. 27.1b

The scan usually begins at the base of the skull and continues upward. Since the hard copies are oriented such that the sections are viewed from caudal, all structures appear as if they were left/right reversed (see p. 14). The small topogram shows you the corresponding position of each image.

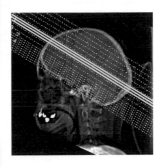

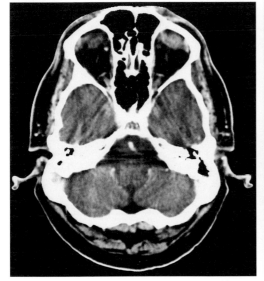

Fig. 27.2a

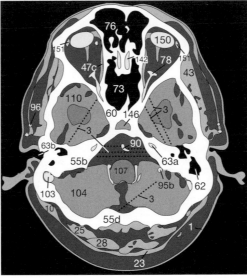

Fig. 27.2b

You should first check for any swellings in the soft tissues which may indicate trauma to the head. Always examine the condition of the basilar artery (**90**) in scans close to the base of the skull and the brainstem (**107**). The view is often limited by streaks of artifacts (**3**) radiating from the temporal bones (**55b**).

When examining trauma patients, remember to use the bone window to inspect the sphenoid bone (**60**), the zygomatic bone (**56**), and the calvaria (**55**) for fractures. In the caudal slices you can recognize basal parts of the temporal lobe (**110**) and the cerebellum (**104**).

Orbital structures are usually viewed in another scanning plane (see pp. 33–40). In Figure 27.1–3 we see only a partial slice of the upper parts of the globe (**150**), the extraocular muscles (**47**), and the olfactory bulb (**142**).

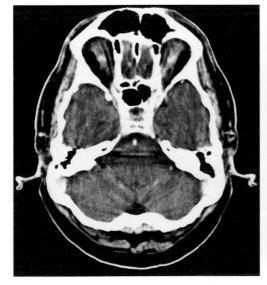

Fig. 27.3a

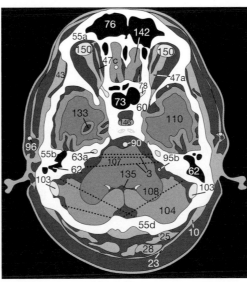

Fig. 27.3b

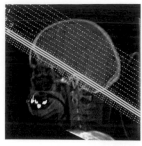

As the series of slices continues dorsally, the crista galli (**162**) and the basal parts of the frontal lobe (**111**) appear. The pons/medulla (**107**) are often obscured by artifacts (**3**). The pituitary gland (**146**) and stalk (**147**) are seen between the upper border of the sphenoid sinus (**73**) and the clinoid process (**163**). Of the dural sinuses, the sigmoid sinus (**103**) can be readily identified. The basilar artery (**90**) and the superior cerebellar artery (**95a**) lie anterior to the pons (**107**). The cerebellar tentorium (**131**), which lies dorsal to the middle cerebral artery (**91b**), shouldn't be mistaken for the posterior cerebral artery (**91c**) at the level depicted in Figure 29.1a on the next page. The inferior (temporal) horns of the lateral ventricles (**133**) as well as the 4th ventricle (**135**) can be identified in Figure 28.3. Fluid occurring in the normally air-filled mastoid cells (**62**) or in the frontal sinus (**76**) may indicate a fracture (blood) or an infection (effusion). A small portion of the roof of the orbit (**✶**) can still be seen in Figure 28.3.

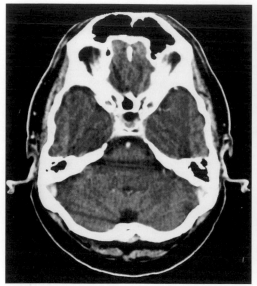

Fig. 28.1a

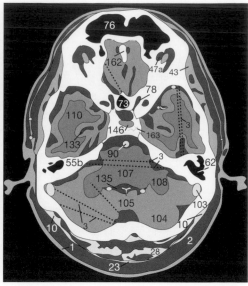

Fig. 28.1b

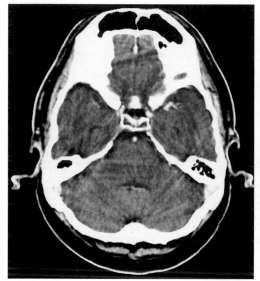

Fig. 28.2a

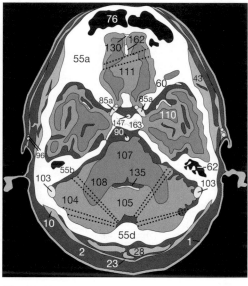

Fig. 28.2b

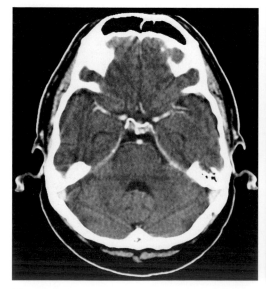

Fig. 28.3a

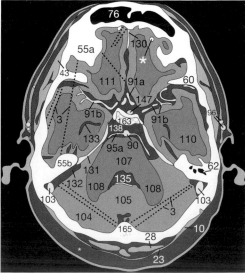

Fig. 28.3b

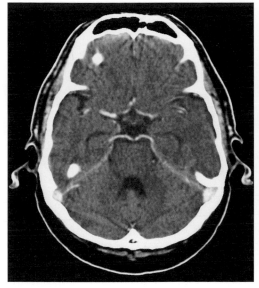

Fig. 29.1a

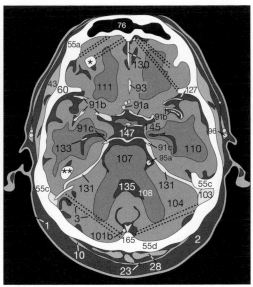

Fig. 29.1b

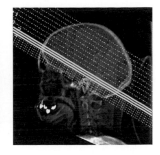

In Figures 28.3a and 29.1a partial volume effects of the orbit (★) or the petrosal bone (★★) might also be misinterpreted as fresh hemorrhages in the frontal (111) or the temporal lobe (110).

The cortex next to the frontal bone (55a) often appears hyperdense compared to adjacent brain parenchyma, but this is an artifact due to beam-hardening effects of bone. Note that the choroid plexus (123) in the lateral ventricle (133) is enhanced after i.v. infusion of CM. Even in plain scans it may appear hyperdense because of calcifications.

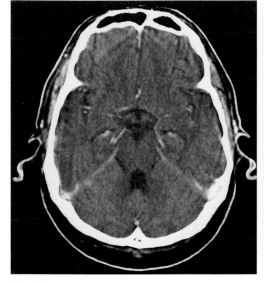

Fig. 29.2a

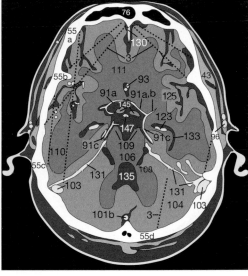

Fig. 29.2b

You will soon have recognized that the CCT images on these pages were taken after i.v. administration of CM: the vessels of the circle of Willis are markedly enhanced. The branches (94) of the middle cerebral artery (91b) are visible in the Sylvian fissure (127). Even the pericallosal artery (93), a continuation of the anterior cerebral artery (91a), can be clearly identified. Nevertheless, it is often difficult to distinguish between the optic chiasm (145) and the pituitary stalk (147) because these structures have similar densities.

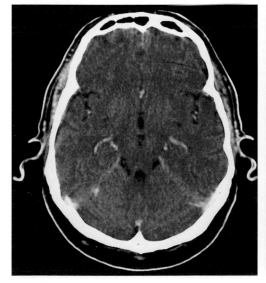

Fig. 29.3a

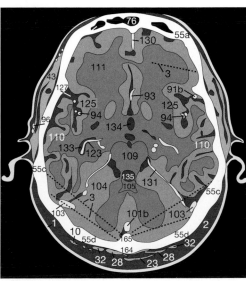

Fig. 29.3b

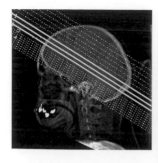

In addition to the above-mentioned cerebral arteries (**93, 94**), the falx cerebri (**130**) is a hyperdense structure. In Figure 30.2a you can see the extension of the hyperdense choroid plexus (**123**) through the foramen of Monro, which connects the lateral ventricles (**133**) with the 3rd ventricle (**134**). Check whether the contours of the lateral ventricles are symmetric.

A midline shift could be an indirect sign of edema. Calcifications in the pineal (**148**) gland and the choroid plexus (**123**) are a common finding in adults, and are generally without any pathologic significance. Due to partial volume effects, the upper parts of the tentorium (**131**) often appear without clear margins so that it becomes difficult to demarcate the cerebellar vermis (**105**) and hemispheres (**104**) from the occipital lobe (**112**).

It is particularly important to carefully inspect the internal capsule (**121**) and the basal ganglia: caudate nucleus (**117**), putamen (**118**), and globus pallidus (**119**) as well as the thalamus (**120**). Consult the number codes in the front foldout for the other structures not specifically mentioned on these pages.

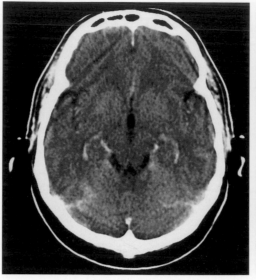

Fig. 30.1a

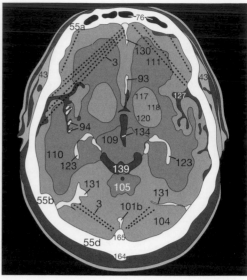

Fig. 30.1b

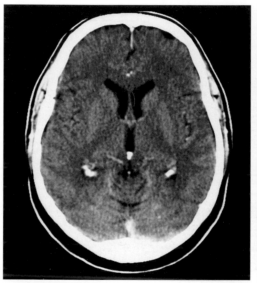

Fig. 30.2a

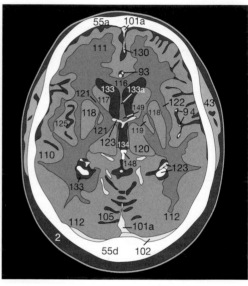

Fig. 30.2b

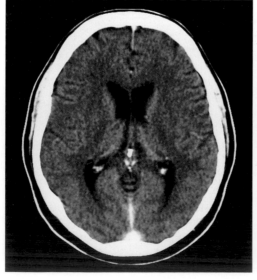

Fig. 30.3a

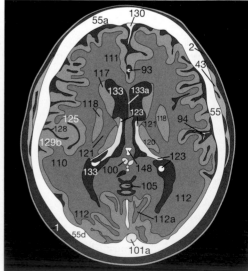

Fig. 30.3b

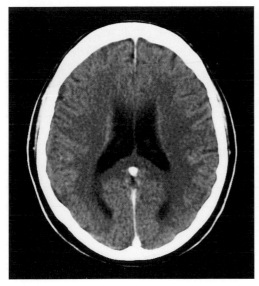

Fig. 31.1a

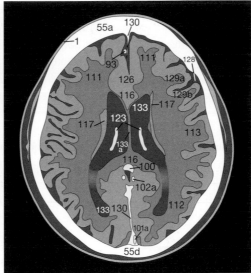

Fig. 31.1b

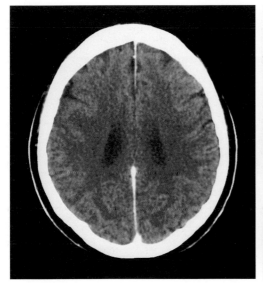

Fig. 31.2a

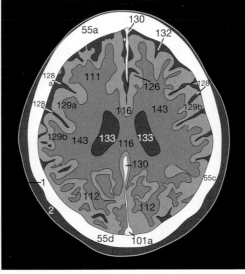

Fig. 31.2b

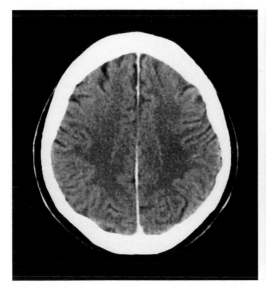

Fig. 31.3a

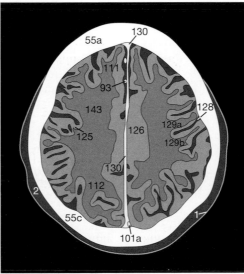

Fig. 31.3b

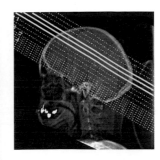

The position of the patient's head is not always as straight as in our example. Even small inclinations may lead to remarkably asymmetric pictures of the ventricular system, though in reality it is perfectly normal. You may see only a partial slice of the convex contours of the lateral ventricles (**133**). This could give you the impression that they are not well defined (Fig. 31.1a).

The phenomenon must not be confused with brain edema: as long as the sulci (external SAS) are not effaced, but configured regularly, the presence of edema is rather improbable.

For evaluating the width of the SAS, the patient's age is an important factor. Compare the images on pages 50 and 52 in this context. The paraventricular and supraventricular white matter (**143**) must be checked for poorly circumscribed hypodense regions of edema due to cerebral infarction.

As residues of older infarctions, cystic lesions may develop. In late stages they are well defined and show the same density as CSF (see p. 58).

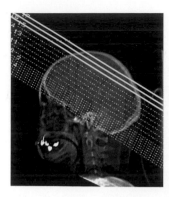

In the upper sections (Figs. 32.1–32.3) calcifications in the cerebral falx (**130**) often appear. You should differentiate this kind of lesion, which has no clinical significance, from calcified meningioma. The presence of CSF-filled sulci (**132**) in adults is an important finding with which to exclude brain edema. After a thorough evaluation of the cerebral soft-tissue window, a careful inspection of the bone window should follow. Continue to check for bone metastases or fracture lines. Only now is your evaluation of a cranial CT really complete.

Test yourself! Exercise **1:**
Note from memory a systematic order for the evaluation of cranial CTs.
If you have difficulties, return to the checklist on page 26.

Note:
-
-
-
-

-
-
-
-

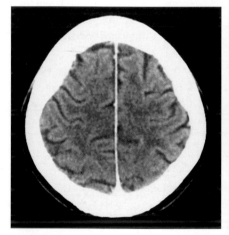

Fig. 32.1a

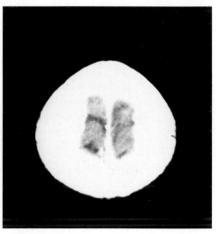

Fig. 32.2a

Fig. 32.3a

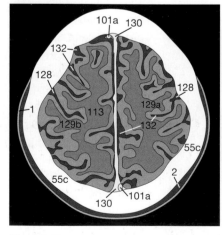

Fig. 32.1b

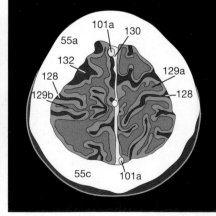

Fig. 32.2b

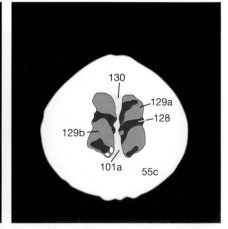

Fig. 32.3b

On the following pages the atlas of normal anatomy continues with scans of the orbits (axial), the face (coronal), and the petrosal bones (axial and coronal). After these you will find the most common anatomic variations, typical phenomena caused by partial volume effects and the most important intracranial pathologic changes on pages 50 to 60.

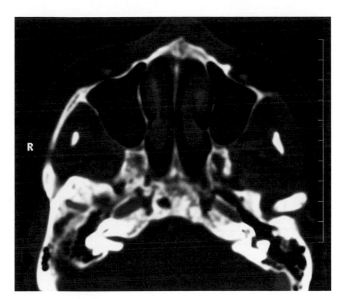

Fig. 33.1a

The face and the orbits are usually studied in thin slices (2 mm) using 2-mm collimation steps or even thinner. The orientation of the scanning plane is comparable to that for CCTs (see p. 26). In the sagittal topogram the line of reference lies parallel to the floor of the orbit at an angle of about 15° to horizontal (Fig. 33.2).

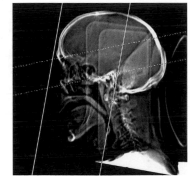

Fig. 33.2

The printouts are usually presented in the view from caudal: all structures on the right side of the body appear on the left, and vice versa.

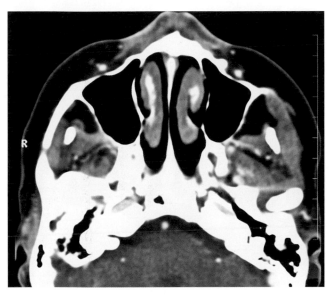

Fig. 33.1b

Alterations in the soft structures of the orbits and the paranasal sinuses can be readily evaluated in the soft-tissue window (Fig. 33.1b). For the detection of a tumor-related erosion of bone or a fracture, the bone window should also be checked (Fig. 33.1a). The following pages therefore present each scan level in both windows. The accompanying drawing (Fig. 33.1c) refers to both. The number codes for all drawings are found in the legend in the front foldout.

On the lower slices of the orbits you will see parts of the maxillary sinus (75), the nasal cavity (77) with the conchae (166), the sphenoid sinus (73), and the mastoid cells (62) as air-filled spaces. If there is fluid or a soft-tissue mass, this may indicate a fracture, an infection, or a tumor of the paranasal sinuses. For examples of such diseases, see pages 58 to 61.
Two parts of the mandible appear on the left side: in addition to the coronoid process (58), the temporomandibular joint with the head of the mandible (58a) is seen on the left. The carotid artery, however, is often difficult to discern in the carotid canal (64), whether in the soft-tissue or bone window.

In the petrous part of the temporal bone (55b), the tympanic cavity (66) and the vestibular system are visible. For a more detailed evaluation of the semicircular canals and the cochlea, images obtained with the petrous bone technique are more appropriate (pp. 44–47). CM was infused intravenously before the examination of the orbits. The branches of both the facial and angular vessels (89) as well as the basilar artery (90) therefore appear markedly hyperdense in the soft-tissue window (Fig. 33.1b).

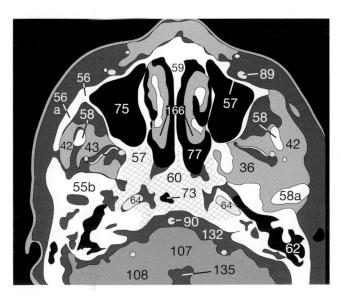

Fig. 33.1c

It is not always possible to achieve a precise sagittal position of the head. Even a slight tilt (Fig. 34.1) will make the temporal lobe (**110**) appear on one side, whereas on the other side the mastoid cells (**62**) can be seen.

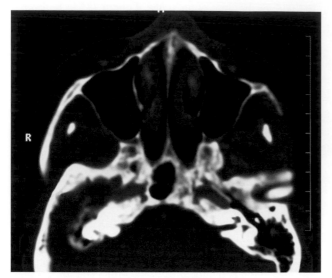

Fig. 34.1a

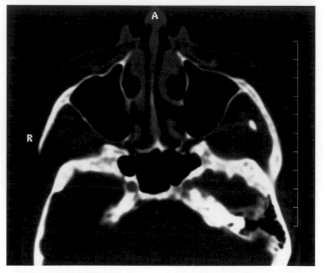

Fig. 34.2a

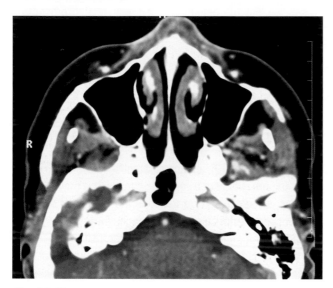

Fig. 34.1b

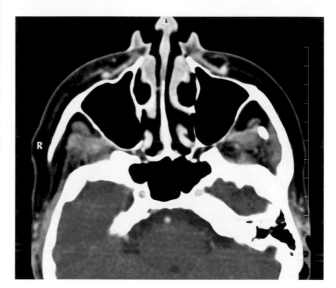

Fig. 34.2b

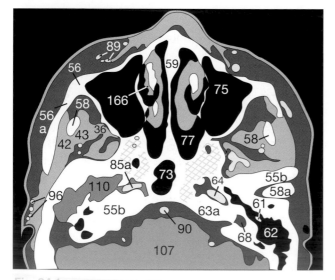

Fig. 34.1c

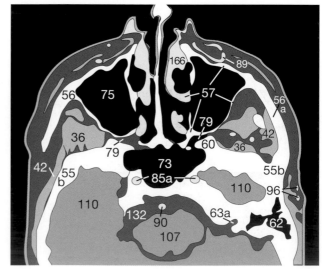

Fig. 34.2c

As experience shows, it is difficult to determine the course of the internal carotid artery **(85a)** through the base of the skull and to demarcate the pterygopalatine fossa **(79)**, through which, among other structures, the greater palatine nerve and the nasal branches of the pterygopalatine ganglion (from CN V and CN VII) pass.

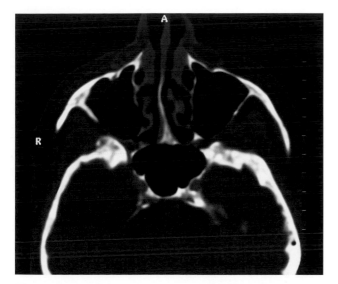

Fig. 35.1a

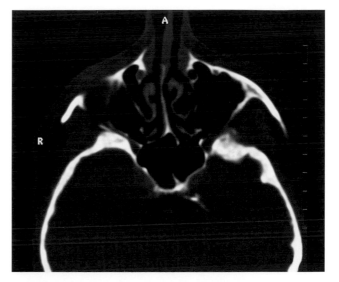

Fig. 35.2a

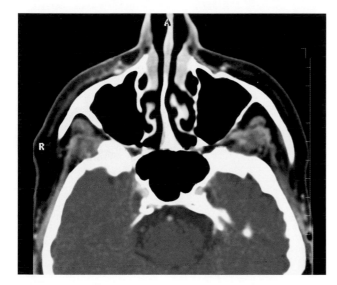

Fig. 35.1b

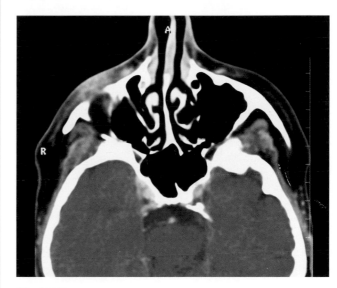

Fig. 35.2b

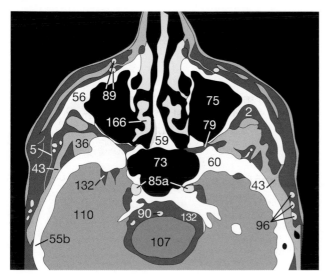

Fig. 35.1c

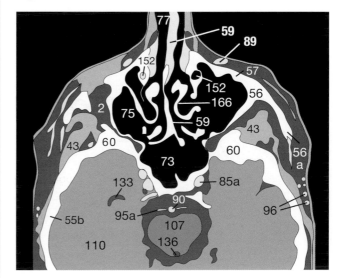

Fig. 35.2c

On the floor of the orbit, the short inferior oblique muscle (**47f**) often seems poorly delineated from the lower lid. This is due to the similar densities of these structures. Directly in front of the clinoid process/dorsum sellae (**163**) lies the pituitary gland (**146**) in its fossa, which is laterally bordered by the carotid siphon (**85a**).

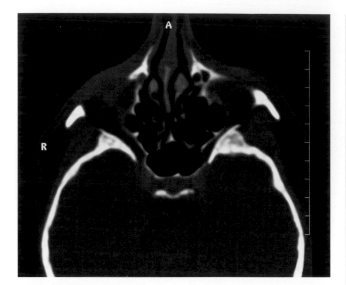

Fig. 36.1a

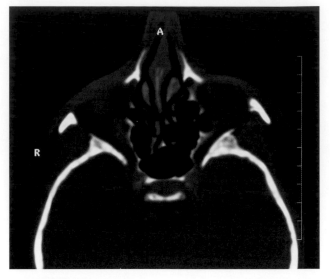

Fig. 36.2a

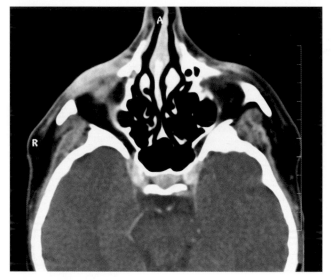

Fig. 36.1b

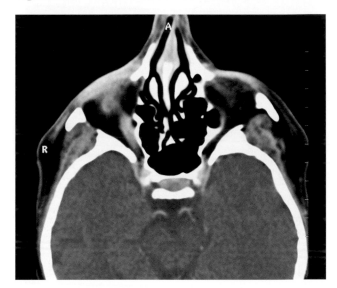

Fig. 36.2b

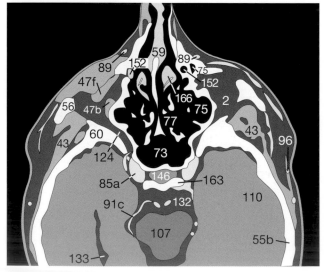

Fig. 36.1c

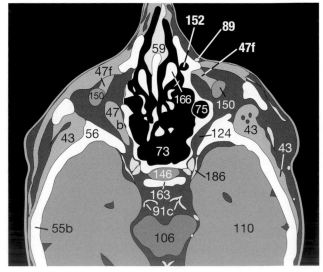

Fig. 36.2c

Small inclinations of the head cause slightly asymmetric views of the globe (**150**) and the extraocular muscles (**47**). The medial wall of the nasolacrimal duct (**152**) is often so thin that it cannot be differentiated. At first sight the appearance of the clinoid process (**163**), between the pituitary stalk (**147**) and the carotid siphon (**85a**) on the left side only, may be confusing in Figure 37.2b.

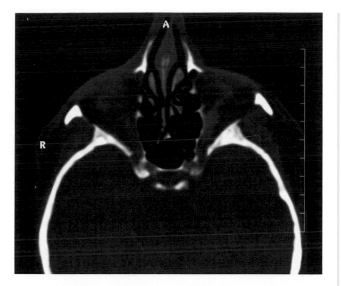

Fig. 37.1a

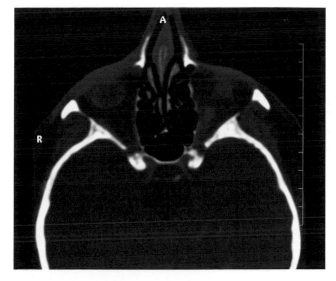

Fig. 37.2a

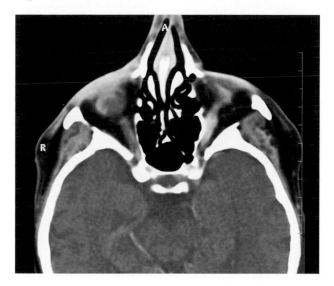

Fig. 37.1b

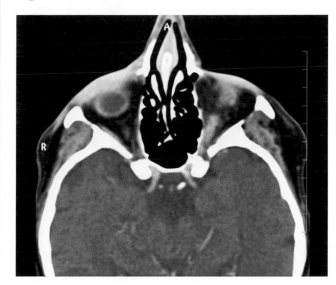

Fig. 37.2b

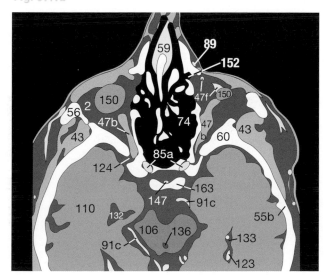

Fig. 37.1c

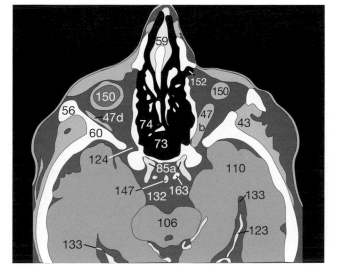

Fig. 37.2c

After intravenous injection of CM, the branches of the middle cerebral artery (**91b**) originating from the internal carotid artery (**85a**) are readily distinguished. The gray shade of the optic nerves (**78**) as they pass through the chiasm (**145**) to the optic tracts (**144**), however, is very similar to that of the surrounding CSF (**132**). You should always check on the symmetry of the extraocular muscles (**47**) in the retrobulbar fatty tissue (**2**).

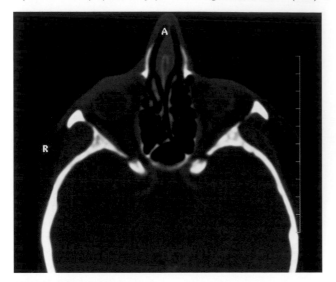

Fig. 38.1a

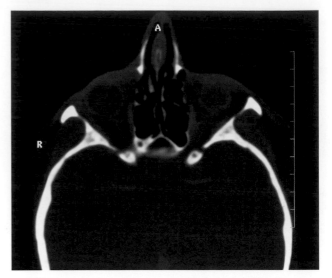

Fig. 38.2a

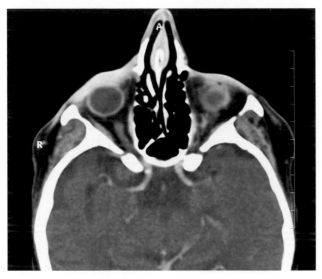

Fig. 38.1b

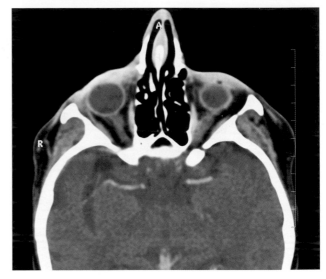

Fig. 38.2b

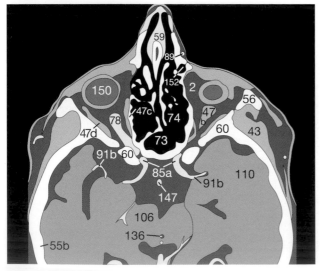

Fig. 38.1c

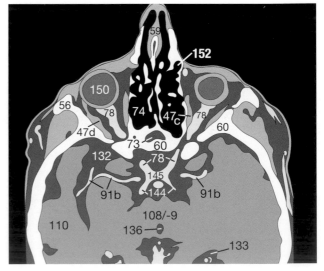

Fig. 38.2c

In the globe (**150**) you can now see the hyperdense lens (**150a**). Notice the oblique course of the ophthalmic artery (★) crossing the optic nerve (**78**) in the retrobulbar fatty tissue (**2**). Figure 39.2b shows a slight swelling (**7**) of the right lacrimal gland (**151**) compared to the left one (see Fig. 40.1b).

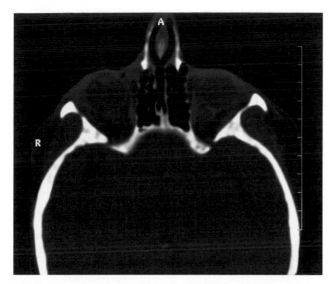

Fig. 39.1a

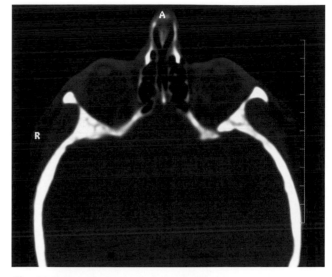

Fig. 39.2a

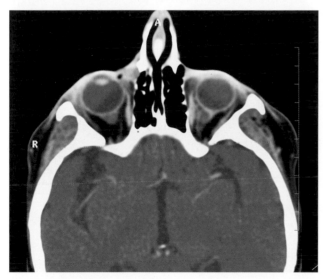

Fig. 39.1b

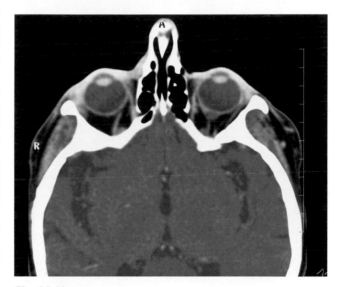

Fig. 39.2b

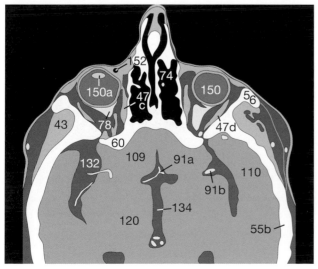

Fig. 39.1c

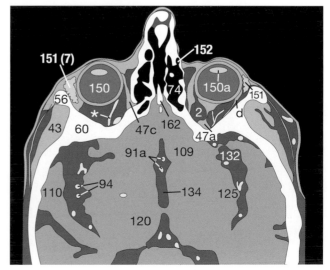

Fig. 39.2c

Figure 40.1b clarifies that in this case there is indeed an inflammation or tumor-like thickening (**7**) in the right lacrimal gland (**151**). The superior rectus muscle (**47a**) appears at the roof of the orbit and immediately next to it lies the levator palpebrae muscle (**46**). Due to similar densities, these muscles are not easily differentiated.

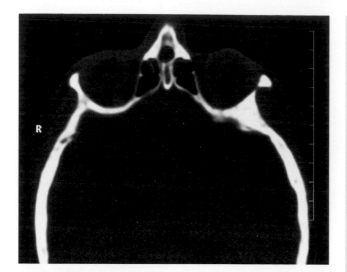

Fig. 40.1a

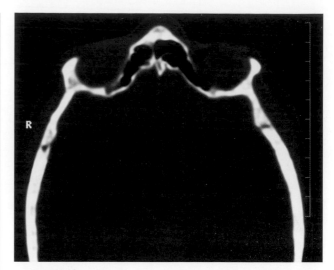

Fig. 40.2a

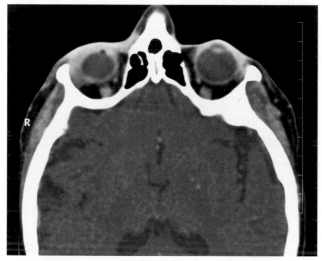

Fig. 40.1b

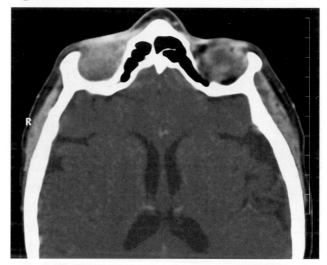

Fig. 40.2b

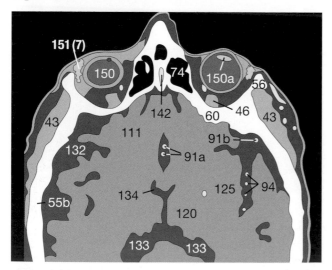

Fig 40.1c

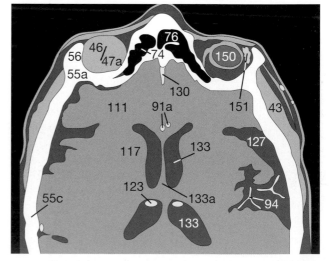

Fig. 40.2c

The axial views of the orbits and the face end here with the appearance of the frontal sinus (**76**). Examples of pathologic changes of the orbits or fractures of facial bones are found on pages 61 to 63.

The possibilites of angling the CT gantry are limited. In order to achieve scans in the coronal plane, the patients were formerly positioned as shown in the planning topogram (Fig. 41.1) in a prone position with the head completely extended. Nowadays coronal images are reconstructed digitally, based upon the threedimensional data set with a narrow collimation in MDCT-units, so that especially trauma patients do not have to be excluded any more for potential lesions of bones or ligaments of their cervical spine. Usually, images are viewed from anterior: the anatomic structures on the patient's right side appear on the left in the images and conversely, as if the examiner were facing the patient.

When looking for fractures, images are usually acquired in the thin-slice mode (slice and collimation, each 2 mm) and viewed on bone windows. Even fine fracture lines can then be detected. A suspected fracture of the zygomatic arch may require additional scans in the axial plane (see p. 34). In Figure 41.2a the inferior alveolar canal (★) in the mandible (**58**) and the foramen rotundum (★★) in the sphenoid bone (**60**) are clearly visible. As for the previous chapter, the code numbers for the drawings are explained in the legend in the front foldout.

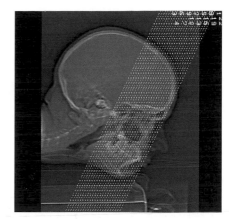

Fig. 41.1

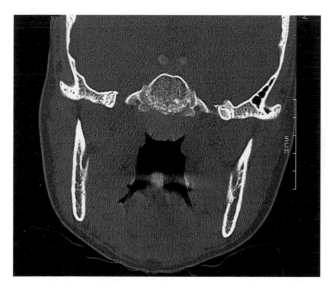

Fig. 41.2a

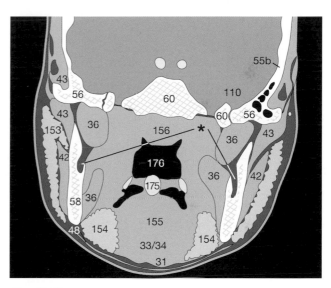

Fig. 41.2b

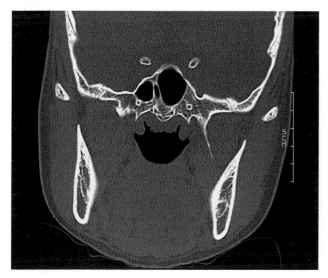

Fig. 41.3a

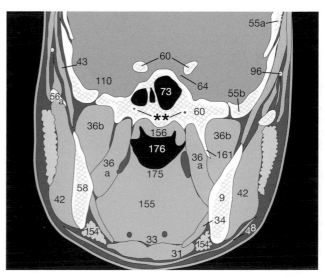

Fig. 41.3b

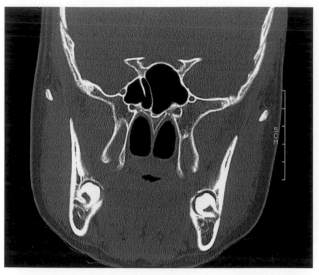

Fig. 42.1a

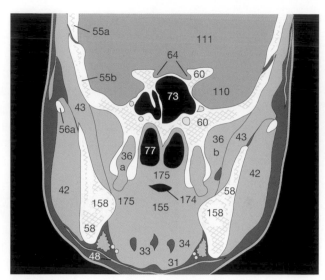

Fig. 42.1b

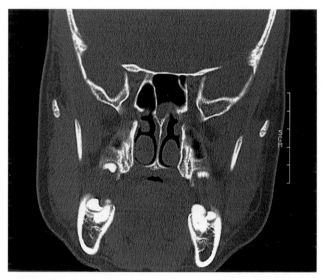

Fig. 42.2a

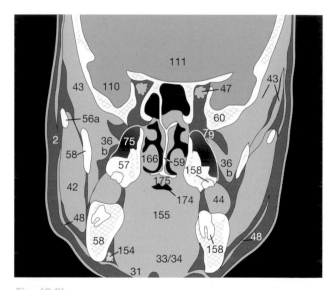

Fig. 42.2b

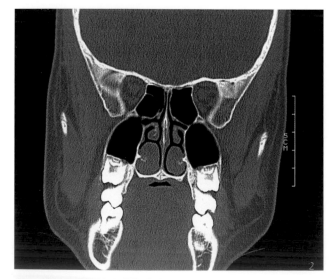

Fig. 42.3a

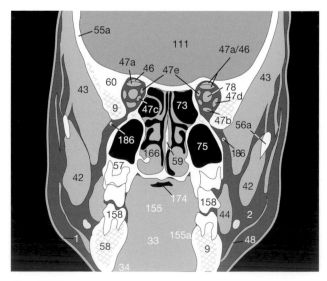

Fig. 42.3b

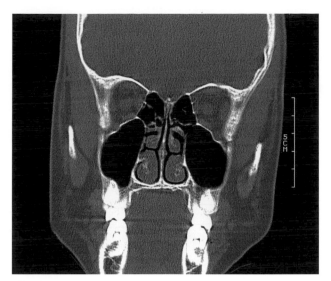

Fig. 43.1a

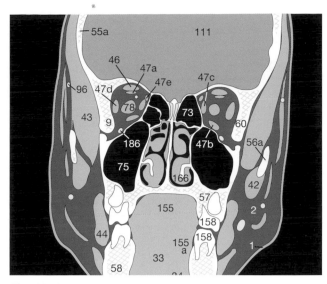

Fig. 43.1b

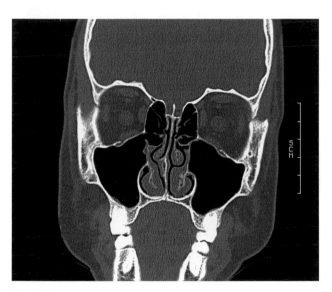

Fig. 43.2a

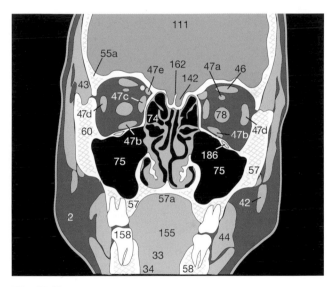

Fig. 43.2b

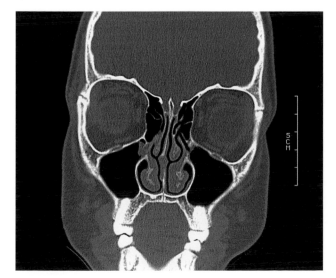

Fig. 43.3a

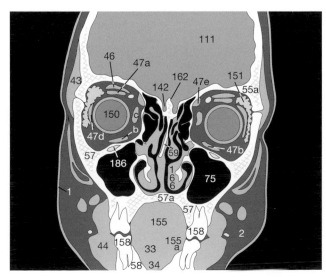

Fig. 43.3b

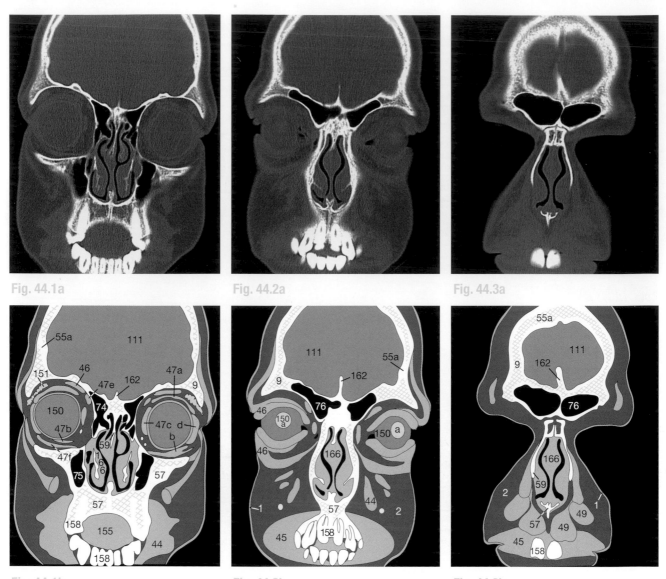

Fig. 44.1a   Fig. 44.2a   Fig. 44.3a

Fig. 44.1b   Fig. 44.2b   Fig. 44.3b

The insertions of the extraocular muscles on the globe (**150**) can also be clearly identified (**47 a–f**) in the anterior slices. The short inferior oblique muscle (**47f**), however, is often seen only in coronal scanning planes, because it does not pass with the others muscles through the retrobulbar fatty connective tissue. The same problem occurs in axial scans of the face (compare with Fig. 36.2b and Fig. 36.2c).

If a case of chronic sinusitis is suspected, it is very important to check whether the semilunar hiatus is open. It represents the main channel for discharging secretions of the paranasal sinuses. In Figure 60.3 you will find examples of anatomic variations which narrow this channel and may promote chronic sinusitis.

Sometimes one discovers a congenitally reduced pneumatization of a frontal sinus (**76**) or an asymmetric arrangement of other paranasal sinuses without any pathologic consequences. You should always make sure that all paranasal sinuses are filled exclusively with air, that they are well defined and present no air-fluid levels. Hemorrhage into the paranasal sinuses or the detection of intracranial bubbles of air must be interpreted as an indirect sign of a fracture – you will find examples of such fractures on page 63.

On the previous pages you have learned about the normal anatomy of the brain, the orbits, and the face. It may be some time ago that you studied the technical basics of CT and about adequate preparation of the patient. Before going on with the anatomy of the temporal bone, it would be good to check on and refresh your knowledge of the last chapters. All exercises are numbered consecutively, beginning with the first one on page 32.

Without doubt, you will improve your understanding of the subject if you tackle the gaps in your knowledge instead of skipping problems or looking at the answers at the end of the book. Refer to the relevant pages only if you get stuck.

Exercise 2: Write down from memory the typical window parameters for images of the lungs, bones, and soft tissues. Note precisely the width and center of each window in HU and give reasons for the differences. If you have difficulties answering this question, go back to pages 16/17 to refresh your memory.

Lung-/pleura window:	**Center**	**Width**	**Grey scale range**
			_____ HU to _____ HU
Bone window			
			_____ HU to _____ HU
Soft-tissue window			
			_____ HU to _____ HU

Exercise 3: Which two types of oral CM do you know? What specific aspects must you consider when administering this kind of CM depending on the clinical problem? Are there any consequences for your list?

Oral CM (name)	**Indication**	**Special schedule**
●		
●		

Exercise 4: What aspects should you always clarify before referring your patients to a CT examination which probably requires the i.v. infusion of CM? The same applies if you consider referring someone to a venogram/angiogram or an IVU (both procedures are carried out with nonionic CM containing iodine). MRI examinations, however, are carried out with gadolinium as the CM. (The answers to questions 3 and 4 can be found on pp. 18 and 19.)

a)

b)

c)

Exercise 5: How would you differentiate between long structures such as vessels, nerves, or certain muscles and nodu- lar structures such as lymph nodes or tumors? (You will find the answer on p. 15.)

Exercise 6: In which vessels might you find turbulence phenomena, caused by the CM injection, that must not be mistaken for a thrombus? (If you don't remember, check back to pp. 21-23.)

Thin-section CT scans (ultra-high resolution CT or UHRCT) are generally used to visualize the petrous bone for evaluating the inner ear. This technique employs slice thicknesses of 0.3 to 1.0 mm with continuous advancement of the couch between successive slices. Better spatial resolution and detail enlargement are achieved by imaging only a reduced FOV in the petrous bone using the thin-section technique as opposed to imaging the entire head. The petrous bone (**55 b**) of each side is visualized separately at high magnification. From experience, this is the best way to visualize small anatomic structures such as the auditory apparatus (**61 a-c**), the cochlea (**68**), or the semicircular duct (**70 a-c**).

The scout topogram film (Fig. 46.1) shows the coronal slices. It is no longer necessary to position the patient prone with the neck hyperextended (see p. 41). The larger tilting angle of the gantry in today's CT systems makes it possible to obtain these slices even in a supine patient.

Note the pneumatization of the mastoid cells (**62**) and the normally thin wall of the external acoustic meatus (**63 b**). Inflammations in these air-filled spaces lead to characteristic effusions and/or mucosal thickening (see Fig. 60.2 a).

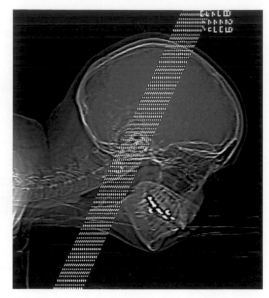

Fig. 46.1

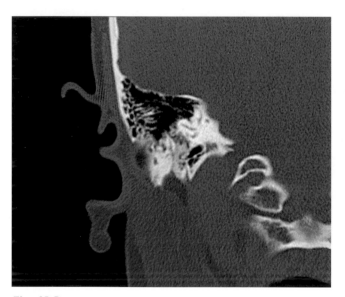

Fig. 46.2a

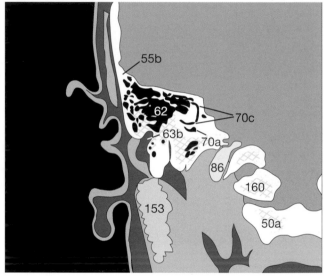

Fig. 46.2b

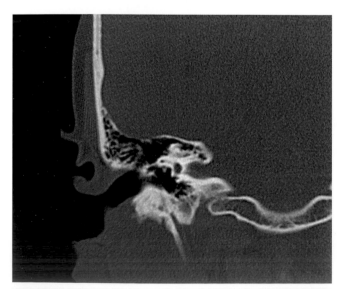

Fig. 46.3a

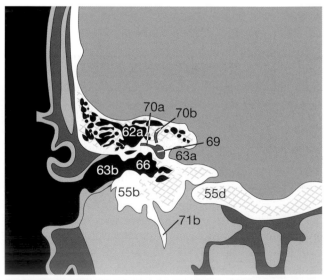

Fig. 46.3b

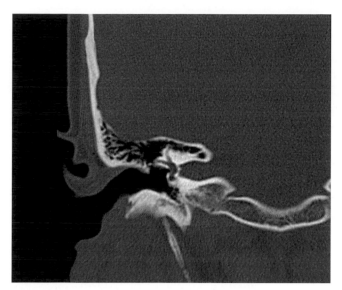

Fig. 47.1a

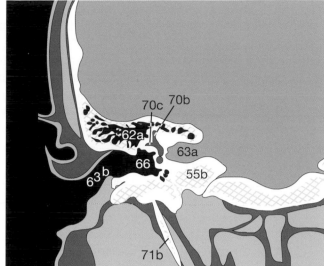

Fig. 47.1b

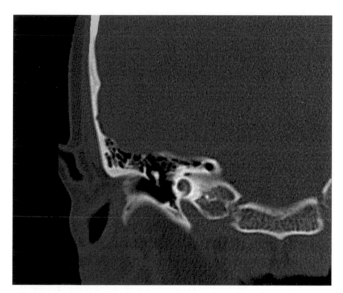

Fig. 47.2a

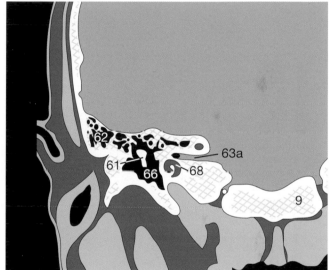

Fig. 47.2b

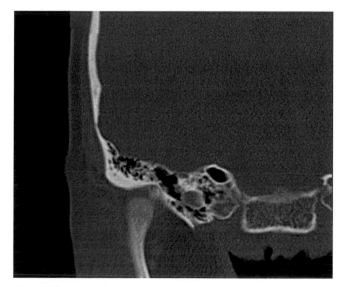

Fig. 47.3a

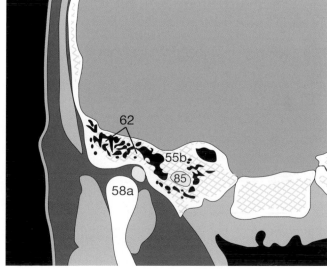

Fig. 47.3b

Analogous to coronal images, axial images are obtained with thin slices without overlap, i.e., 2 mm thickness and 2 mm increment and viewed on bone windows. The cerebellar hemispheres (**104**), the temporal lobe (**110**), and the soft tissues of the galea are therefore barely identifiable. Apart from the ossicles (**61a–c**) and the semicircular canals (**70a–c**), the internal carotid artery (**64**), the cochlea (**68**), and the internal (**63a**) and external auditory canals (**63b**) are visualized. The funnel-shaped depression in the posterior rim of the petrosal bone (Fig. 48.2a) represents the opening of the perilymphatic duct (**★★** = aqueduct of the cochlea) into the subarachnoid space. In Figure 49.1a note the localization of the geniculate ganglion of the facial nerve (**★**) ventral to the facial canal. The topogram (Fig. 48.1) shows an axial plane of section, obtained with the patient lying supine.

Test Yourself!   Exercise 7:   Think about differential diagnoses involving effusion in the middle ear (**66**), the outer auditory canal, or the mastoid cells (**62**) and compare your results with the cases shown on pages 60 and 62 to 63.

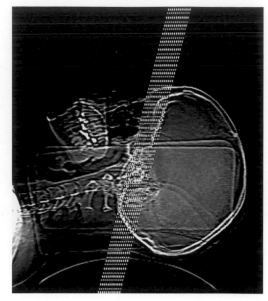

Fig. 48.1

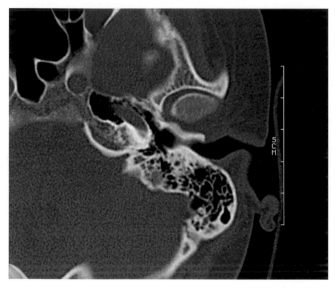

Fig. 48.2a

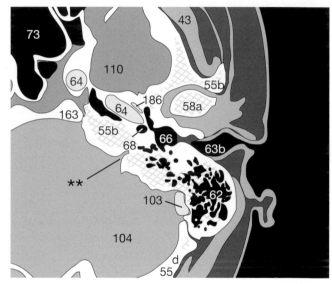

Fig. 48.2b

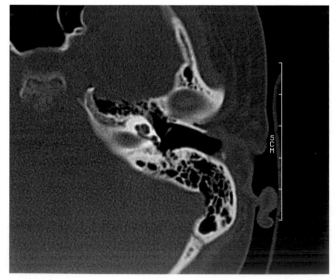

Fig. 48.3a

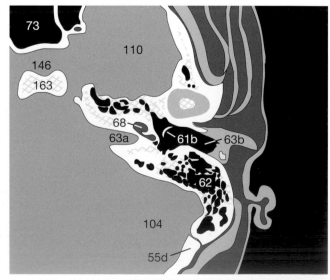

Fig. 48.3b

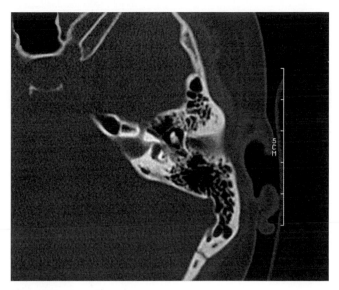

Fig. 49.1a

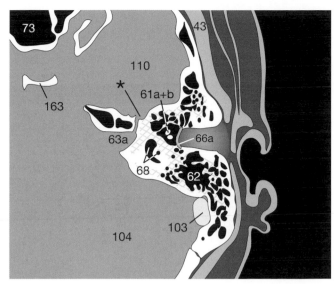

Fig. 49.1b

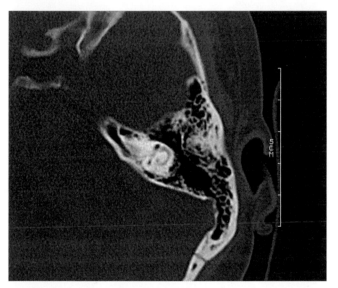

Fig. 49.2a

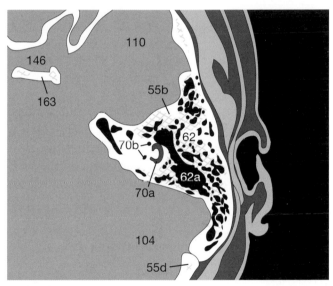

Fig. 49.2b

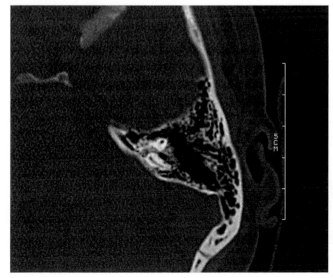

Fig. 49.3a

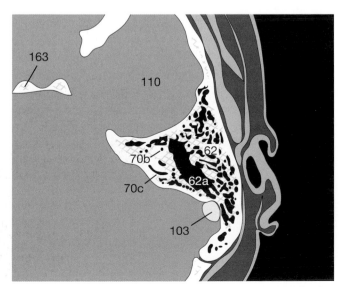

Fig. 49.3b

Do you remember the systematic sequence for evaluating CCT scans? If not, please go back to the checklist on page 26 or to your own notes on page 32.

After evaluating the soft tissues it is essential to examine the inner and outer CSF spaces. The width of the ventricles and the surface SAS increases continuously with age.

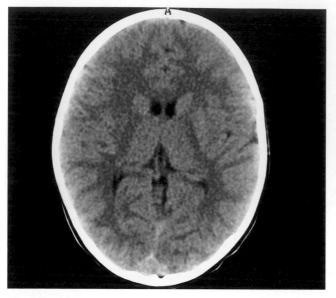

Fig. 50.1a

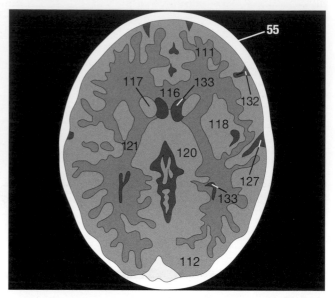

Fig. 50.1b

Since the brain of a child (Fig. 50.1a) fills the cranium (**55**), the outer subarachnoid space is scarcely visible, but with increasing age the sulci enlarge (Fig. 50.2a) and CSF (**132**) becomes visible between cortex and calvaria. In some patients this physiologic decrease in cortex volume is especially obvious in the frontal lobe (**111**). The space between it and the frontal bone (**55a**) becomes quite large. This so-called fron-

tally emphasized brain involution should not be mistaken for pathologic atrophy of the brain or congenital microcephalus. If the CT scan in Figure 50.1a had been taken of an elderly patient, one would have to consider diffuse cerebral edema with pathologically effaced gyri. Before making a diagnosis of cerebral edema or brain atrophy you should therefore always check on the age of the patient.

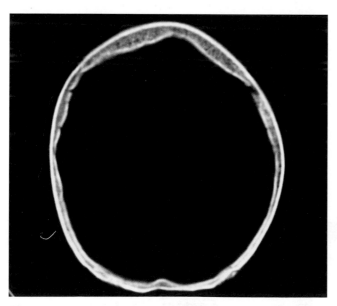

Fig. 50.2a

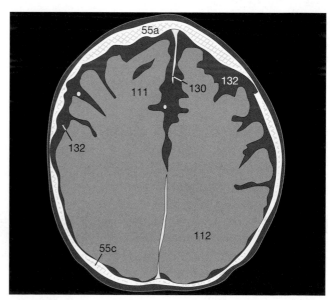

Fig. 50.2b

Figure 50.2a shows an additional variation from the norm. Especially in middle-aged female patients you will sometimes find hyperostosis of the frontal bone (**55a**) (Steward-Morel-Syndrome) without any pathologic significance. The frontal

bone (**55a**) is internally thickened on both sides, sometimes with an undulating contour. In cases of doubt, the bone window can help to differentiate between normal spongiosa and malignant infiltration.

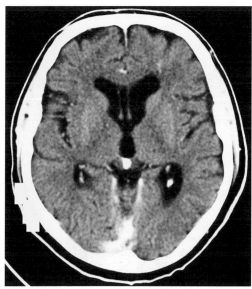

Fig. 51.1a

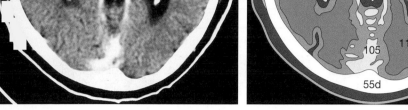

Fig. 51.1b

An incomplete fusion of the septum pellucidum (**133a**) can, as another variation, lead to the development of a so-called cavum of the septum pellucidum. Please review the normal scans in Figures 30.2a, 30.3a, and 31.1a for comparison. Usually only the part of the septum located between the two anterior horns of the lateral ventricles (Fig. 51.1a) is involved, less frequently the cavum extends all the way to the posterior horns (Fig. 51.2a).

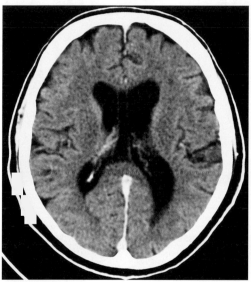

Fig. 51.2a

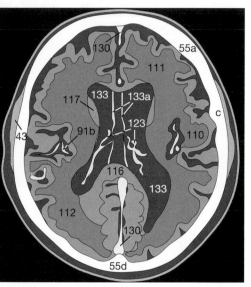

Fig. 51.2b

In the plane of Figure 51.1, just medial of the head of the caudate nucleus (**117**), you can evaluate both foramina of Monro (**141**) which function as a route for the choroid plexus (**123**) and the CSF from the lateral ventricles (**133**) to the 3rd ventricle (**134**). Refresh your anatomic skills by naming all other structures in Figure 51.1 and checking your results in the legend.

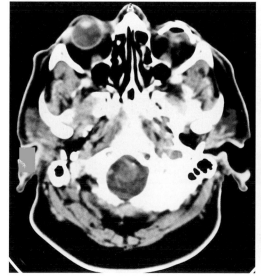

Fig. 51.3a

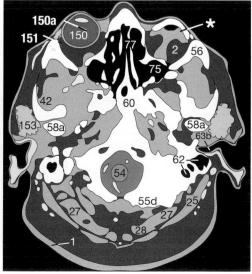

Fig. 51.3b

The radiologist will rarely be confronted with an eye prosthesis (★) after enucleation of a globe (**150**). In patients with a history of orbital tumor, a local relapse, i.e. in the retrobulbar space (**2**) has to be ruled out in check-up CT scans. The CT scan of the orbit in Figure 51.3a showed minor postoperative change without any evidence of recurrent tumor.

One of the most important rules of CT scan interpretation is to always compare several adjacent planes (see pp. 14–15). If the head is tilted even slightly during the scan procedure, one lateral ventricle (**133**) for example, can appear in the image plane (**d$_S$**), whereas the contralateral ventricle is still outside the plane (Fig. 52.1). Only its roof will appear.

The computer therefore calculates a blurred, hypodense area which could be mistaken for a cerebral infarction (Fig. 52.2a). By comparing this plane with the adjacent one below it (Fig. 52.3a), the situation becomes clear, since the asymmetric contours of the imaged ventricles are now obvious.

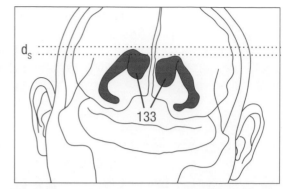

Fig. 52.1

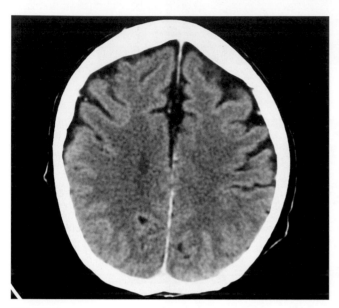

Fig. 52.2a

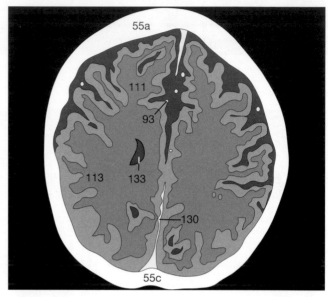

Fig. 52.2b

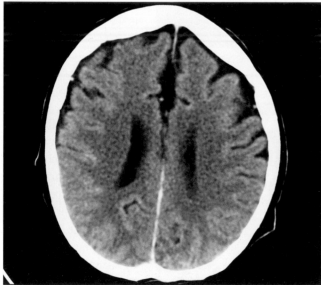

Fig. 52.3a

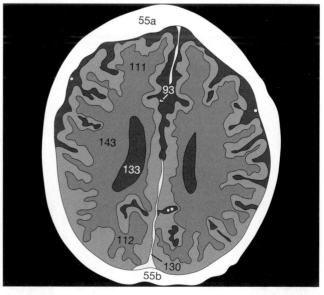

Fig. 52.3b

This example illustrates the importance of the correct placement of the patient's head. The exact position of the nose in an a.p. projection is obtained by using the gantry positioning lights. Involuntary movements of the head can be kept at a minimum by soft padding. In ventilated or unconscious patients an additional immobilization of the head with suitable bandings may be necessary.

One of the first steps in interpreting CCTs is the inspection of the soft tissues. Contusions with subcutaneous hematomas (**8**) may indicate skull trauma (Fig. 53.1a) and call for a careful search for an intracranial hematoma. Many injured patients cannot be expected to have their heads fixed for the duration of the CT scan, and this leads to considerable rotation. Asymmetric contours (★ in Fig. 53.1b) of the roof of the orbit (**55a**), the sphenoid bone (**60**), or the petrosal bone (not asymmetric in the illustrated examples!) are therefore frequent occurrences and may lead to misinterpretations of the hyperdense bone as a fresh intracranial hematoma.

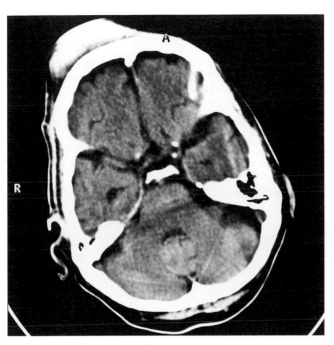

Fig. 53.1a

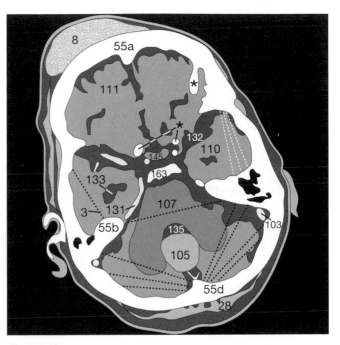

Fig. 53.1b

The question of whether it is just an asymmetric projection of the skull base or a real hematoma can be answered by comparing adjacent sections (Fig. 53.2a). In this example the bones of the skull base caused the hyperdense partial volume effect. Despite the obvious right frontal extracranial contusion, intracranial bleeding could not be confirmed. Please note the considerable beam hardening (bone) artifacts (**3**) overlapping the brain stem (**107**). Such artifacts would not appear in MR images of these levels.

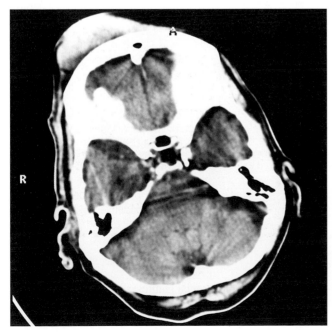

Fig. 53.2a

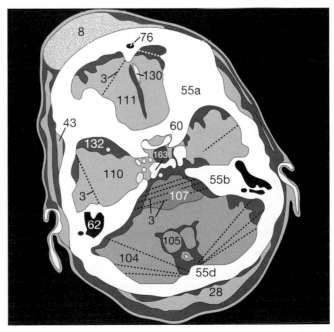

Fig. 53.2b

After having discussed that partial volume effects due to asymmetric projections (i.e., **55b** in Fig. 54.2b) may be misinterpreted as acute hematomas, this chapter will point out the characteristics of the different types of intracranial hemorrhage.

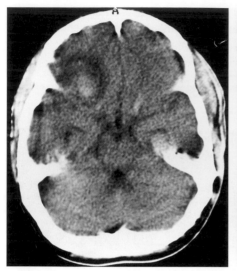

Fig. 54.1a

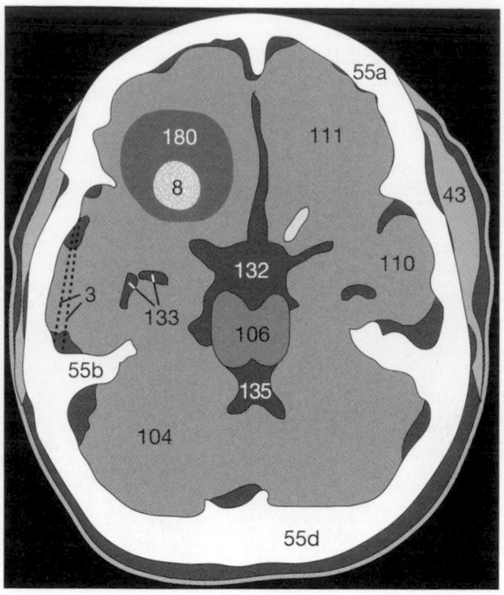

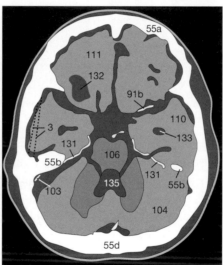

Fig. 54.1b

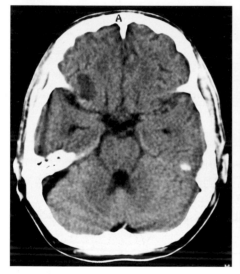

Fig. 54.2a

Fig. 54.2b

Bleeding Caused by a Contusion

As a direct consequence of skull trauma, cerebral contusion bleeding may occur (Fig. 54.1a). An acute hemorrhage (**8**) appears as a hyperdense mass which may be accompanied by surrounding edema (**180**) and displacement of adjacent brain tissue. In anemic patients the hematoma is less dense and may therefore appear isodense to normal brain.

If the vascular wall is damaged only secondarily by hypoperfusion mediated by edema, hemorrhage may not occur until hours or, more rarely, days after skull trauma. A CCT obtained immediately after skull trauma which does not show any pathologic changes is therefore not a good predictor since delayed cerebral bleeding cannot be ruled out. A follow-up scan should be obtained if the patient's condition deteriorates. After complete resorption of a hematoma (Fig. 54.2a), a well-defined defect isodense with CSF remains (**132**).

Contusion frequently leads to an epidural, subdural, or subarachnoid hemorrhage and may leak into the ventricles (Fig. 55.1a). Possible complications of such leakage or of a subarachnoid hemorrhage are disturbed CSF circulation caused by obstruction of the pacchionian granulations, the foramen of Monro, or of the 4th ventricle. An hydrocephalus with increased intracranial pressure and transtentorial herniation of the brain may result.

Epidural and subdural hematomas can also lead to major displacement of brain tissue and to midline shifts. Quite frequently this in turn causes obstruction of the contralateral foramen of Monro resulting in unilateral dilation of the lateral ventricle on the side opposite the bleeding (Fig. 56.3). The characteristics useful in differential diagnosis of the various types of intracranial bleeding are listed in Table 54.1.

Type of bleeding	Characteristics
Subarachnoid bleeding	Hyperdense blood in the subarachnoid space or the basal cisterna instead of hypodense CSF
Subdural bleeding	Fresh hematoma: crescent-shaped, hyperdense bleeding close to the calvaria with ipsilateral edema; hematoma is concave toward hemisphere; may extend beyond cranial sutures
Epidural bleeding	Biconvex, smooth ellipsoidal in shape; close to calvaria; does not exceed cranial sutures; usually hyperdense, rarely sedimented

Table 54.1

If there is intraventricular extension of intracranial hemorrhage (Fig. 55.1a), physiologic calcification of the choroid plexus (**123**), in the lateral (**133**) and 3rd ventricles (**134**), as well as those of the habenulae and the pineal (**148**), must be distinguished from fresh, hyperdense blood clots (**8**). Please note the edema (**180**) surrounding the hemorrhage (Fig. 55.1a).

If the patient has been lying supine, a horizontal fluid–fluid level caused by blood sedimenting in the posterior horns of the lateral ventricles may be seen (Fig. 55.2a). The patient is in danger of transtentorial herniation if the ambient cistern is effaced (Fig. 55.2b). In this case the 3rd ventricle is completely filled with clotted blood (➡ in Fig. 55.2a, b), and both lateral ventricles are markedly dilated. CSF has leaked into the paraventricular white mater (⇨). In addition, a lower section of this patient shows subarachnoid hemorrhage into the SAS (↙, ↘ in Fig. 55.2b).

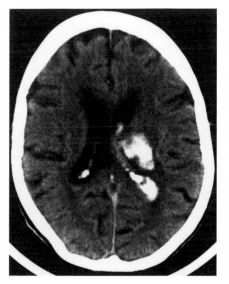

Fig. 55.1a

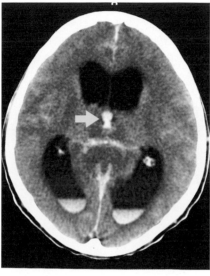

Fig. 55.2a

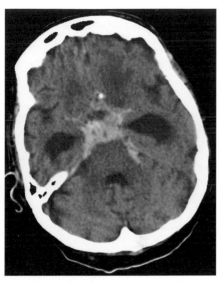

Fig. 55.3a

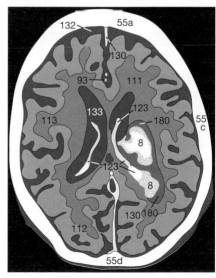

Fig. 55.1b

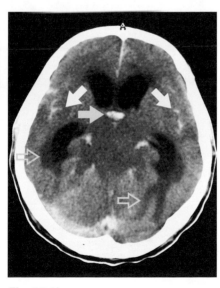

Fig. 55.2b

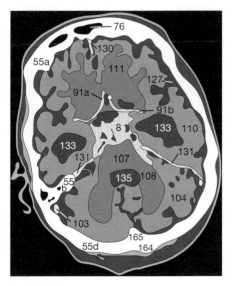

Fig. 55.3b

Subarachnoid Hemorrhage

An obstructive hydrocephalus, as caused by subarachnoid hemorrhage (**8** in Fig. 55.3a, b), may easily be identified because the temporal horns (**133**) of the lateral ventricles appear distended. In such cases it is important to have a closer look at the width of the SAS over the cerebral surface: blunted cerebral gyri usually indicate a diffuse cerebral edema. In the present case though, the width of the Sylvian fissure (**127**) and the surface SAS are normal. Acute edema is therefore not present (yet).

Since the surface SASs are very narrow in younger patients, it is possible to miss a subarachnoid hemorrhage in children. The only identifiable sign may be a small hyperdense area adjacent to the falx (**130**). In adults a small subarachnoid hemorrhage also causes only a minor, circumscribed area of hyperdensity (**8** in Fig. 56.1a). At the time of this CT scan the bleeding was so slight that it had not yet caused any displacement of brain tissue.

Subdural Hematoma

Bleeding into the subdural space results from cerebral contusions, damaged vessels in the pia mater, or from torn emissary veins. The hematoma initially appears as a long, hyperdense margin close to the skull (**8** in Fig. 56.2a). In contrast to an epidural hematoma, it is usually somewhat irregular in shape and slightly concave toward the adjacent hemisphere. This kind of bleeding is not confined by cranial sutures and may spread along the entire convexity of the hemisphere.

Subdural hematomas can also cause marked displacement of brain tissue (Fig. 56.3a) and lead to disturbances in CSF circulation and to incarceration of the brain stem in the tentorial notch. It is therefore not as important, for treatment purposes, to distinguish between a subhematoma or an epidural hematoma as it is to ascertain the extent of the hemorrhage. Hematomas with the propensity to expand, especially if edema is a threat, should therefore be drained or treated surgically.

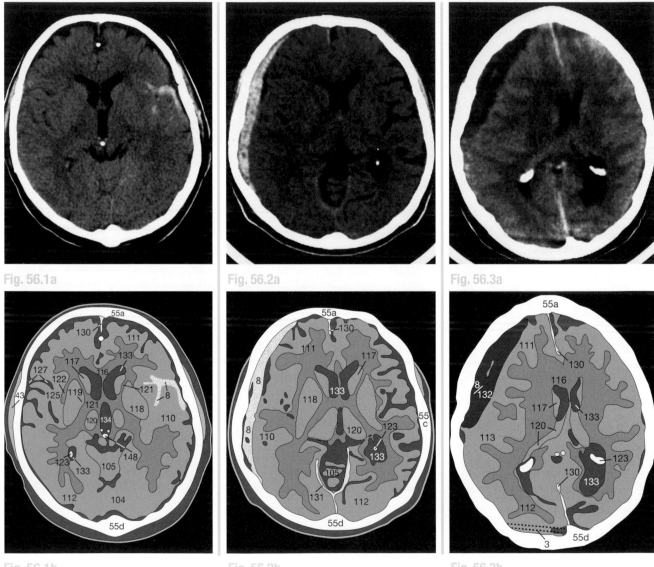

Fig. 56.1a

Fig. 56.2a

Fig. 56.3a

Fig. 56.1b

Fig. 56.2b

Fig. 56.3b

Chronic subdural hematomas (**8** in Fig. 56.3a) may appear homogeneously hypodense or show inhomogeneous density with sedimentation of blood. The danger involved in a small, venous bleed is the symptom-free interval and the slow onset of somnolence up to the development of a coma. Therefore, a patient with suspected bleeding after cranial trauma should always be kept under observation in order to detect any clinical deterioration.

Extradural Hematomas

Bleedings into the extradural spaces are usually caused by dam-age to the middle meningeal artery, and rarely by venous bleeding from the sinuses or the pacchionian bodies. Predisposed areas are temporoparietal regions or sometimes the posterior cranial fossa, in which case there is severe danger of tonsillar herniation. Arterial hemorrhage lifts the dura from the inner surface of the cranium (**55**) and then appears as a biconvex, hyperdense area with a smooth border to the adjacent hemisphere. The hematoma does not extend beyond the sutures between the frontal (**55a**), temporal (**55b**), parietal (**55c**), or occipital (**55d**) bones. In small extradural hematomas (**8**) the biconvex shape is not distinct (Fig. 57.1a), making it difficult to differentiate the finding from a subdural hematoma.

It is important to distinguish between a closed skull fracture with an intact dura, and a compound skull fracture with the danger of secondary infection. An unequivocal sign of a compound skull fracture (Fig. 57.2a) is the evidence of intra-cranial air bubbles (**4**), which prove that there is a connection between intracranial spaces and the paranasal sinuses or the outside. It is difficult to determine whether the bilateral, hyperdense hematomas (**8**) in Figure 57.2 are extradural or subdural. In this case the distortion of the midline was caused by the right-sided, perilesional edema (left side of Fig. 57.2a) since it was shifted toward the left (the side of the hematoma).

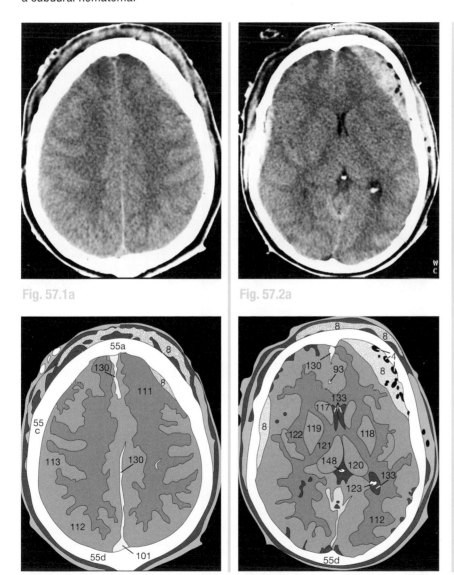

Fig. 57.1a

Fig. 57.2a

Fig. 57.1b

Fig. 57.2b

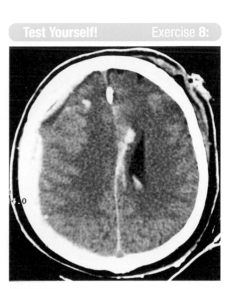

Test Yourself!   Exercise **8:**

Fig. 57.3

Space for your suggested answer:

Test Yourself!   Exercise **8:**

When looking at the image of another patient (Fig. 57.3), you will note several pathologic changes. Use the free space below the picture to note how many different types of bleeding (if any) you can distinguish and what other pathology/complications you suspect. You will find the answers at the end of the book, but remember: be a good sport and don't cheat, think first!

Apart from cardiovascular and malignant diseases, cerebral infarctions are among the most frequent causes of death. A thrombus occludes a cerebral artery, which leads to irreversible necrosis in the area of blood supply. Vascular occlusion develops in association with atherosclerotic changes of cerebral arteries or, less frequently, as a result of arteritis. A further cause are blood clots from the left heart or thrombotic plaques from the carotid bifurcation which embolize into a cerebral vessel.

In case of embolization, diffusely situated, small, hypodense zones of infarction in both basal ganglia and hemispheres are typical. Old emboli result in small, well-defined areas (**180**) which eventually appear isodense to the CSF (**132**). Such areas are called lacunal infarcts (Fig. 58.1a). A diffuse pattern

of defects calls for color flow Doppler imaging or carotid angiography and an echocardiogram to exclude atrial thrombus.

Please remember that in a suspected stroke it might take up to 30 hours to distinguish clearly the accompanying edema as a hypodense lesion from unaffected brain tissue. A CT scan should be repeated if the initial scan does not show any pathologic changes even though the patient is symptomatic and if symptoms do not resolve (resolution of symptoms points to a **t**ransient **i**schemic **a**ttack, **TIA**). In case of a TIA: no abnormalities are visible in the CT scan.

In contrast to the TIA, the **p**rolonged **r**eversible **i**schemic **n**eurologic **d**eficit (**PRIND**) is often associated with hypodense zones of edema in the CT scan.

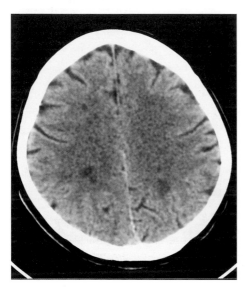

Fig. 58.1a

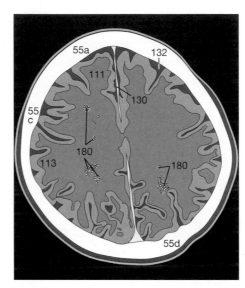

Fig. 58.1b

If the area of infarction corresponds to the distribution of a cerebral artery, one should con-sider an occlusion of the corresponding blood vessel. In classical infarctions of branches of the middle cerebral artery, ischemia will cause a hypodense area of edema (←, ↙ in Fig. 58.2a).

Depending on the size, the infarction may have severe mass effect and cause midline shift. Smaller areas of infarction do not usually show any significant midline shift. If the arterial walls are damaged, bleeding may occur and appear as hyperdense areas coating the neighboring gyri.

The unenhanced follow-up CT scan in Figure 58.2b shows an additional bleed into the head of the right caudate nucleus (⇐) and right putamen (↖). In this case the infarction is 2 weeks old and necrotic tissue has been mostly resorbed and replaced by CSF.

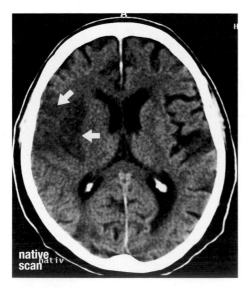

Fig. 58.2a

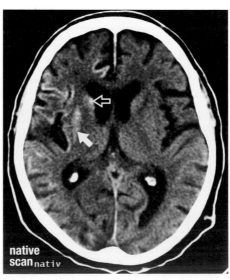

Fig. 58.2b

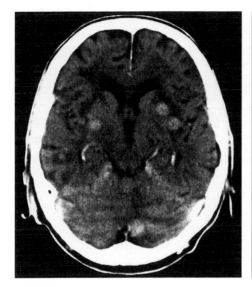

Fig. 59.1a

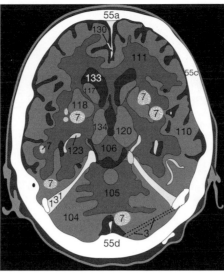

Fig. 59.1b

Whereas differential diagnosis (DD) of intracranial hemorrhage and infarction may be obtained without the use of CM, detection of cranial metastases (**7**) is definitely improved by the administration of i.v. CM. Even small areas in which the blood-brain barrier is disturbed become visible (Fig. 59.1a).Large metastases sometimes cause surrounding edema (**180**) which could be misinterpreted as infarct-related edema on unenhanced images if the metastasis appears isodense to the adjacent tissue. After i.v. CM the lesion in the left hemisphere (**7**) is clearly demarcated (Fig. 59.2a). Did you also spot the second, smaller metastasis within the right frontal lobe, which also shows some surrounding edema (**180**)?

The differential diagnosis of brain tumors is made much easier by the injection of i.v. CM. In the unenhanced image (Fig. 59.3a), the temporoparietal glioblastoma on the left (**7**) which has a central necrosis (**181**) could have been mistaken for cerebral infarction. The post-CM image, however, reveals the typical appearance of a glioblastoma with an irregular rim enhancement of its margin (Fig. 59.3c).

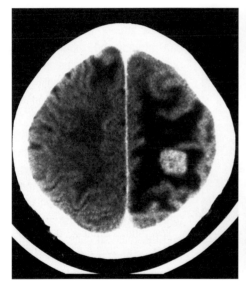

Fig. 59.2a

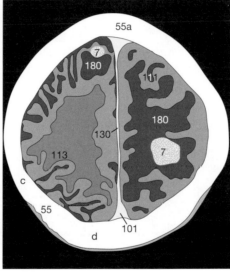

Fig. 59.2b

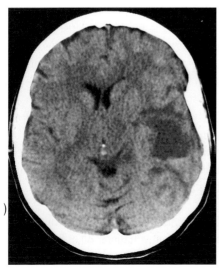

Fig. 59.3a

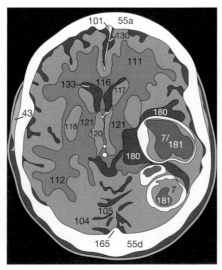

Fig. 59.3b

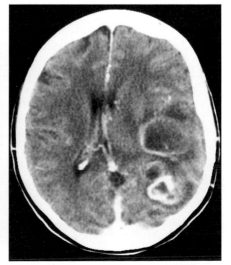

Fig. 59.3c

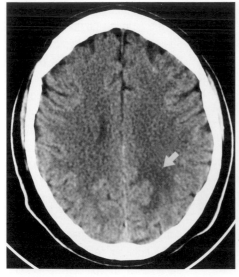

Fig. 60.1a

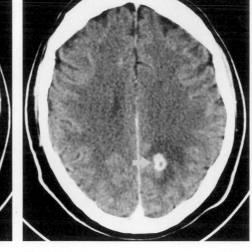

Fig. 60.1b

Another example of the advantages of i.v. CM is the demonstration of inflammatory processes, since the accompanying defect in the bloodbrain barrier will not show on an unenhanced image. Figure 60.1a shows hypodense edema ( ) in an unenhanced section of a patient suffering from aortic valve endocarditis. Contrast medium (Fig. 60.1b) confirmed the finding by enhancing the inflammatory process ( ). Bacteria from the aortic valve caused this septic embolism in the left occipital lobe.

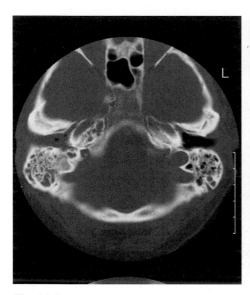

Fig. 60.2a

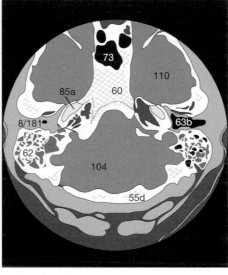

Fig. 60.2b

Inflammation of the paranasal sinuses and of the middle ear can already be diagnosed in native images as effusions **(8)**, for example in the normally air-filled mastoid cells **(62)**. Swelling of the mucous membranes of the external auditory canal **(63b)** is visible without the need for CM. Figure 60.2a shows bilateral otitis externa and media, which is more severe on the right side where it involves the antrum and the mastoid cells. With progressing abscess formation, an image on bone windows should be obtained in order to detect possible bone erosion.

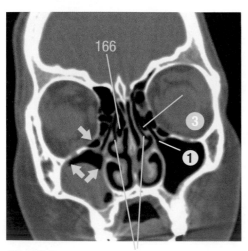

Fig. 60.3

A retention cyst, which often appears in one of the paranasal sinuses, should be considered in the differential diagnosis of advanced inflammations. They typically have a broad base on the wall of a paranasal sinus, extend into its lumen, and have a roundish convex shape (, in Fig. 60.3).

Such cysts are only of significance if they obstruct the infundibulum (**1**) of the maxillary sinus or the semilunar canal (**2**), causing an accumulation of secretions. In patients with chronic sinusitis, it is therefore important to check for an unobstructed lumen of the semilunar canal (**2**) or for variations which may restrict mucociliary transport of secretory products.

Haller's cells ( ), a pneumatized middle concha (166), and a pneumatized uncinate process (**3**) are among the most frequent variations. All of these variations can obstruct the semilunar canal and cause chronic, relapsing sinusitis.

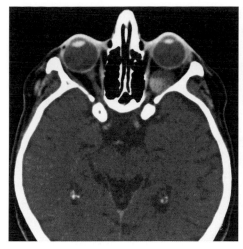

Fig. 61.1a

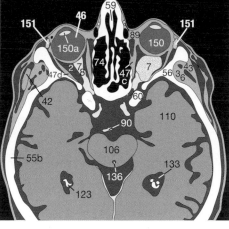

Fig. 61.1b

You have already seen pathologic changes in the lacrimal gland (pp. 39/40) and the CT morphology of an eye prosthesis (p.51). Every mass within the orbit should, of course, be diagnosed early and treated effectively because of the possibly severe consequences to vision. In order not to miss tumor invasion into the walls of the orbit, bone windows should also be obtained. In Figure 61.1a there is a hemangioma (**7**) within the retrobulbar fat (**2**), which is not necessarily an indication for operation because of its benign character. In this case it causes a minor proptosis.

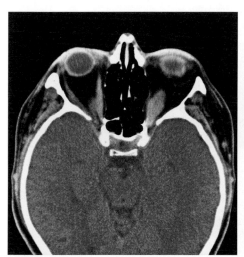

Fig. 61.2a

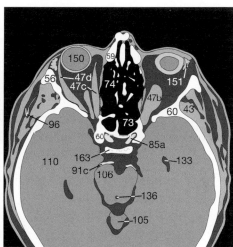

Fig. 61.2b

Endocrine Ophthalmopathy

Minimal discrete changes can be missed during the reporting of a CT scan: endocrine ophthalmopathy often appears as part of Graves' disease and can, in its early stage, only be diagnosed on the basis of a thickening of the external ocular muscles, e.g. the inferior rectus muscle (**47b** in Figs. 61.2a, 61.3a).

Myositis should be considered in the differential diagnosis. If this early sign is not detected, the disease of the orbital tissue, which is most probably an autoimmune disease, may progress in the absence of therapeutic intervention. Therefore, you should always examine the symmetry of the external ocular muscles (**47**) when looking at an orbital CT scan.

There will often be a typical temporal pattern of involvement. The first finding is an increase in the volume of the inferior rectus muscle (**47b**). The disease will continue and affect the medial rectus muscle (**47c**), the superior rectus muscle (**47a**), and finally all the other external ocular muscles.

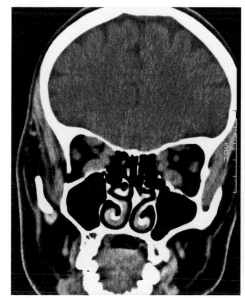

Fig. 61.3a

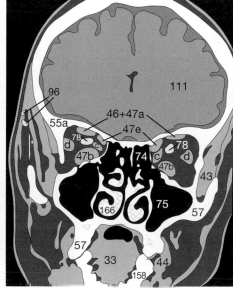

Fig. 61.3b

In contrast to benign retention cysts (p. 60), malignant tumors of the paranasal sinuses often lead to destruction of the facial bones and may invade the orbit, the nasal cavity (**77**), or even the cranial fossa. It is therefore useful to examine both the soft tissue and bone windows. For planning a resection, different CT planes might be necessary. The following example shows a tumor of the paranasal sinuses (**7**) in an axial (Fig. 62.1a) and a coronal view (Fig. 62.2a). Originating from the mucous membranes of the right maxillary sinus (**75**), the tumor has infiltrated the nasal cavity (**77**) and the ethmoid cells.

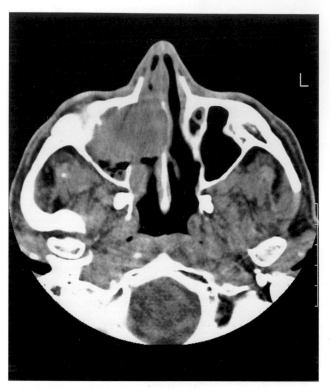

Fig. 62.1a

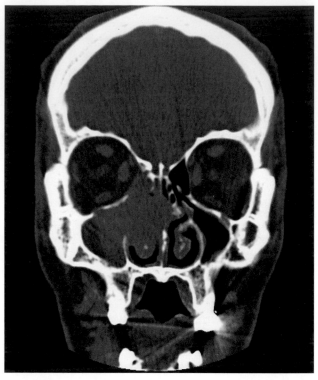

Fig. 62.2a

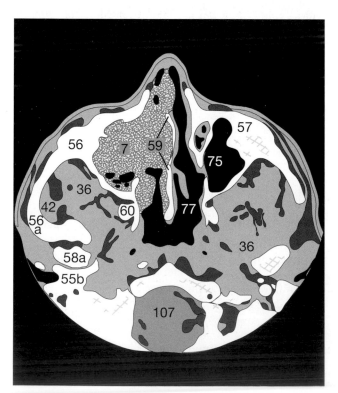

Fig. 62.1b

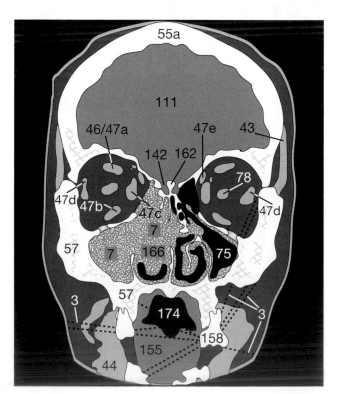

Fig. 62.2b

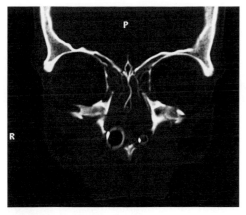

Fig. 63.1a

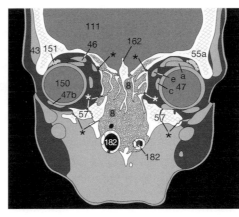

Fig. 63.1b

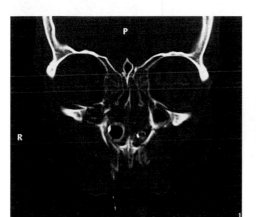

Fig. 63.2a

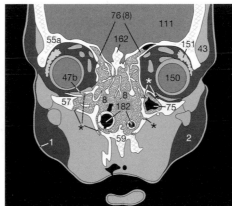

Fig. 63.2b

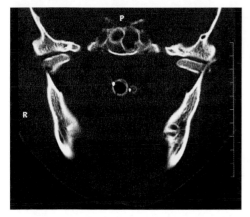

Fig. 63.3a

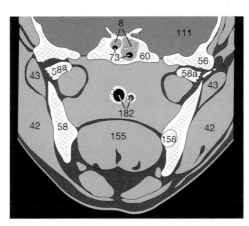

Fig. 63.3b

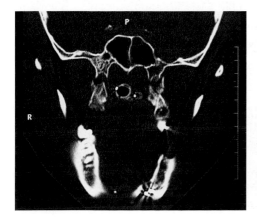

Fig. 63.4a

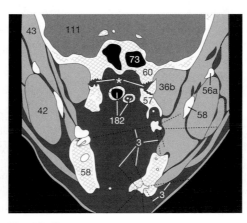

Fig. 63.4b

The most common reason for doing a coronal CT scan is, apart from determining the extent of chronic sinusitis, the diagnosis of fractures: in fractures of the orbital floor (Figs. 63.1a, 63.2a) any accompanying herniation of retrobulbar fat (**2**) or the inferior rectus muscle (**47b**) into the fracture site (✱) or even into the subjacent maxillary sinus (**75**) should be determined preoperatively. Diagnosis of the fracture in Figure 63.2a is easier because there are dislocated bone fragments. In addition, it is important to detect indirect signs of fracture, such as very fine, step-like contours of the bones and secondary bleeding (**8**) into the nasal cavity (**77**) or the frontal (**76**) and maxillary sinuses (**75**). Another important question is whether or not the head of the mandible (**58a** in Fig. 63.3a) is fractured or the maxillary bone (**57**) has been fractured and displaced (✱) from the sphenoid (**60**) bone (Fig. 63.4a). In this case, severe bleeding (**8**) required intubation (**182**) and a nasogastric tube (**182**).

Fractures of the facial skull (Le Fort [33])

Type I: Straight across the maxillary bones and the maxillary sinuses (Guérin's fracture)

Type II: Across the zygomatic process of the maxilla, into the orbit, and through the frontal process of the maxilla to the contralateral side; maxillary sinus not involved

Type III: Involving the lateral wall of the orbit and the frontal process of the maxilla to the contralateral side; ethmoid cells and zygomatic arch usually involved, sometimes also affecting the base of the skull.

Whenever there is no contraindication, CT examinations of the neck are carried out after i.v. administration of CM. Malignant and inflammatory processes can be depicted more accurately with the aid of CM. Adequate enhancement of cervical vessels requires higher doses of CM than, for example, in CTs of the head. In spiral CT, the injection of CM must be precisely timed to the acquisition of data. There are specific recommendations and suggested schemes for CM injection at the end of the manual.

Selection of the Image Plane
In an analogous manner to head CT, a sagittal planning topogram (scanogram) at lower resolution is obtained first. The transverse (axial) levels and gantry angulation are determined from this topogram (Fig. 64.1). Usually sections of the neck are obtained using a 4–5 mm thickness. The axial images are obtained and printed as viewed from caudally so the right lobe of the thyroid is imaged to the left of the trachea, the left lobe to the right.

Images should be obtained with a small-scan field-of-view to optimize detail in smaller structures in the neck. As the thoracic inlet is approached during the scanning, the scan field-of-view is increased to include possible abnormalities in the clavicular fossa and the axilla.

Artifacts caused by dental prostheses (**3**) usually obscure surrounding structures (✶) in only one or two levels (Fig. 64.2a). It may be necessary to carry out a second acquisition at another angle (Fig. 64.2b) to reveal areas hidden by artifact (✶).

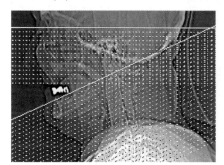

Fig. 64.1

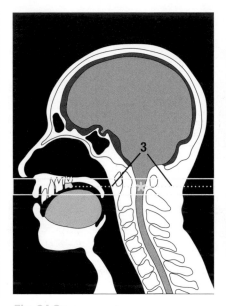

Fig. 64.2a

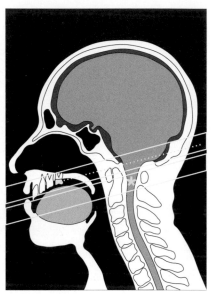

Fig. 64.2b

Systematic Sequence for Readings
We have already recommended a systematic approach with which to read CT scans of the head (see p. 26). For cervical CTs there is also no 'one and only' approach. The checklist presented here was developed through experience and is just one of many options for the beginner. Each examiner is free to set up his or her own checklist and strategy.

During neck imaging, separate hard copies at bone windows are rarely printed owing to cost. The radiologist must remember to check images at bone windows on the screen for fractures or lytic lesions.

Checklist for Reading Cervical CT Images

➡ Symmetry of neck musculature?
⇨ Condition and clarity of fat?
➡ Normal perfusion of vessels?
⇨ Thromboses or atherosclerotic stenoses?
➡ Symmetry and definition of salivary glands?
⇨ Thyroid parenchyma homogeneous and without nodules?
➡ Any focal pathologic enhancement with CM?
⇨ Narrowing of the tracheal lumen?
➡ Assessment of lymph nodes? Number and size?
⇨ Cervical vertebrae examined in bone window?
➡ Vertebral canal patent or narrowed?

The radiologist quickly reaches the limits of CT resolution (perhaps also of his/her anatomic knowledge) when trying to identify all of the different neck muscles. We have therefore reduced the amount of detail in the accompanying drawings so that smaller muscles are grouped. Single muscles have little clinical relevance and thus the legends to these images refer to combined muscle groups, e.g. the scalene muscles, the erector spinae muscles. Readers who want more anatomic detail should consult the relevant literature [5, 31].

Cervical images usually begin at the base of the skull and continue caudally to the thoracic inlet. The cranial sections

(Figs. 65.1 - 65.3) therefore include the maxillary sinus (**75**), the nasal cavity (**77**), and the pharynx (**176**). Dorsal to the pharynx lie the longus capitis and longus cervicis muscles (**26**), which extend caudally. Lateral to the mandible (**58**), beginning in Figure 65.2a, the parotid gland (**153**) is situated next to the large cervical vessels and vagus nerve (also p. 66). In front of the pons/medulla oblongata (**107**), the vertebral arteries (**88**) join to form the basilar artery (**90**).

The spread of inflammatory processes within the cervical connective tissue spaces is restricted within compartments defined by the cervical fascia [30]. The different layers of the cervical fascia are explained on the following page (Fig. 66.4).

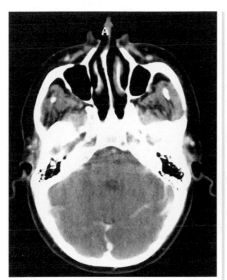

Fig. 65.1a

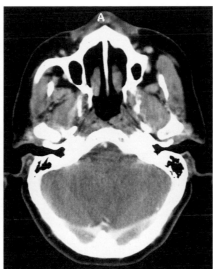

Fig. 65.2a

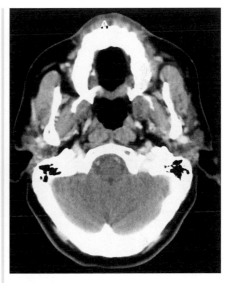

Fig. 65.3a

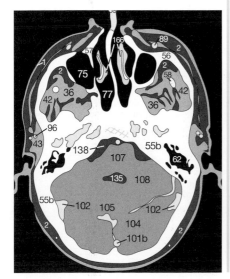

Fig. 65.1b

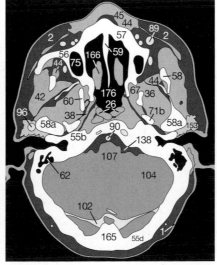

Fig. 65.2b

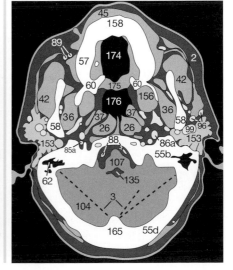

Fig. 65.3b

Further caudally the following cervical muscles become visible beneath the trapezius muscle (**23**): medial lie the semispinalis capitis (**28**) and longissimus capitis muscles (**27**), and more laterally the splenius capitis muscle (**25**). The parotid gland (**153**) is situated cranial and posterior to the submandibular gland (**154**) next to the mandible (**58**). The pharynx (**176**) is surrounded by Waldeyer's ring of tonsillar tissue (**157, 156**). Note that the carotid bulb is situated between Figures 67.4a and 68.2a; it is the point at which the common carotid artery (**85**) bifurcates into internal (**85a**) and external (**85b**) carotid branches. Under the tongue (**155**) the floor of the mouth is organized in layers. From cranial to caudal are: the genioglossus muscle (**33**), further laterally the geniohyoid muscle (**34**), and the anterior belly of the digastric muscle (**31**). The thin superficial muscle is the platysma (**48**).

Compartments of the Neck

If infections or inflammatory processes originate in the suprasternal (+) or pretracheal spaces between the superficial fascia (*) and the dorsal layer of the pretracheal fascia (**), they cannot spread into the mediastinum because both fascias insert into the sternum (**56** in Fig. 66.4). At the level of the parotid gland there is a similar barrier consisting of the sagittal septum which splits a retropharyngeal from a parapharyngeal space. Inflammations originating further dorsal, between the pretracheal (**) and the prevertebral (***) fascias, can spread caudally into the mediastinum.

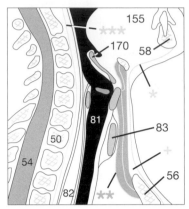

Fig. 66.4a

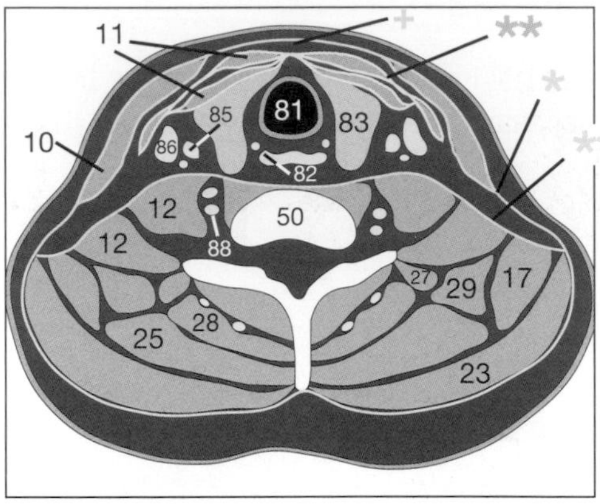

Fig. 66.4b

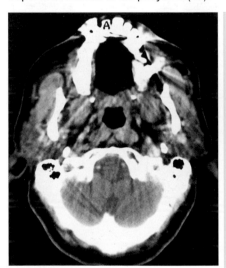

Fig. 66.1a

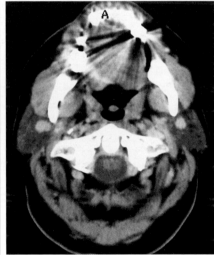

Fig. 66.2a

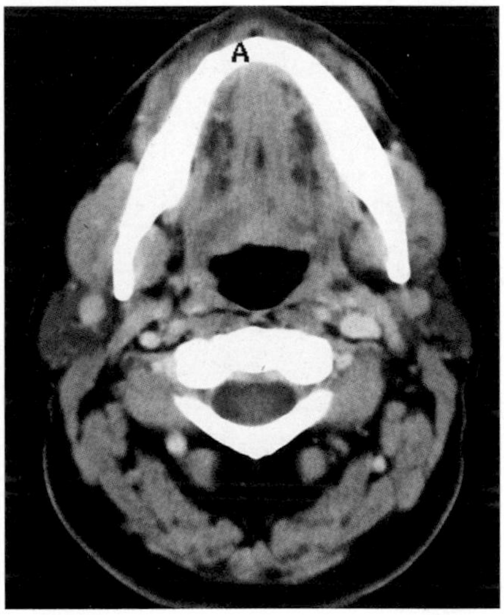

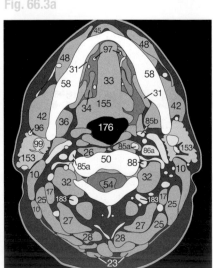

Fig. 66.3a

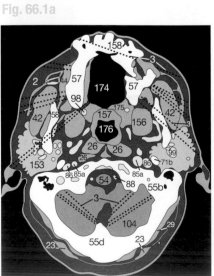

Fig. 66.1b

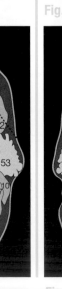

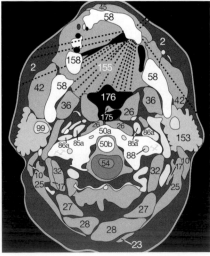

Fig. 66.2b

Fig. 66.3b

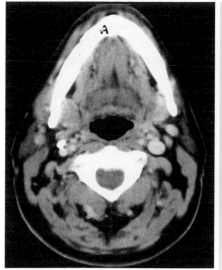

Fig. 67.1a

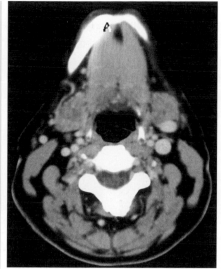

Fig. 67.2a

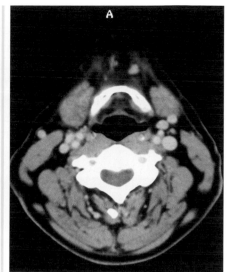

Fig. 67.3a

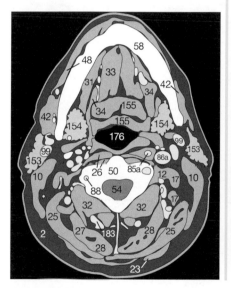

Fig. 67.1b

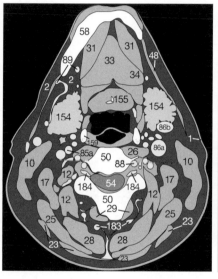

Fig. 67.2b

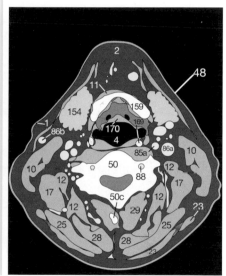

Fig. 67.3b

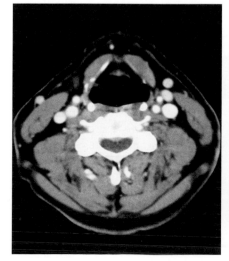

Fig. 67.4a

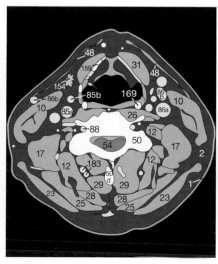

Fig. 67.4b

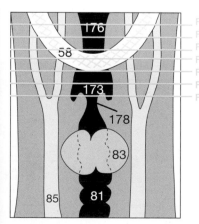

Fig. 67.5

The bifurcation of the common carotid artery (**85**) is an area of predilection for atherosclerotic plaques (Fig. 68.1a) which may be complicated by thrombus deposition (*****). Note the positions of the cricoid (**167**) and arytenoid cartilages (**168**) at the rima glottidis (**178**). In these normal individuals, CM enhances the density not only of the internal (**86a**), the external (**86b**), and the anterior jugular veins (**86c**), but also of the vertebral artery (**88**) in the transverse foramina of the cervical vertebrae. Always check for degenerative changes at the margins of the bodies of cervical vertebrae (**50**) or for herniated discs which might narrow the spinal canal containing the cervical cord (**54**). On either side of the trachea (**81**) lie the two lobes of the thyroid gland (**83**), which should have a smooth outline and have homogeneous parenchyma (Fig. 68.3a).

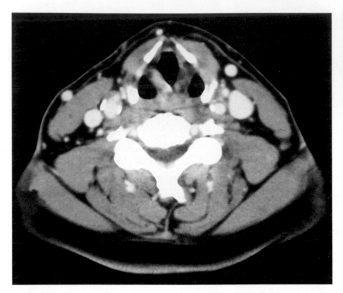

Fig. 68.1a

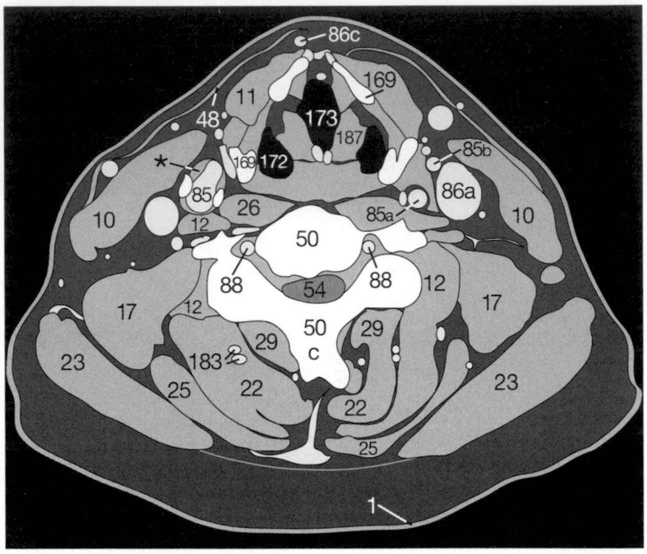

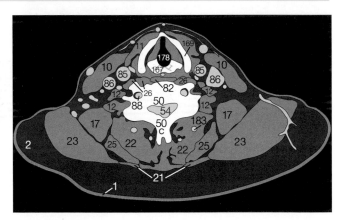

Fig. 68.1b

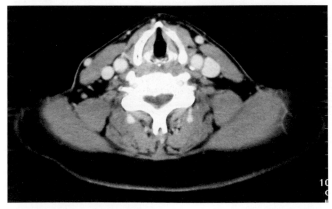

Fig. 68.2a

Fig. 68.2b

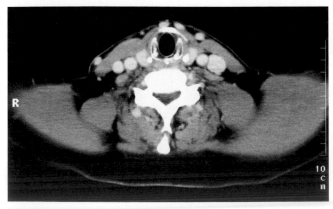

Fig. 68.3a

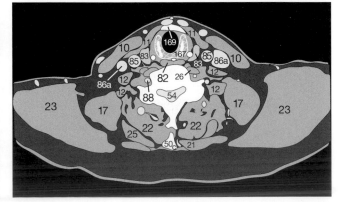

Fig. 68.3b

Because of its iodine content, the thyroid gland (**83**) appears hyperdense compared with surrounding muscles both before and, even more so, after the administration of CM (Figs. 69.1–69.3). Beginners occasionally mistake the esophagus (**82**), dorsal to the trachea (**81**), for swollen lymph nodes or a tumor. In case of doubt, comparison with other sections is helpful: usually a small, hypodense area indicates air in the lumen of the esophagus in an adjacent section. As a rule, the cervicothoracic junction is examined with the arms elevated to minimize artifacts due to bones. The muscles of the pectoral girdle as well as the shoulder joints therefore appear in unfamiliar positions.

The following chapter deals with neck pathology and includes a short "Test Yourself"; images and drawings of normal anatomy extending further caudally are continued on page 74.

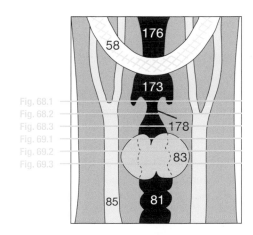

Fig. 68.1
Fig. 68.2
Fig. 68.3
Fig. 69.1
Fig. 69.2
Fig. 69.3

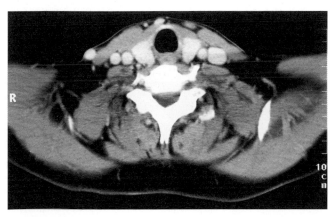

Fig. 69.1a

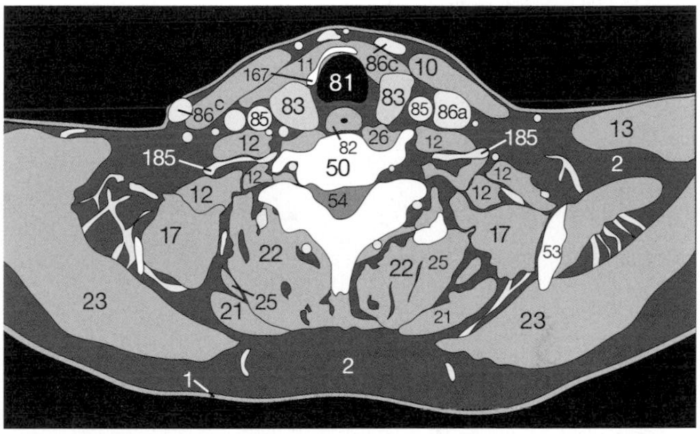

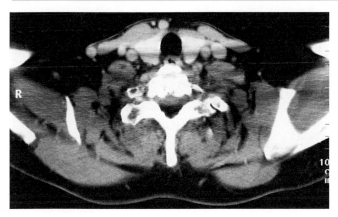

Fig. 69.1b

Fig. 69.2a

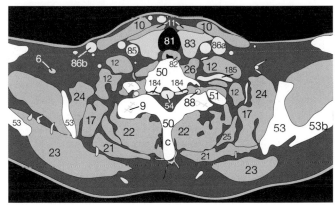

Fig. 69.2b

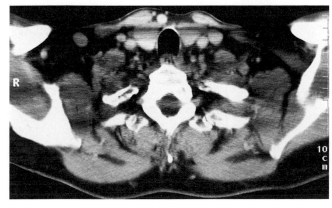

Fig. 69.3a

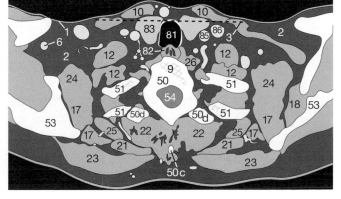

Fig. 69.3b

Enlarged cervical LNs (Fig. 70.1a) appear conspicuously as isolated nodular masses (**6**) that cannot be followed into adjacent levels (see p. 15). Large lymphomas (**7**) or conglomerate LN masses (Fig. 70.1a) often develop central necrosis (**181**). It is sometimes difficult to distinguish them from abscesses with central necrosis (**181**) as shown, for example, in Figure 70.2a. Abscesses typically infiltrate the surrounding adipose tissue with a streaky pattern of edema (**180**) so that structures such as arteries, veins, or nerves (on the left side of the neck in Fig. 70.2a) become difficult to identify. In immune-suppressed patients, abscesses can become remarkably large. Compare the scans in Figures 70.3a (unenhanced) and 70.3b (enhanced): after injection of CM, the outer wall of the abscess (✱) as well as the central septa have become enhanced. These appearances are so similar to large hematomas or necrotic tumors that a differential diagnosis may be difficult without a detailed clinical history.

Note also the atherosclerotic plaques or thromboses in the lumen of the carotid artery (**85**) as in Figure 70.1a.

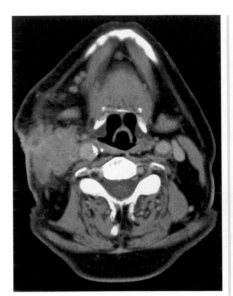

Fig. 70.1a

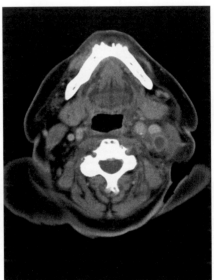

Fig. 70.2a

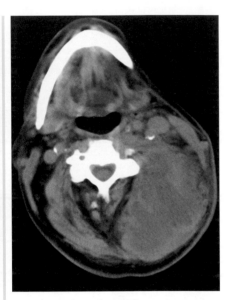

Fig. 70.3a (unenhanced)

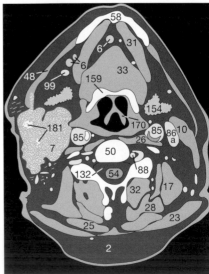

Fig. 70.1b

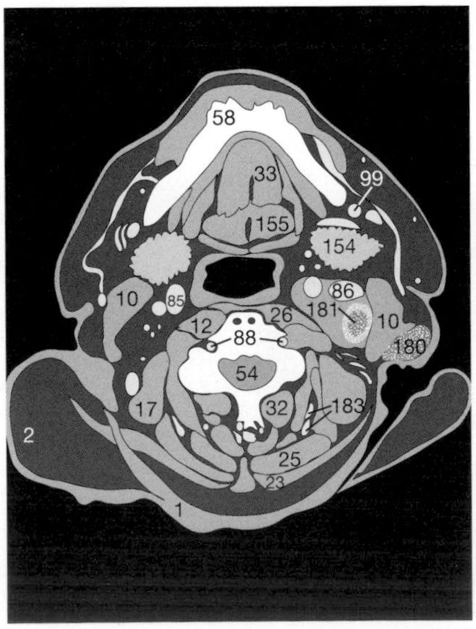

Fig. 70.2b

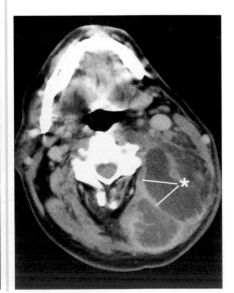

Fig. 70.3b (enhanced)

The parenchyma of the thyroid gland (83) should appear sharply demarcated and have an homogeneous pattern in CT scans. The average transverse diameter of each lobe is 1-3 cm, 1-2 cm sagittally and 4-7 cm in craniocaudal direction. The total volume of the thyroid gland varies between 15 and 25 ml in adults. If the thyroid is enlarged, check for tracheal compression or stenosis (81) and the caudal border of the goiter should be determined.

A benign struma (83) may extend into retrosternal regions and laterally displace supra-aortic vessels (85, 87, 88) (Fig. 71.2).

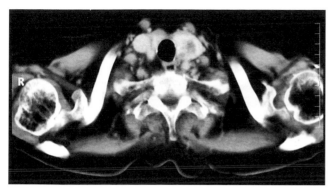

Fig. 71.1a

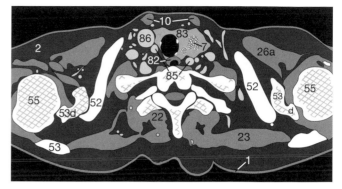

Fig. 71.1b

The parenchymal structure of a thyroid carcinoma (7) appears inhomogeneous, and the contours are not easily distinguished from the remaining normal parenchyma (83) (Fig 71.1a).

In advanced stages of carcinoma (Fig. 71.3), cervical vessels and nerves are completely surrounded by tumor, and areas of necrosis (181) appear. The tracheal walls (81) are compressed and may become infiltrated. After partial resection of a struma (Fig. 71.4), some thyroid tissue (83) may still be seen close to the trachea. In this case the left internal jugular vein was also removed and the lumen of the right one (86a) is therefore larger than normal.

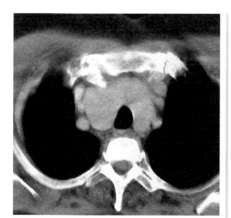

Fig. 71.2a

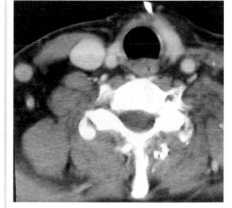

Fig. 71.3a

Fig. 71.4a

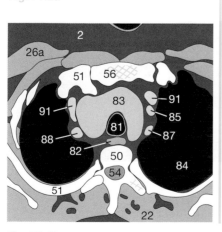

Fig. 71.2b

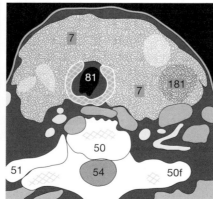

Fig. 71.3b

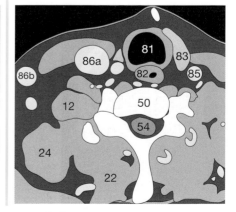

Fig. 71.4b

After having discussed normal anatomy of caudal cervical sections (p. 67), normal thoracic anatomy is presented. From this page on, you will find the number codes for the drawings in the rear foldout.

Selection of Image Plane
As a rule, the sections of the thorax are chosen in the transverse or axial plane at thicknesses and steps of 4 to 8 mm. Sections 7 mm thick will overlap by 1 mm, for example, when the patient table is advanced in 5 mm steps. A small topogram (Fig. 75.1) accompanying each sheet of images shows the position of the sections relative to the major anatomic structures of the region. In order not to miss any pathologic changes within the lung (review p. 13), it has become accepted practice to make a hard copy of both soft-tissue and lung windows or to provide a CD with the image data. Each image can therefore be viewed at two different window settings. Again the large number of images necessitates a systematic technique for evaluation so as not to waste time looking randomly back and forth between them.

Systematic Sequence for Readings
The beginner often forgets to check the soft tissues of the thoracic wall because the examination of the mediastinum and the lungs is automatically considered more important. These tissues should therefore be evaluated first. Common sites of abnormality are the breasts and fat in the axilla (**2**). After this–also using soft-tissue windows–the mediastinum is checked for pathologic masses. The easiest approach is to orient yourself relative to the arch of the aorta (**89b**), which can be recognized even by the inexperienced (Fig. 77.3). From this point cranially, the major branches are identified to exclude pathologic masses in the upper mediastinum next to the brachiocephalic trunk (**88**), the left common carotid artery (**85**), the subclavian artery (**87**), as well as the brachiocephalic veins (**91**), superior vena cava (**92**), trachea (**81**), or more dorsally, the esophagus (**82**).

Caudally, the most common sites for enlarged LNs are: at the aortopulmonary window, directly below the bifurcation of the trachea (**81a**), in the perihilar tissue, posterior to the crura of the diaphragm (=retrocrural) next to the descending aorta (**89c**). The presence of a few LNs smaller than 1.5 cm in diameter in the aortopulmonary window may be considered normal [19, 41]. Anterior to the aortic arch (**89b**) LNs of normal size are rarely seen in the CT. The evaluation of the soft-tissue window is complete when the heart (any coronary sclerosis, dilations?) and the lung hila (vessels well defined and not lobulated or enlarged) have been checked. Only now should the radiologist turn to the lung or pleural window.

Since the pleural window is very wide, the marrow of the spinal column as well as the parenchyma of the lung can be examined. It is therefore possible to evaluate bone structure in addition to the pulmonary vasculature. When examining the lung vessels, look for a gradual reduction in their diameter as you proceed from the hilum to the periphery. Pulmonary oligemia is normal only along the margins of the lobes and in the periphery. It is essential to differentiate between cross-sectioned vessels and solid masses by comparing adjacent levels (cf. p. 15). More or less spherical solid masses may indicate intrapulmonary metastases. The checklist will help you read thoracic CTs systematically.

The simultaneous presentation of two window settings in one hard copy (both the lung and the soft-tissue window) has not proved practical because pathologic abnormalities which have density levels between the two would be overlooked. Consult the lung chapter on pages 84ff. for scans in the lung window.

Checklist for Thorax Readings

1. On the soft-tissue window:

• **soft tissues, especially:**
  - axillary LNs
  - breast (malignant lesions?)

• **mediastinum in four regions:**
  - from the aortic arch cranially (LNs?, thymoma / struma?)
  - hilar region (configuration and size of vessels, lobulated and enlarged?)
  - heart and coronary arteries (sclerosis?)
  - four typical sites of predilection for LNs:
    • anterior to aortic arch (normal: almost none or < 6 mm)
    • in the aortopulmonary window (normal: < 4 LNs < 15 mm)
    • subcarinal (normal: < 10 mm; DD: esophagus)
    • next to descending aorta (normal: < 10 mm; DD: azygos)

2. On the lung window:

• **Parenchyma of the lung:**
  - normal branching pattern and caliber of vessels?
  - vascular oligemia only at interlobar fissures? bullae?
  - any suspicious lung foci? inflammatory infiltrates?

• **Pleura:** - plaques, calcification, pleural fluid, pneumothorax?

• **Bones (vertebrae, scapula, ribs):**
  - normal structure of marrow?
  - degenerative osteophytes?
  - focal lytic or sclerotic processes?
  - stenoses of the spinal canal?

The parenchyma of the thyroid gland (**83**) should appear homogeneous and clearly defined from the surrounding fat (**2**). Asymmetry in the diameter of the jugular vein (**86**) is seen quite often and has no pathologic significance. Orthogonally sectioned branches of the axillary (**93**) and lateral thoracic (**95**) vessels must be distinguished from axillary LNs.

If the arms are elevated, the supraspinatus muscle (**19**) lies medial to the spine of the scapula (**53b**) and the infraspinatus muscle (**20**). Usually the pectoralis major (**26a**) and minor (**26b**) muscles are separated by a thin layer of fat.

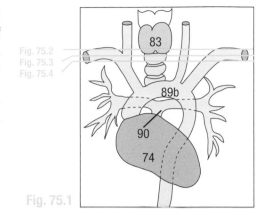

Fig. 75.1

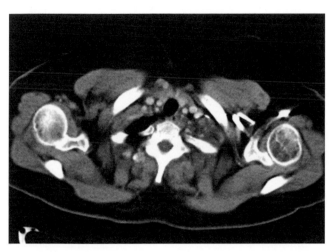

Fig. 75.2a

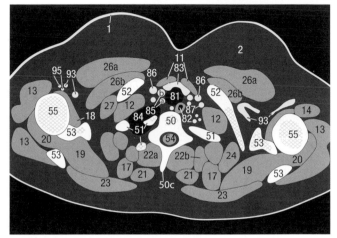

Fig. 75.2b

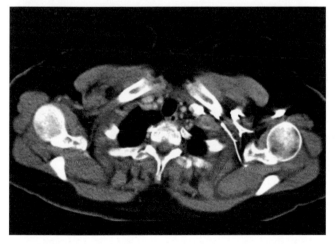

Fig. 75.3a

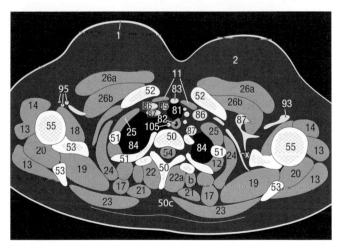

Fig. 75.3b

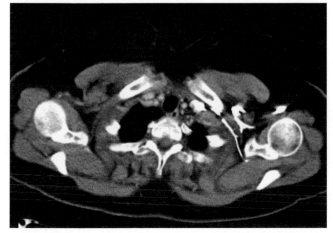

Fig. 75.4a

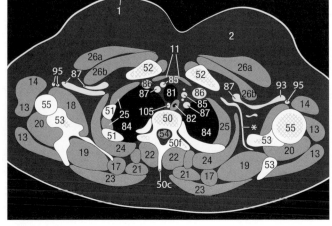

Fig. 75.4b

Artifacts (**3**) will be observed at the level of the thoracic inlet if CM is present in the subclavian vein (**87**) at the time of data acquisition (cf. Fig. 23.3).

Thoracic CTs are also viewed from caudally. The left lung (**84**) appears on the right side of the image and vice versa. Beginning at the aortic arch (**89b** in Figs. 77.2/3), the layout of the aortic arch vessels should be thoroughly familiar to you. At the section in Figure 76.1, the left subclavian artery (**87**) is seen most posteriorly and can be followed in cranial direction in the images on page 75. In front of the subclavian artery lie the left

common carotid artery (**85**) and the brachiocephalic trunk (**88**). More to the right and anteriorly are the brachiocephalic veins (**91**), which form the superior vena cava (**92**) at the levels of Figures 76.3 to 77.1. In the fat of the axilla (**2**), normal LNs (**6**) are often recognizable by their typical indented shape: the hilum contains fat. At a different angle, the hypodense hilum will appear in the center of an oval. Healthy LNs are well defined and should not exceed 1 cm in diameter in this location (Figs. 76.1 and 76.3).

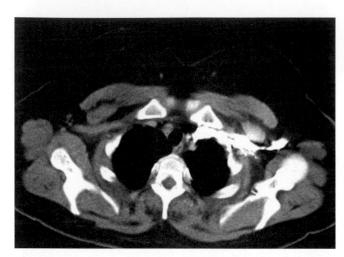

Fig. 76.1a

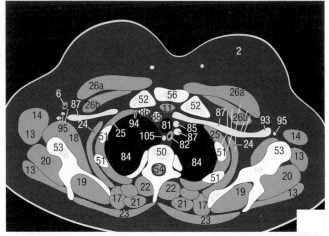

Fig. 76.1b

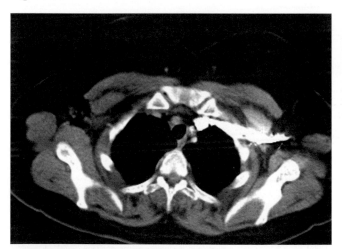

Fig. 76.2a

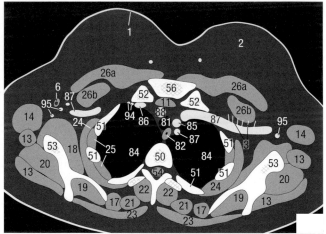

Fig. 76.2b

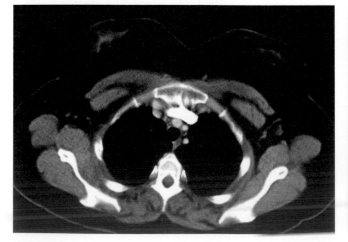

Fig. 76.3a

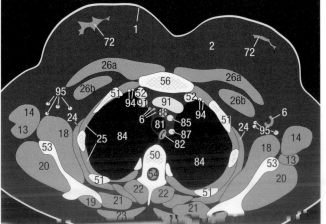

Fig. 76.3b

The azygos vein (**104**) lies dorsal to the trachea (**81**) next to the esophagus (**82**). Directly above the right main bronchus, it arches anteriorly into the superior vena cava (**92**). Be sure not to confuse the paravertebral azygos vein (**104**), the hemiazygos vein (**105**) or accessory hemiazygos (**105a**) with paraaortic LNs (Fig. 77.3).

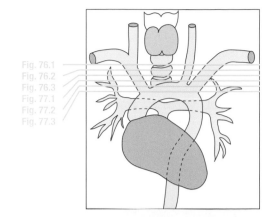

Fig. 76.1
Fig. 76.2
Fig. 76.3
Fig. 77.1
Fig. 77.2
Fig. 77.3

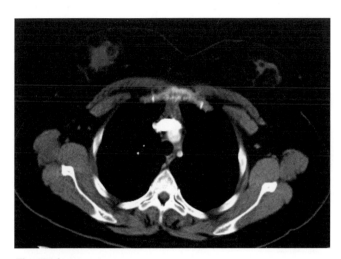

Fig. 77.1a

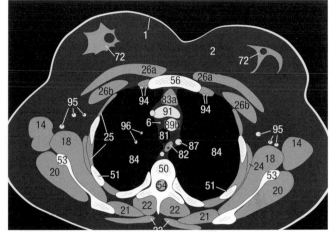

Fig. 77.1b

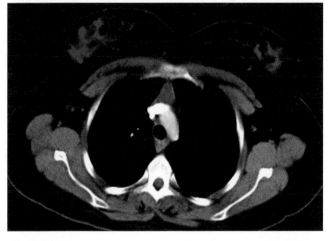

Fig. 77.2a

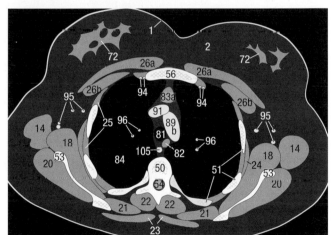

Fig. 77.2b

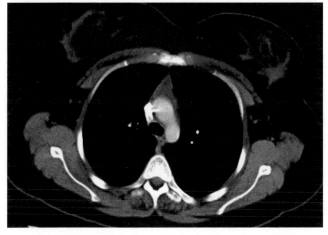

Fig. 77.3a

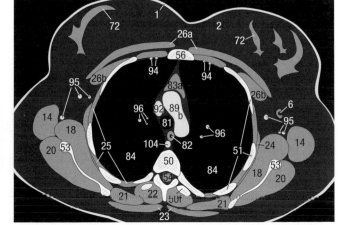

Fig. 77.3b

Immediately caudal to the arch of the aorta (**89b**) is situated the pulmonary trunk (**90**), which divides into the right (**90a**) and left (**90b**) pulmonary arteries (Fig. 78.2). At the level of Figure 78.1 there is the aortopulmonary window, a site of predilection for mediastinal LNs (**6**). Also check for enlarged LNs or malignant masses in the subcarinal position between the two main bronchi (**81b**) close to the pulmonary vessels (**96**) (Fig. 78.3). Near the internal thoracic (mammary) vessels (**94**) lies the regional lymphatic drainage of the medial parts of the breasts, whereas the lymphatic drainage of the lateral portions of the breasts is primarily to the axillary nodes.

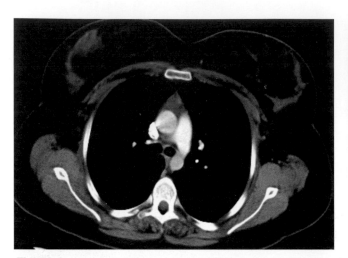

Fig. 78.1a

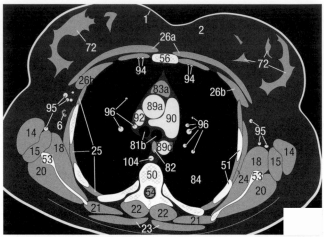

Fig. 78.1b

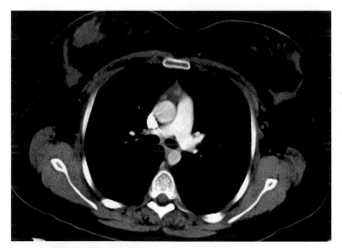

Fig. 78.2a

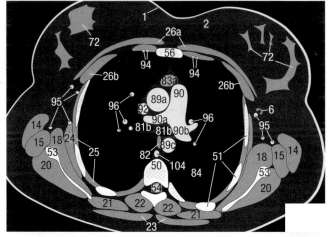

Fig. 78.2b

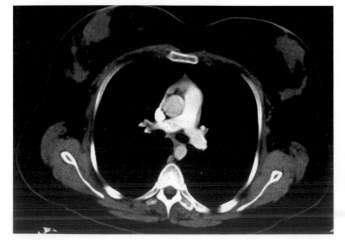

Fig. 78.3a

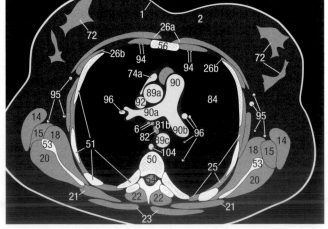

Fig. 78.3b

The glandular tissue (**72**) in the fat of the breasts of the anterior thoracic wall is easily differentiated from skin tumors because of the symmetry (Figs. 79.1-3). The main coronary arteries (**77**) are also distinguishable in the epicardial fat (Figs. 79.2/3). Develop a clear mental picture of the positions of the azygos vein (**104**) and the esophagus (**82**) next to the descending aorta (**89c**) so that you will later be able to recognize any pathologic LNs close to these structures.

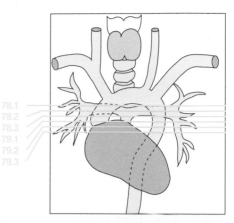

Fig. 78.1
Fig. 78.2
Fig. 78.3
Fig. 79.1
Fig. 79.2
Fig. 79.3

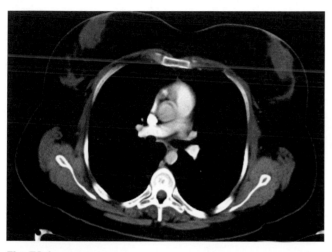

Fig. 79.1a

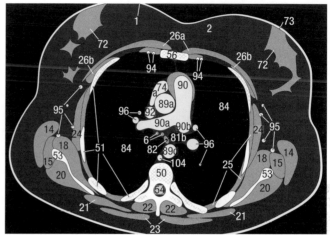

Fig. 79.1b

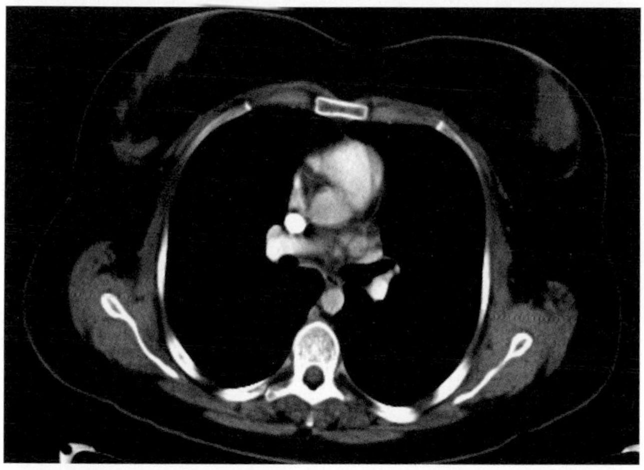

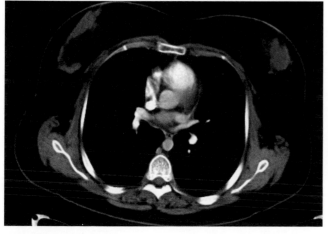

Fig. 79.2a

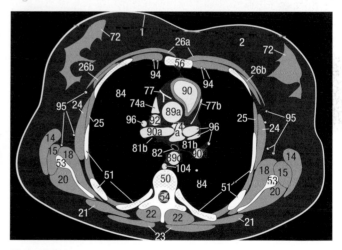

Fig. 79.2b

Fig. 79.3a

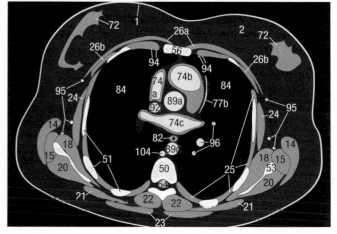

Fig. 79.3b

The left atrium (**74c**) is the most posterior chamber of the heart, whereas the outlet of the left ventricle (**74d**) and the ascending aorta (**89a**) lie in the center of the heart. The right atrium (**74a**) lies on the right lateral side and the right ventricle (**74b**) anteriorly behind the sternum (**56**). Only the larger central branches of the pulmonary vessels (**96**) can be seen on the soft-tissue window. The smaller, more peripheral lung vessels are better judged on the lung window (not shown here).

Note the junction between the hemiazygos vein (**105**) and the azygos vein (**104**), which must not be confused with a paravertebral lymphoma (Fig. 80.3).

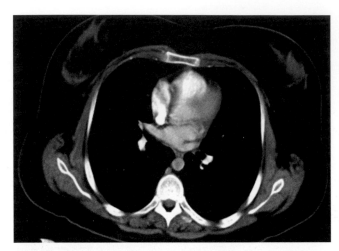

Fig. 80.1a

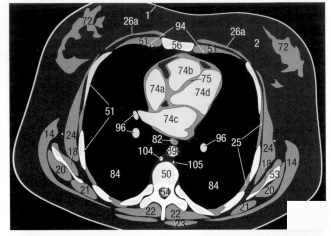

Fig. 80.1b

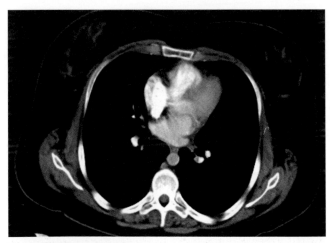

Fig. 80.2a

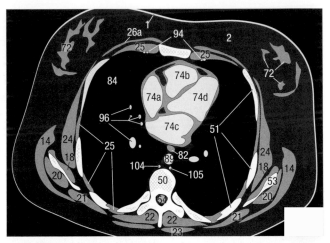

Fig. 80.2b

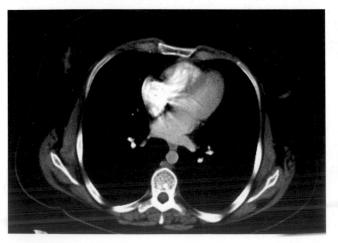

Fig. 80.3a

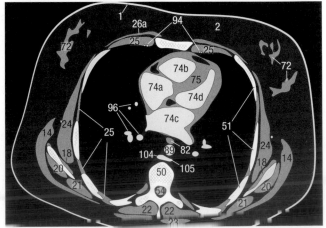

Fig. 80.3b

The sections on previous and this page show the opening of the coronary sinus (**76**) into the right atrium (**74a**) and sequential sections of the coronary arteries (**77**). The hypodense epicardial fat (**79**) must not be mistaken for fluid within the pericardial space. The internal thoracic artery, also known as the internal mammary artery (**94**), is more and more frequently used in bypass operations. It is surgically anastomosed with the anterior descending branch of the left coronary artery.

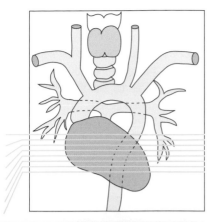

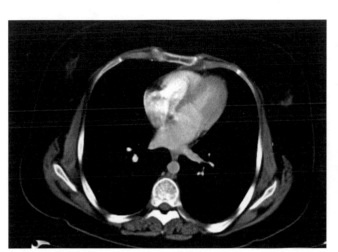

Fig. 81.1a

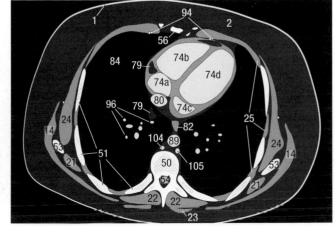

Fig. 81.1b

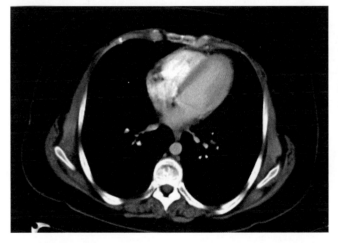

Fig. 81.2a

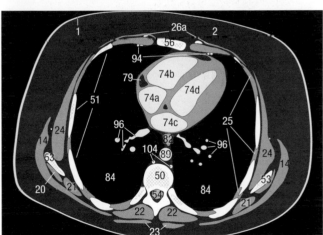

Fig. 81.2b

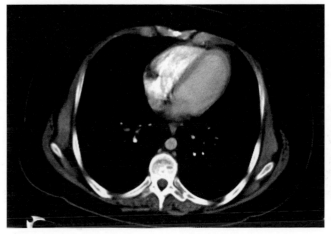

Fig. 81.3a

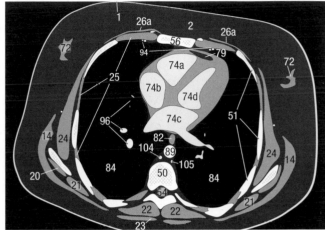

Fig. 81.3b

The inferior vena cava (**80**) is seen more caudally (Figs. 82.1–3), and finally the diaphragm (**30**) appears together with the upper parts of the liver (**122**). Many radiologists who suspect the presence of a bronchial carcinoma (BC) obtain images to the caudal edge of the liver (see p. 83) because a BC often metastasizes to the liver and the adrenal glands. The caliber of lung vessels near the periphery of the diaphragm is so small that they are not visible on the soft-tissue window, as in the present images. The pattern of the pulmonary vasculature should therefore be examined on the lung windows, which include the negative density values of the Hounsfield scale. Only after this step has been carried out is the evaluation of a chest CT complete.

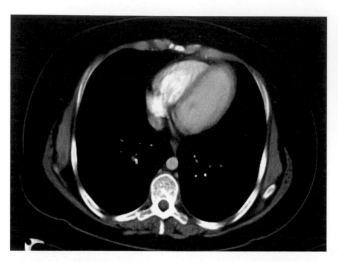

Fig. 82.1a

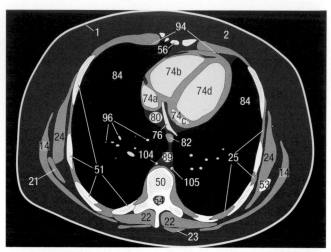

Fig. 82.1b

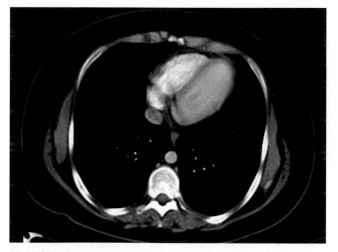

Fig. 82.2a

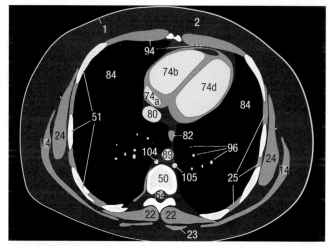

Fig. 82.2b

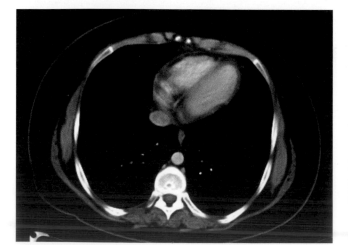

Fig. 82.3a

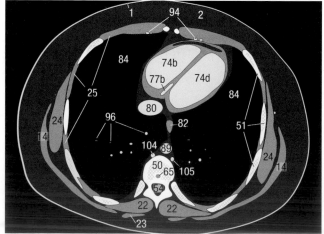

Fig. 82.3b

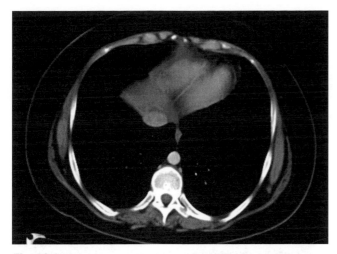

Fig. 83.1a

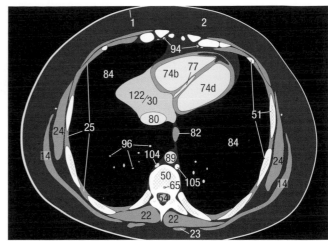

Fig. 83.1b

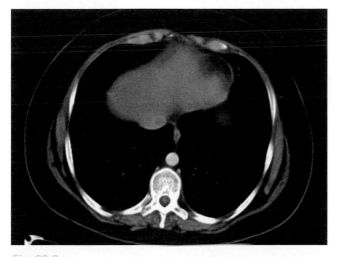

Fig. 83.2a

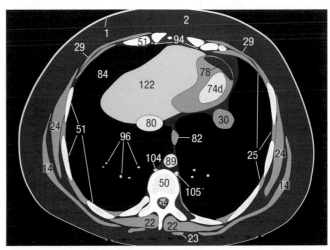

Fig. 83.2b

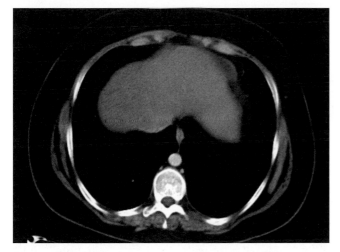

Fig. 83.3a

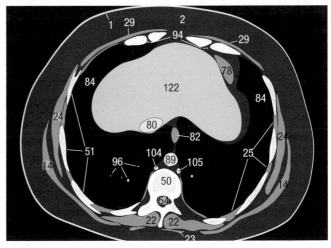

Fig. 83.3b

Test Yourself! Exercise 19:

Write down a concise but complete sequence of all criteria for interpreting a thoracic CT. Then compare your notes with the checklist on page 74 and repeat this exercise from time to time until you remember every criterion.

Segments of the Lung

It is especially important to be able to identify the segments of the lungs in CT images if bronchioscopy is planned for biopsy or to remove a foreign body. The right lung has 10 segments.

In the left lung, the apical and posterior upper lobe segments have a common bronchus and there is no 7th segment (paracardiac [medial basal] segment of the lower lobe).

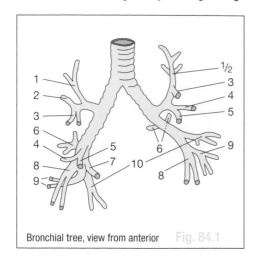

Bronchial tree, view from anterior   Fig. 84.1

Upper lobe	1	apical
	2	posterior
	3	anterior
Middle lobe	4	lateral (superior lingula)
	5	medial (inferior lingula)
Lower lobe	6	superior/apical
	7	paracardiac/medial basal
	8	anterior basal
	9	lateral basal
	10	posterior basal

The parenchyma next to the interlobular fissures (——) appears avascular.

The borders of the segments (– – –) are usually not visible in sections of normal thickness and can only be identified by the branches of the pulmonary veins (**96**) which pass along these borders.

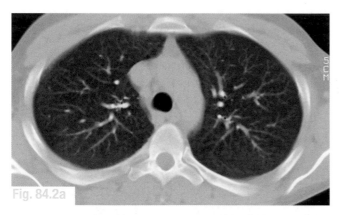

Fig. 84.2a

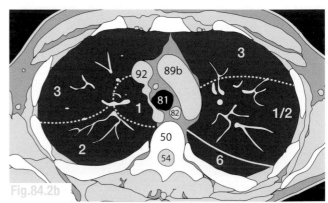

Fig. 84.2b

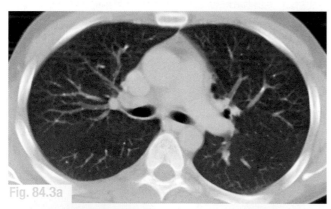

Fig. 84.3a

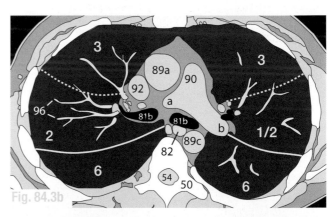

Fig. 84.3b

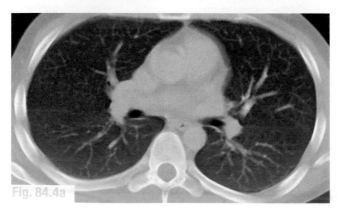

Fig. 84.4a

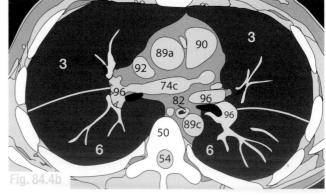

Fig. 84.4b

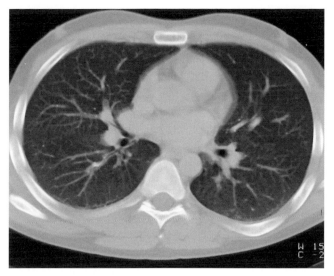

Fig. 85.1a

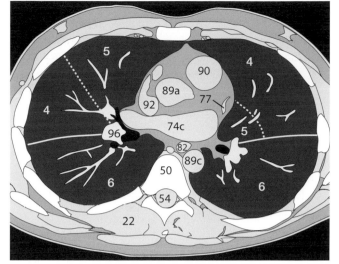

Fig. 85.1b

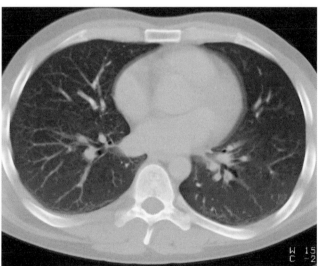

Fig. 85.2a

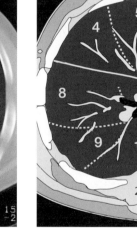

Fig. 85.2b

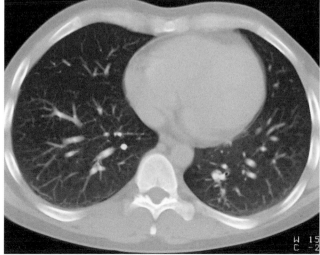

Fig. 85.3a

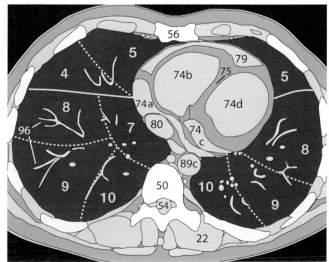

Fig. 85.3b

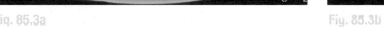

High-Resolution Technique

HRCT stands for high-resolution computed tomography using thin sections and a high spatial resolution reconstruction algorithm. Even conventional CT scanners can acquire images of narrower slice thickness than the standard 5-8 mm. The image acquisition parameters can be adjusted on the console to a thickness of 1-2 mm if necessary.

In the SCT technique, thinner sections can also be computed at a pitch factor of 1:1 after acquisition (see also p. 8). However, it is not always worth reconstructing slices of less than 1 mm thickness because the low signal-to-noise ratio reduces image quality.

HRCT is therefore not the method of choice for routine chest examination because radiation dosage is much higher if more sections are acquired. Longer examination times and higher hard-copy film cost ("slice pollution") are also arguments against using HRCT. Only structures with naturally high levels of contrast such as areas surrounding bone will be well demonstrated.

High-Resolution Effects on Image Quality

Figure 86.1 shows a conventional scan of a pulmonary lesion (7) surrounded by a zone of edema or an infiltrate (185). At a d_S setting of 10 mm this zone closely resem-bles the poorly ventilated area at the back of the posterior lobe (178).

HRCT distinguishes these areas of increased density more clearly (Fig. 86.2) because voxel averaging does not have any appreciable effect (see also p. 14).

The DD includes bronchial carcinoma, metastasis of breast cancer resulting in lymphangitis carcinomatosa, and atypical pneumonia.

These images show a rare complication after catheterization of the right heart. The catheter was positioned too peripherally and caused hemorrhage (173) into adjacent parts of the lung. Follow-up 3 weeks later showed complete recovery.

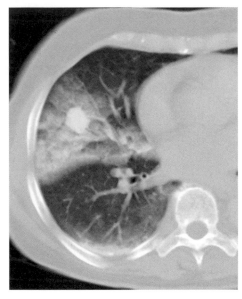

Fig. 86.1a

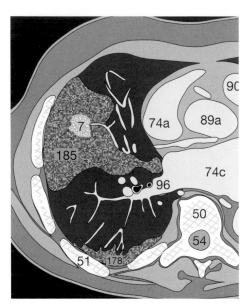

Fig. 86.1b

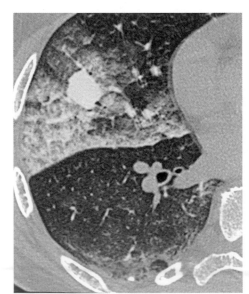

Fig. 86.2a

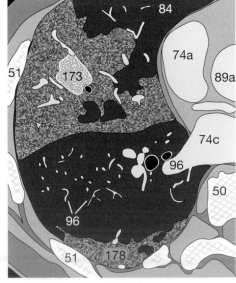

Fig. 86.2b

Indications

One of the many advantages of the HRCT technique is that older scar tissue can be distinguished from acute inflammation, for example in immune-suppressed patients or bone marrow recipients. Older scar tissue (**186**) is always well defined (Fig. 87.1), whereas fresh infiltrates are surrounded by a zone of edematous tissue (**185**) as in Figure 87.2. HRCT is often the only method with which to determine whether chemotherapy should be continued in a lympho-

ma patient who is in the aplastic phase on therapy or whether chemotherapy must be discontinued because of fungal pneumonia. Fresh infiltrates (**178**) can sometimes be seen next to older scar tissue (**186**) (Fig. 87.3).

Because the slices are extremely thin, the horizontal interlobular fissure (★) may appear as a bizarre ring or crescentic (Figs. 87.1 and 87.2).

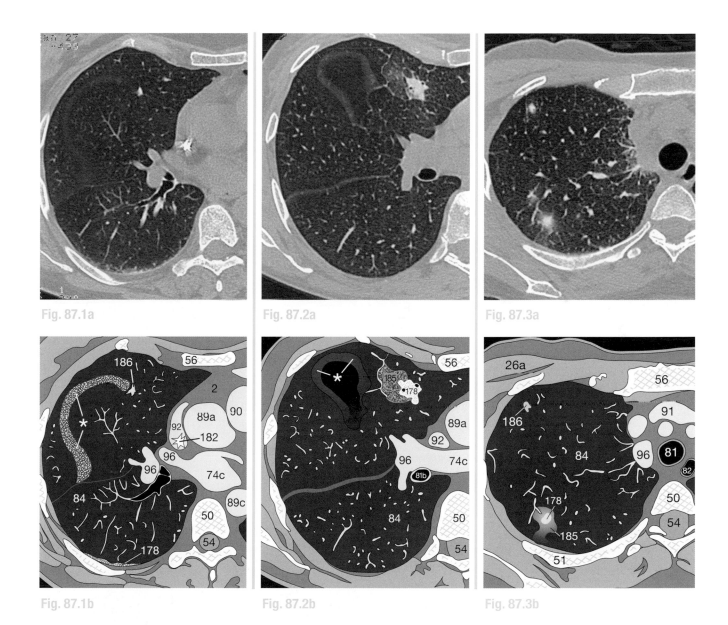

Fig. 87.1a   Fig. 87.2a   Fig. 87.3a

Fig. 87.1b   Fig. 87.2b   Fig. 87.3b

Minor areas of collapse, which are usually found close to the pleura posteriorly in the lung, must be differentiated from flat sections of fissures (**178** in Fig. 87.1). In doubtful cases, it may be helpful to repeat a scan in the prone position. Areas of collapse and poor ventilation may then disappear or be seen anteriorly. Pulmonary abnormalities due to an infiltrate or to a pneumoconiosis would be unchanged.

Among the many anatomic variations of the thorax, an atypical course of the azygos vein (**140**) is relatively common. It can pass from the posterior mediastinum through the right apical lobe to the superior vena cava (**92**). It is located within a fold of the pleura and therefore separates the azygos lobe from the remainder of the right upper lobe. This variation is usually discovered incidentally on a conventional chest X-ray (↗ in Fig. 88.1) and has no clinical significance. Figures 88.2 to 88.4 show the anomalous path of the vessel as it appears in CT images.

Atypical positions or branching of the aortic arch (**89**) vessels are rarer. An example is the right subclavian artery, known as the "lusorian artery", which can resemble a lesion in the upper mediastinum.

Note that normal breast tissue, surrounded by fat (**2**), may have very irregular contours (**72** in Fig. 88.4). When using lung windows, you should not only look for solid round lesions and inflammatory infiltrates, but also recognize any thinning or even absence of lung vessels.

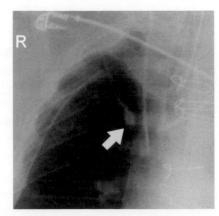

Fig. 88.1

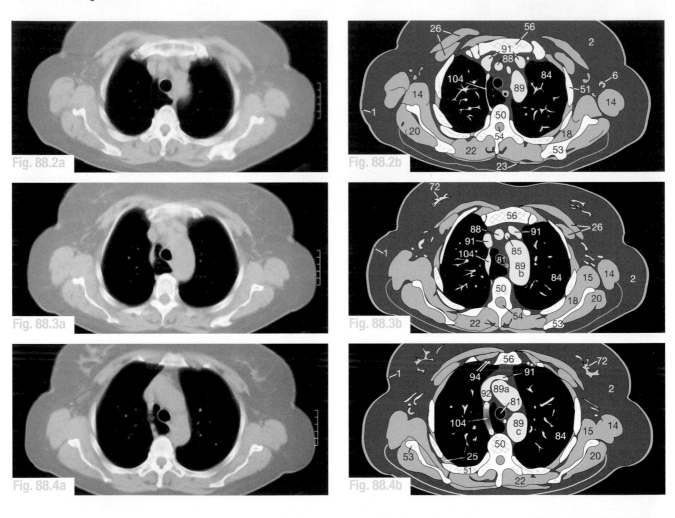

Fig. 88.2a

Fig. 88.2b

Fig. 88.3a

Fig. 88.3b

Fig. 88.4a

Fig. 88.4b

However, attenuation of vessels is not always a sign of emphysema. Asymmetry in the bronchovascular pattern develops after a part of the lung has been resected. In the patient imaged in Figure 88.5, the left upper lobe had been removed and the remaining lung tissue has compensated and filled the entire left thoracic cavity (right half of the image). There are fewer lung vessels per unit volume and an ipsilateral shift of the mediastinum. These changes are accompanied by a slight elevation of the diaphragm. At the time of this follow-up CT, the patient was healthy and had neither emphysema nor recurrent tumor.

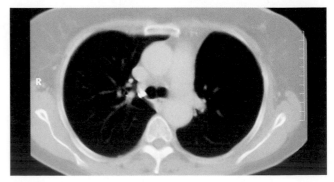

Fig. 88.5

According to the sequence in the checklist on page 74, one should now turn to soft-tissue windows in order to examine the soft tissues of the chest wall. Most abnormalities will be located in the axillae and in the female breast.

Alterations in Lymph Nodes

Normal axillary LNs (**6**) are usually oval and less than 1 cm in dimension. They often have a hypodense center or are horse-shoe-shaped as in Figure 89.1, a feature known as the "hilum fat sign". The architecture of a normal LN is characterized by vessels entering the hilum, which contains hypodense fat. Many abnormal LNs have lost their normal contours and are rounder or irregular. Such LNs all appear solid and lack the hilum fat sign, as seen in those in the left axilla in Figure 89.2. For direct comparison, two lymph nodes on the other side in the same image are normal.

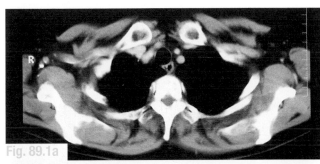

Fig. 89.1a

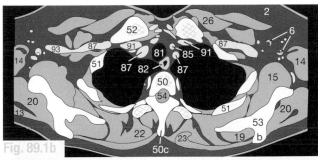

Fig. 89.1b

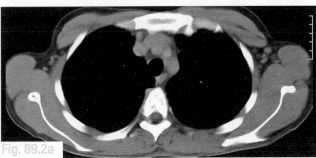

Fig. 89.2a

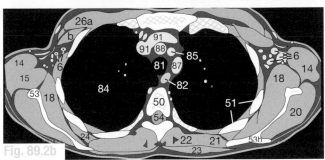

Fig. 89.2b

Larger metastatic LNs (**7**) are usually poorly defined and difficult to differentiate from surrounding fat (**2**). They often have central areas of necrosis (**181**), so that the differential diagnosis of an abscess with central liquefaction must be considered (Fig. 89.3). If axillary lymph node metastases have been treated operatively or with radiotherapy, the date and treatment should be noted on the referral sheet for follow-up CT. Postoperative healing processes and scarring (**186**) change the morphology of LNs (Fig. 89.4), so they resemble abnormal nodes (see above). Again the lack of clinical information makes diagnosis unnecessarily difficult for the radiologist.

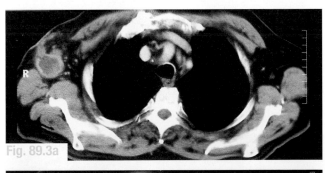

Fig. 89.3a

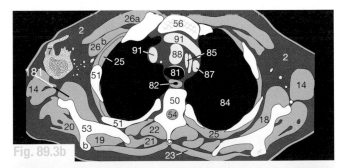

Fig. 89.3b

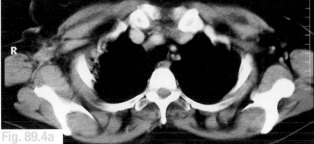

Fig. 89.4a

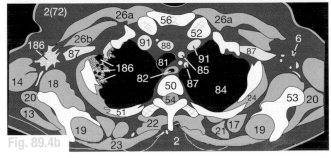

Fig. 89.4b

Breast

The normal parenchyma (72) of the female breast has very irregular contours and slender, finger-like extensions into the surrounding fat (2) (cf. Fig. 88.4). Bizarre shapes can often be seen (Fig. 90.1). Advanced stages of breast cancer (7) have a solid, irregular appearance (Fig. 90.1). The malignant tissue crosses the fascial planes or infiltrates the thoracic wall, depending on size. Baseline CT after mastect my (Fig. 90.2) should help in the early identification of recurrent tumor. The diagnosis of recurrent tumor is made more difficult by fibrosis after radiation, postoperative scar tissue, and the absence of surrounding fat. Special attention must therefore be paid to the regional LNs (cf. pp. 74, 89) and th bones, so that metastases (7) in the vertebrae (50) (Fig. 90.2) are not overlooked. The bone window must be examined in such cases.

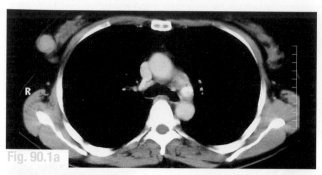

Fig. 90.1a

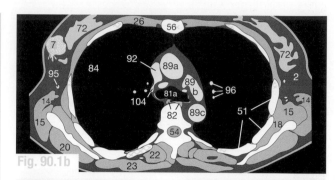

Fig. 90.1b

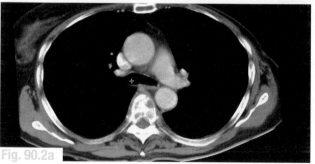

Fig. 90.2a

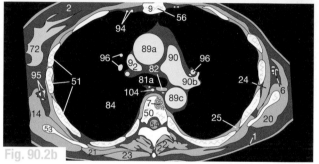

Fig. 90.2b

Thoracic Skeleton

Osteolysis within the thoracic skeleton is not uncommon and is usually due to either metastases or a plasma cell tumor. In Figure 90.3, a metastasis (7) from a thyroid carcinoma has destroyed part of the left clavicle (52). Osteolysis can, however, also be caused by an enchondroma or an eosinophilic granuloma, for example of a rib. In addition to destructive processes (cf. Fig. 22.3), degenerative processes involving sclerosis and osteophyte formation of bone must be differentiated from osteosclerotic metastases, which are typical of, for example, prostate carcinoma (cf. p. 145).

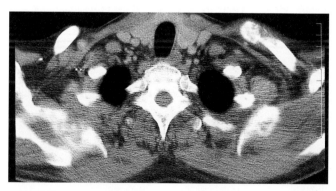

Fig. 90.3a

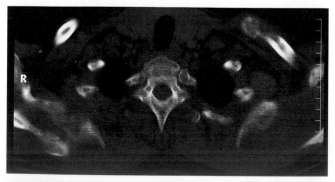

Fig. 90.3b

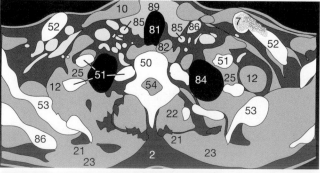

Fig. 90.3c

Before being able to detect lesions and lymphadenopathy, you must know the normal anatomy. If you are a preclinical student, you should firstly study normal sectional anatomy. It is in your own interests to work through the following pages only when you are sufficiently familiar with the previous chapters.

Tumors

A benign increase in fat (**2**) due to cortisone therapy is occasionally observed in the anterior mediastinum (Fig. 91.1). In doubtful cases, densitometry is helpful in the DD (cf. p. 15). In this example, the average density within the region of interest (ROI), which is positioned in possible fatty tissue, is −89.3 HU with a standard deviation of about 20 HU (cf. Table 16.1). As a rule, the size of an ROI in cm² (AR) is also provided (Fig. 91.1). The DD of such a mass would include retrosternal goiter and thymoma.

In children and young adults, the density of the thymus is about +45 HU. As a result of involution, the density of the organ decreases with age from the third decade onward until it has dropped to the density typical of fat (−90 HU). The left lobe of the thymus is often larger than the right and can reach the aortopulmonary window. A lobe should not be thicker than 1.3 cm in adults; up to the age of 20, 1.8 cm is considered normal.

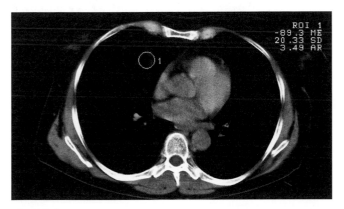

Fig. 91.1a

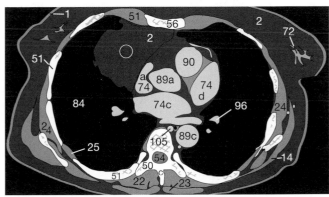

Fig. 91.1b

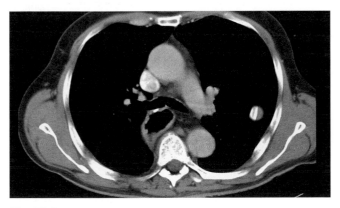

Fig. 91.2a

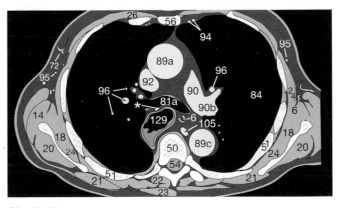

Fig. 91.2b

Malignant thickening of the walls of the esophagus must be differentiated from gastric conduits following esophageal surgery (Fig. 91.2). Possible enlargement of LNs (**6**) next to the stomach (**129**) must be excluded by follow-up CTs. Occasionally postoperative metal clips cause artifacts (★), which make assessment of the mediastinum more difficult. Following esophageal resection, parts of the colon (⇒) may become drawn up into the anterior mediastinum (Fig. 91.3). Comparison with adjacent sections quickly shows that this structure is not an emphysematous bulla, but is a tubular organ containing a lumen.

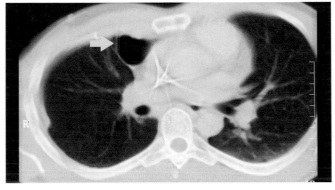

Fig. 91.3

Enlarged Lymph Nodes

Normal LNs are often found at the level of the aortopulmonary window. They are mainly oval or irregular, less than 10 mm across [19], and sharply delineated from mediastinal fat (**2**). LNs (**6**) in this area are not usually considered suspicious until they exceed 1.5 cm in diameter. The demonstration of a "hilum fat sign" (cf. p. 89) is not obligatory, but does suggest a benign nature (Fig. 92.1).

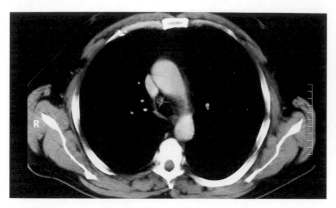

Fig. 92.1a

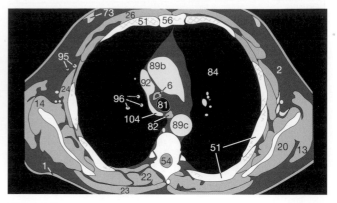

Fig. 92.1b

If more than three LNs are seen in the aortopulmonary window or if a single LN is abnormally enlarged, the DD includes not only a metastasis from a bronchial carcinoma, but also a lymphoma (Fig. 92.2).

Enlarged mediastinal, and especially hilar, LNs are also characteristic of sarcoidosis (Boeck's disease) (**6** in Fig. 92.3). In Figure 92.2, there are intrapulmonary metastases (**7**) as well. Did you notice them? Other sites of predilection for abnormal LNs are anterior to the aortic arch, beneath the bifurcation of the trachea (subcarinal), and the para-aortic and retrocrural regions.

Normal size (diameter) of thoracic LNs [19, 41]:

- anterior mediastinum   < 6 mm
- aortopulmonary window   < 15 mm
- hilar   < 10 mm
- subcarinal   < 10 mm
- para-aortic   < 7 mm

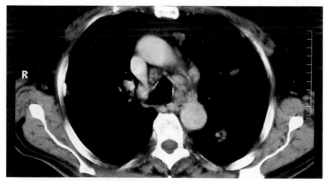

Fig. 92.2a

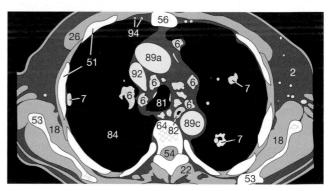

Fig. 92.2b

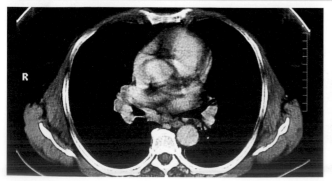

Fig. 92.3a

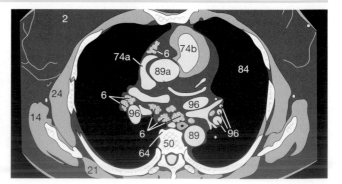

Fig. 92.3b

Vascular Pathologies

Inflow phenomena of CM injected through an arm vein (cf. p. 21) and anomalous vessels (cf. p. 88) in the mediastinum have already been discussed. Incompletely mixed CM must be distinguished from a possible thrombus (**173**) in the lumen of the brachiocephalic vein (**91**). Such a thrombus can adhere to a central venous catheter (**182** in Fig. 93.1).

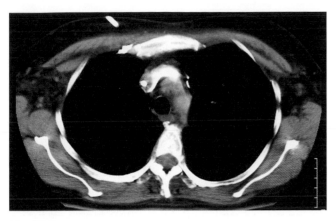

Fig. 93.1a

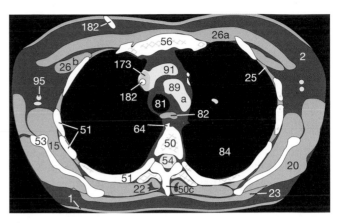

Fig. 93.1b

Atherosclerotic plaques (**174**) in the aorta (**89**) are often accompanied by thrombotic deposits (**173** in Fig. 93.3). They promote aortic elongation and dilation and can ultimately lead to an aneurysm (**171**). Dilation of the thoracic aorta is considered to be an aneurysm if the lumen is wider than 4 cm. Recording the measurements of distances and sizes (Fig. 93.2) makes it easier to assess any progressive dilation in follow-up CTs. It is important to check for any involvement of the branches of the great vessels or for the presence of a dissection flap (**172** in Fig. 93.4). Three types of dissection can be diagnosed according to the extent of the dissection flap (see de Bakey [20]).

A true aneurysm with a diameter of more than 6 cm, with a more saccular than fusiform shape or with an eccentric lumen, has a higher incidence of rupture. The consequences of rupture include a mediastinal hematoma, a hemothorax, or pericardial tamponade.

Dissecting Aneurysms of the Aorta
(according to de Bakey [20])

Type I (approx. 50%)
Ascending aorta; may extend to abdominal bifurcation

Type II (approx. 15%)
Only ascending aorta, extending to brachiocephalic trunk

Type III (approx. 25%)
Torn intima distal to left subclavian artery

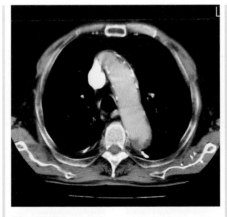

Fig. 93.3a

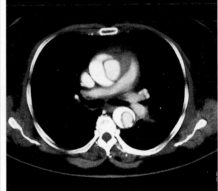

Fig. 93.4a

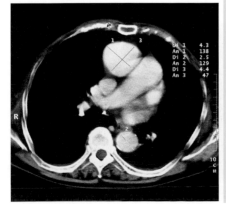

Fig. 93.2

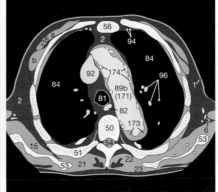

Fig. 93.3b

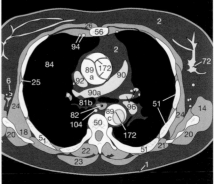

Fig. 93.4b

Pulmonary Embolism

If a large embolus has detached from a thrombus in a deep vein of the leg, it will be visible as a hypodense area ( ) within the involved pulmonary artery on contrast-enhanced images (Fig. 94.1). After large pulmonary emboli, the affected segments or lobes ( ) usually become poorly ventilated and atelectasis occurs. The pulmonary vessels become attenuated, which can be demonstrated in conventional x-rays. The CT-angiographic detection of pulmonary emboli is described on page 186 in more detail.

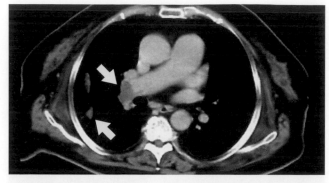

Fig. 94.1

Heart

You have already familiarized yourself with the normal anatomy of the heart on pages 79 to 81. Dilation resulting from valvular incompetence or from cardiomyopathies, as well as intracardiac filling defects can be recognized in CT images. If CM has been injected, it is possible to detect atrial thrombus or a thrombosed ventricular aneurysm. The image in Figure 94.2 illustrates a case of global cardiac failure with markedly dilated atria ( ) and incidental thoracic vertebral degenerative osteophytes( ).

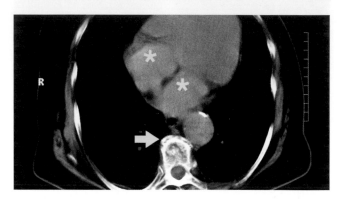

Fig. 94.2

Pericardial effusions may occur with viral infections, uremia, the collagen vascular diseases, a heart attack, or tuberculosis, among other causes. A pericardial effusion (**8**) appears as a broad rim of low-density fluid (between 10 and 40 HU) surrounding the heart (Fig. 94.3). Only fresh blood would have a higher level of density. Massive effusions as seen in Figure 94.3 not only compress the adjacent lungs (**178**), but also compromise heart function.

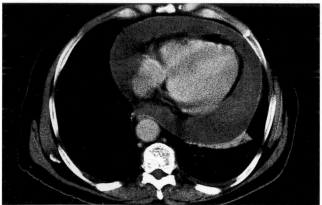

Fig. 94.3a

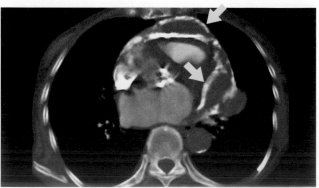

Fig. 94.3b

Effusions may lead to pericardial fibrosis or calcification ( ), which in turn causes constrictive pericarditis (Fig. 94.4). Note that in such cases the vena cava, the azygos vein, or even the atria may be markedly dilated as a sign of cardiac insufficiency.

Atherosclerosis of the coronary arteries causes calcification that is well demonstrated by thin, hyperdense lines in the epicardial fat. At present, however, a complete assessment of the degree of stenosis requires angiography.

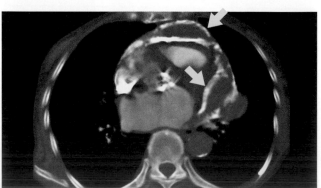

Fig. 94.4

Focal Intrapulmonary Lesions

When multiple lung metastases are far advanced, the lesions can even be recognized in the topogram (Fig. 95.1a). Depending upon the age and vascularization of the metastases, they appear as spherical nodules of varying sizes (Fig. 95.1b). The more irregular the contours of the lesions (for example, stellate or spiculated), the more likely they are to be malignant. If, however, they are solitary and have central calcification (like a popcorn), or peripheral calcification, the lesions are most likely to be a benign hamartoma or granuloma.

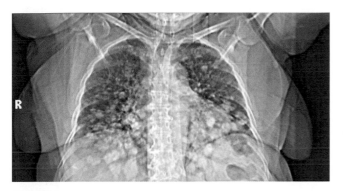

Fig. 95.1a

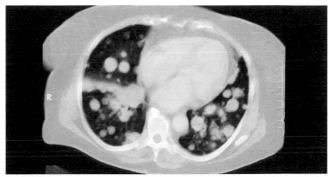

Fig. 95.1b

Pulmonary metastases are not visible in conventional x-rays unless they are larger than 5 or 6 mm in diameter. In CT images, however, they can be detected at 1 to 2 mm in diameter. If metastases are located in the periphery, it is easy to differentiate them from blood vessels cut in crosssection.

Small metastases located close to the hilum are much more difficult to distinguish from vessels. In such cases, the detailed analysis of high-resolution scans (HRCT) may be the best method.

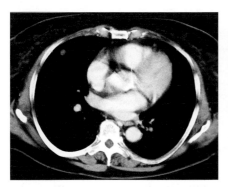

Fig. 95.2a

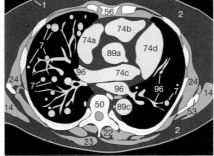

Fig. 95.2b

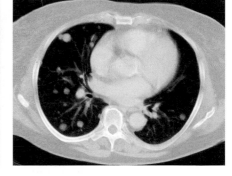

Fig. 95.2c

The correct choice of image display (window) is essential: Small focal lesions (**7**) of the lung (**84**) do not appear on soft-tissue windows (Fig. 95.2a) or may be mistaken for normal vessels (**96**). Lung windows (Fig. 95.2c) should always be used for examining lung parenchyma. In the case below (Fig. 95.3a), the multiple small metastases (**7**) close to the pleura would have been overlooked if lung windows had not been used (Fig. 95.3c). These examples demonstrate the importance of viewing each image on long and soft-tissue windows.

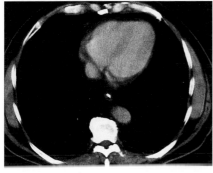

Fig. 95.3a

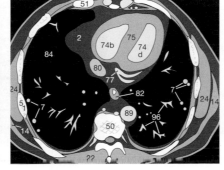

Fig. 95.3b

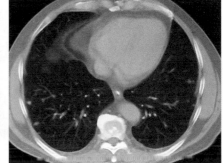

Fig. 95.3c

As a result of changes in the behavior of smokers, the incidence of bronchial carcinomas (BC), especially among women and young people, has increased. In addition to the histologic diagnosis and grading of carcinoma, the location of the lesion is an important prognostic factor: a BC of considerable size (**7**) in the periphery of the lung (Fig. 96.1) will almost certainly

be visible on a conventional chest x-ray. More advanced BCs located centrally are usually not operable and may obstruct the bronchial lumen, resulting in distal collapse (**178**). Figure 96.2 illustrates an advanced case in which the tumor has areas of central necrosis (**181**) and the lung is surrounded by a pleural effusion (**8**).

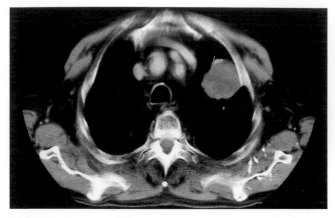

Fig. 96.1a

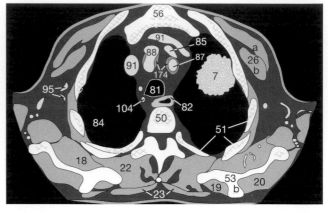

Fig. 96.1b

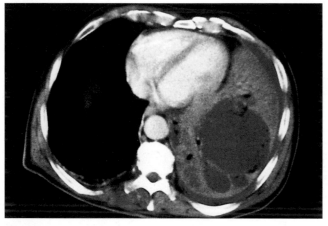

Fig. 96.2a

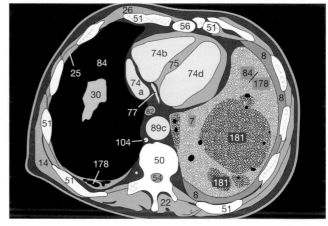

Fig. 96.2b

Lymphangitis carcinomatosa (**7** in Fig. 96.3) spreads from the hilum or the visceral pleura into the interstitial tissue of the lung by way of the lymphatic vessels. Obstruction of these vessels by cancer cells leads to lymphatic

congestion (**185**). At first, the upper lobes remain clear, but as the disease progresses these also become infiltrated. The larger lymphatics and LNs gradually become infiltrated by metastatic disease.

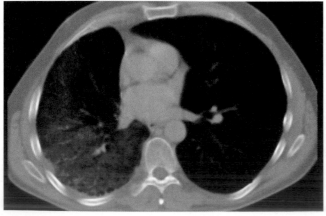

Fig. 96.3a

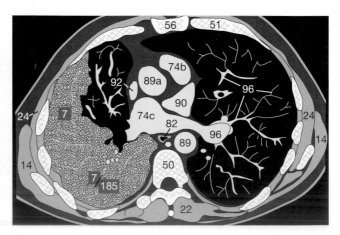

Fig. 96.3b

Sarcoidosis

The changes of sarcoidosis (Boeck's disease) must be differentiated from multiple metastases in the lung: epithelial granulomas usually infiltrate the hilar lymph nodes (**6**) bilaterally (Fig. 97.1) and then spread within the perivascular tissue and along the lymphatics into the periphery of the lung. Multiple small pulmonary nodules and various degrees of interstitial fibrosis may be present. Large granulomas (**7**), as seen in Figure 97.2, may resemble intrapulmonary metastases.

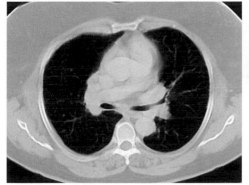

Fig. 97.1a

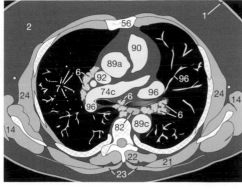

Fig. 97.1b

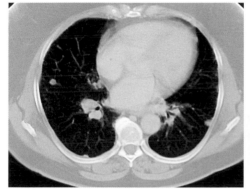

Fig. 97.2a

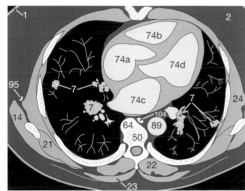

Fig. 97.2b

Tuberculosis

If a larger mass cavitates (**181**), the DD will include, for example, a bronchial carcinoma with central necrosis or cavitary tuberculosis. Figure 97.3 illustrates the latter in an atypical location in an HIV+, immune-compromised patient. Note also the emphysematous changes in the tissue at the periphery of the lesion (**176**).

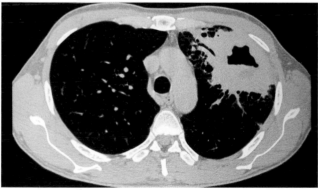

Fig. 97.3a

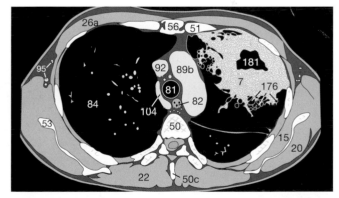

Fig. 97.3b

Aspergillus

Superinfection with Aspergillus may occur within a pre-existing cavity in immune-compromised patients. The spores of A. fumigatus are common in plant material and soil. Often the cavity is not completely filled with the aspergillus ball so that a small crescent of air can be recognized (⬉ in Fig. 97.4). Aspergillosis may also lead to allergic bronchial asthma or provoke exogenous allergic alveolitis.

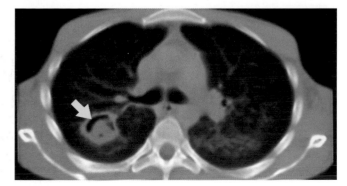

Fig. 97.4

Pleura

Massive pleural effusions (8), as seen in the case illustrated in Figure 98.1, compress the lung (84) and may cause large areas of atelectasis (178) affecting individual segments or even an entire lobe. Effusions appear as collections of homogeneous fluid of near-water density within the pleural spaces. Effusions usually accompany infections, lung congestion due to right heart failure, as well as venous congestion due to mesothelioma and peripheral bronchial carcinoma.

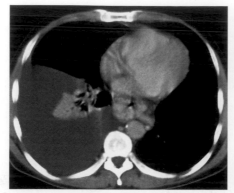 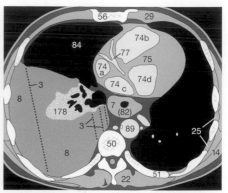

Fig. 98.1a   Fig. 98.1b

Pleural drainage by the insertion of a catheter (182) is indicated if atelectasis (178) affects large portions of the lung (Fig. 98.2). In the case shown in Figure 98.2, the drainage tube was blocked by fibrin-rich fluid. The lung can only be re-inflated if the fibrin clot is cleared or the catheter is replaced.

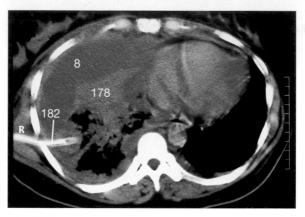

Fig. 98.2

Foreign bodies are rarely found in the pleural spaces (166 in Fig. 98.3), but must be considered after thoracotomy (chest surgery). Images on lung windows (Fig. 98.3c) clearly show the inflammation and collapse (178) surrounding a lost swab.

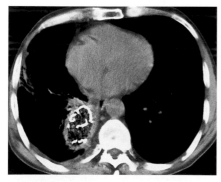 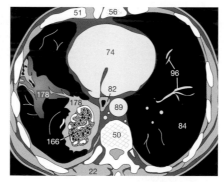 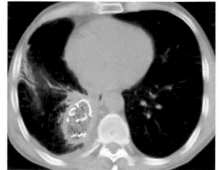

Fig. 98.3a   Fig. 98.3b   Fig. 98.3c

Asbestos-Related Lung Disease

Asbestos-related lung disease has a fine reticulonodular pattern of increased densities scattered throughout the lung tissue, especially at interlobular septa (⬆ and ⬈ in Fig. 98.4). Typical pathologic features in the pleura are thickening and plaques (186 in Fig. 98.4). Fibrosis and scar emphysema appear in later stages of the disease. The spindle-shaped or more triangular areas of increased attenuation are often difficult to distinguish from those characteristic of bronchial carcinomas.

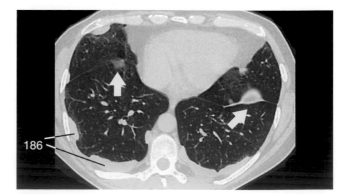

Fig. 98.4

Silicosis

Multiple, well-defined nodules appear in the interstitial connective tissue in response to phagocytosed particles of silica. The upper lobes of the lung are most commonly affected. Signs of fibrosis, which may progress to a honeycomb pattern, can best – and at earlier stages – be detected with HRCT (using 2-mm rather than 10-mm slice thickness; Fig. 99.1). The finer, smaller nodules can be found scattered throughout the lung; larger opacities, which may cavitate, are located within areas of denser fibrosis (↗ in Fig. 99.2). Enlarged mediastinal or hilar lymph nodes (Fig. 99.3) often develop an eggshell pattern of calcification. As the disease progresses, fibrosis and scar emphysema increase (← in Fig. 99.1).

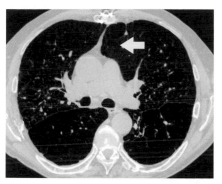

Fig. 99.1

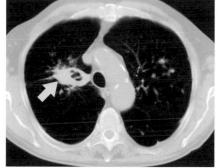

Fig. 99.2

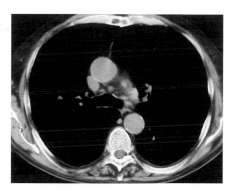

Fig. 99.3

Emphysema

Progressive emphysema with accompanying bullae (**176** in Fig. 99.4b) or bronchiectasis with associated inflammatory infiltrates (**178** in Fig. 99.5) are not visible on soft-tissue window images in the early stages. These infiltrates are more easily seen and detected sooner on thin section images using lung windows [25–27].

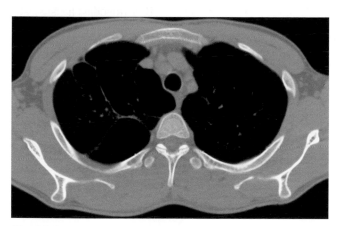

Fig. 99.4a

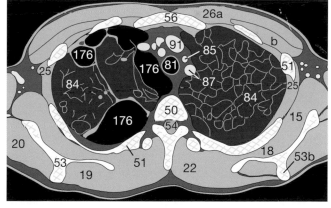

Fig. 99.4b

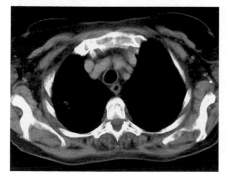

Fig. 99.5a

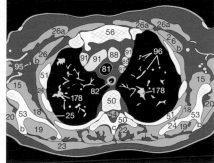

Fig. 99.5b

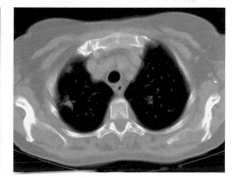

Fig. 99.5c

The pathogenesis of interstitial fibrosis of the lung (Fig. 100.1) cannot always be established and is referred to as idiopathic pulmonary fibrosis. This is particularly true when it affects middle-aged women. The pattern of fibrosis resembles that illustrated on the previous pages with the exception that emphysematous changes typically begin in subpleural regions. Fibrosis of the lung can accompany any of the collagen vascular diseases in the advanced stages and lead to similar morphologic changes, for example in scleroderma (Fig. 100.2) or polyarteritis nodosa (Fig. 100.3).

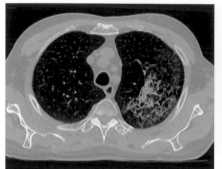

Fig. 100.1

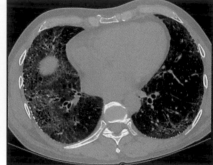

Fig. 100.2

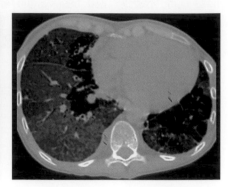

Fig. 100.3

Test Yourself!

You should try to answer all the questions on this and the following page before turning to the back of the book for the answers so as not to spoil the fun of tackling each one.

Exercise 20:
Do you recognize any abnormalities in Figure 100.4 or is it a scan of normal anatomy? Discuss your DD.

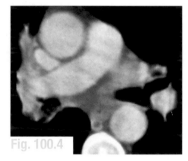

Fig. 100.4

Exercise 21:
How would you interpret the dense area in the left lung in Figure 100.5? Discuss your DD and make a list of additional information that you need and the steps necessary in order to be certain about the lesion.

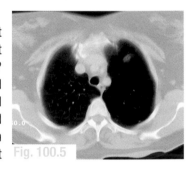

Fig. 100.5

Exercise 22: A 62-year-old patient presented with intense back pain and was examined by CT. What is your diagnosis of the changes seen in Figure 100.6? Can you classify the type of change and the degree of severity?

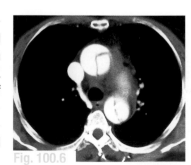

Fig. 100.6

Exercise 23: Describe in detail the pathologic changes visible in Figure 100.7 and the steps in your DD.

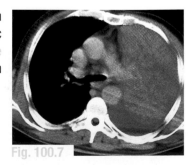

Fig. 100.7

Exercise 24:
What further diagnostic procedures would you recommend for the case illustrated in Figure 101.1? What do you suspect the lesion to be? What other changes do you recognize?

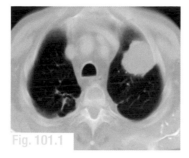

Fig. 101.1

Exercise 25:
Detecting even minor changes may be decisive in order to arrive at the correct diagnosis. What do you see in Figure 101.2?

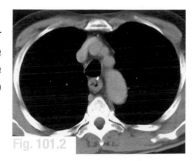

Fig. 101.2

Exercise 26:
A patient in her 26th week of pregnancy complained of shortness of breath. Her physician initially thought it was because of a high diaphragm. Two weeks later she was examined by CT. Make careful note of all abnormal changes you see in Figure 101.3 and the steps in your DD.

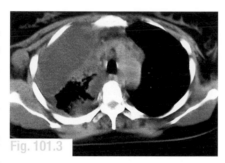

Fig. 101.3

Exercise 27:
A 56-year-old woman with a history of smoking presented with unintended weight loss and severe attacks of coughing which had already lasted for 3 months. She had no previous illnesses. Does Figure 101.4 illustrate normal anatomy, a normal variant, or an abnormality?

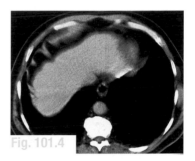

Fig. 101.4

Exercise 28:   Do Figures 101.5a and 101.5b illustrate normal anatomy, an anomaly, or a lymphoma? Discuss your opinion.

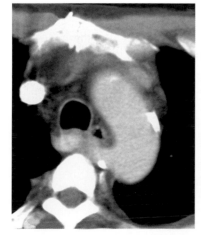

Fig. 101.5a

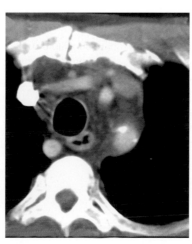

Fig. 101.5b

In general, all soft-tissue organs should appear uniform and be well defined, except when partial volume effects occur (cf. p.14) or during the early arterial phase of CM enhancement in a helical scan (cf. pp.120 and 126). Structures such as blood vessels and bowel loops should be clearly defined in intra-abdominal fat. The same applies to the fat in muscles.

Poorly defined connective-tissue spaces may indicate edema or an inflammatory or malignant infiltration. If the anatomy cannot be clearly resolved, additional information can be gained by measuring the density of specific areas or by comparing unenhanced with CM-enhanced scans (cf. pp. 15 and 121).

Again, the proposed checklist is not intended to be "prescriptive", but to give an useful tool for the novice in order to reduce the number of missed pathological findings.

Selection of Image Plane

The sections of the abdomen are also acquired transversally (=axially). If the table advance is set at 8 mm with a slice thickness of 10 mm, there will be an overlap of 1 mm on each side of the section. In recent years, there is a trend towards thinner slices with a slice thickness between 5 and 8 mm.

The small topograms on the following pages (based on Fig. 102.1) clearly show the slice positions as related to the anatomy of major structures for each series of images.

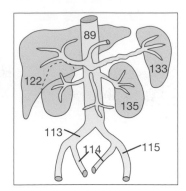

Fig. 102.1

Systematic Sequence for Readings

Analogous to interpreting chest CTs, we suggest you begin with the tissues of the abdominal wall. Considerable time is saved if you consistently look at them from cranial to caudal. For beginners a systematic inspection of each organ or system from cranial to caudal is recommended, so that you do not need to concentrate on too many structures at once. The proposed procedure encompasses two or three passages through the images. As you become experienced, you may wish to devise your own method. Experienced readers are more easily able to detect all pathologic changes in one passage from cranial to caudal.

It is sensible to evaluate internal organs that lie in the same transverse plane. The uniformity of the parenchyma, the size and the smooth surface of liver and spleen should be checked together. The same is true for the assessment of the pancreas and the adrenal glands: they also lie at the same level (cf. pp. 104/105). If the entire urinary system is to be examined, it saves time to inspect the reproductive organs and bladder in the lesser pelvis before looking at the cranial parts of the GIT, or the regional lymph nodes and the retroperitoneal vessels (see checklist on the right).

Finally, the presence of sclerotic and lytic bone lesions and the state of the spinal canal should be checked (cf. p.155).

Checklist for Abdominal Readings

Abdominal wall:	(especially periumbilical and inguinal regions) hernias, enlarged lymph nodes?
Liver and spleen:	homogeneous parenchyma without focal lesions? well-defined surfaces?
Gallbladder:	well-defined, thin wall? calculi?
Pancreas, adrenals:	well-defined, size normal?
Kidneys, ureter, and bladder	symmetric excretion of CM? obstruction, atrophy, bladder wall smooth and thin?
Reproductive organs:	uniform prostate of normal size? spermatic cord, uterus, and ovaries?
GIT:	well defined? normal thickness of walls? stenoses or dilations?
Retroperitoneum:	vessels: aneurysms? thromboses? enlarged lymph nodes?
	mesenteric (normally < 10 mm)
	retrocrural (normally < 7 mm)
	para-aortic (normally < 7 mm)
	parailiacal (normally < 12 mm)
	parainguinal (normally < 18 mm)
Bone window:	lumbar spine and pelvis: degenerative lesions? fractures? focal sclerotic or lytic lesions? spinal stenoses?

The images of the abdominal organs include the costodia-phragmatic recesses of the lungs (**84**), which extend quite far caudally, laterally, and dorsally. Liver (**122**) and spleen (**133**) parenchyma usually appear homogeneous without focal lesions in the venous phase of CM enhancement: branches of the hepatic veins (**103**) can be distinguished. In order to assess the gastric wall (**129a**), the stomach

(**129**) can be filled with water, which acts as a low-density CM, after an i.v. injection of Buscopan. The diaphragm (**30**) between the thoracic and abdominal cavities has an attenuation similar to the parenchyma of the liver and spleen and can therefore not be differentiated from these organs if its thin dome is sectioned obliquely.

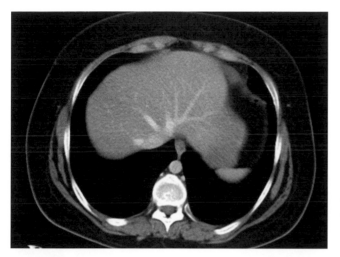

Fig. 103.1a

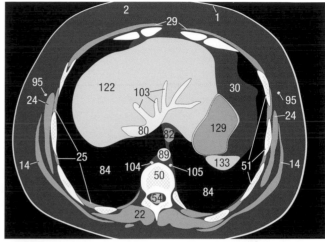

Fig. 103.1b

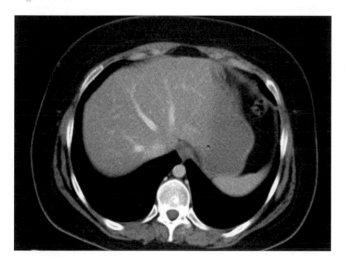

Fig. 103.2a

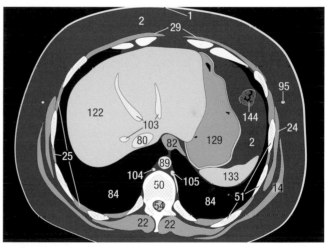

Fig. 103.2b

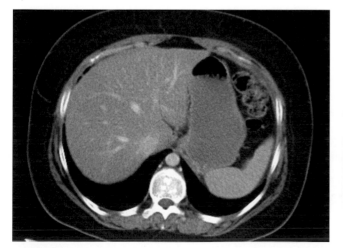

Fig. 103.3a

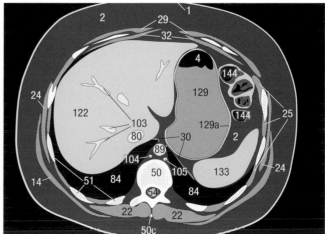

Fig. 103.3b

The right adrenal gland usually lies cranial to the upper pole of the kidney (**135**), whereas the left adrenal gland lies ventral to the upper pole of the kidney. Consequently, the two adrenal glands (**134**) are seen on the same sections.

Note the position of the diaphragm (**30**) between the lung (**84**) and the inferior vena cava (**80**). The vessels on the lesser curvature of the stomach (**109**) and the gastric walls (**129a**) are usually well defined and clearly demarcated in the surrounding fat and connective tissue (**2**).

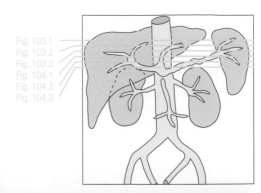

Fig. 103.1
Fig. 103.2
Fig. 103.3
Fig. 104.1
Fig. 104.2
Fig. 104.3

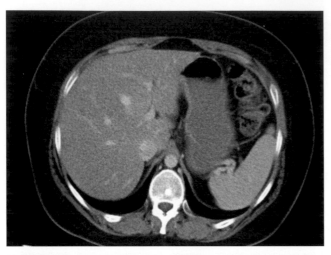

Fig. 104.1a

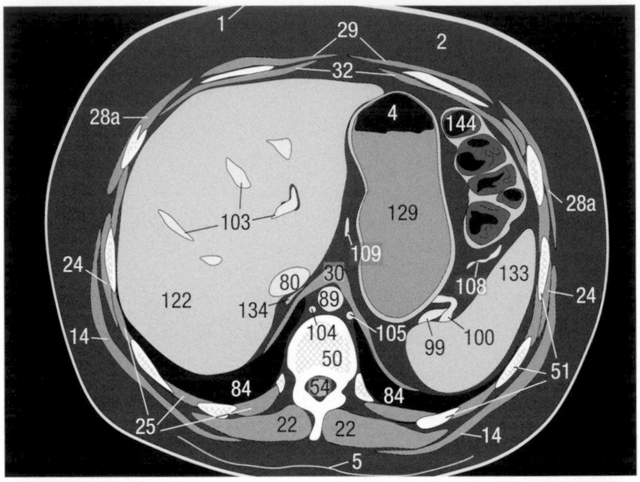

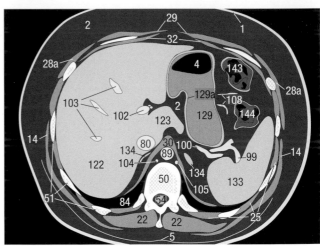

Fig. 104.1b

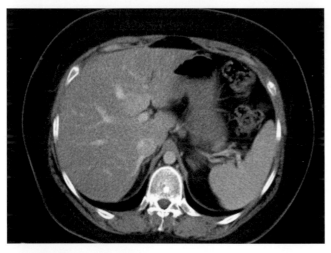

Fig. 104.2a

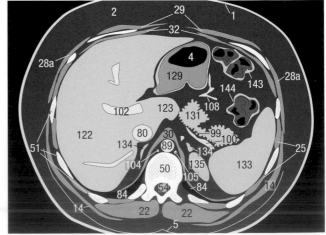

Fig. 104.2b

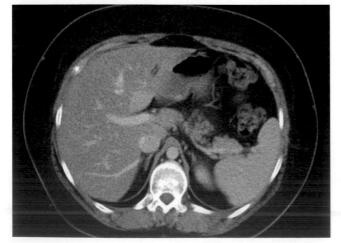

Fig. 104.3a

Fig. 104.3b

Typically the pancreas (**131**) has well-defined parenchyma with an irregular outline. The head and uncinate process of the pancreas extend quite far caudally (down to Fig. 107.3).

The left adrenal gland (**134**) is often Y-shaped, whereas the right adrenal gland may look like an arrow or a comma.

Note the origin of the celiac trunk (**97**) and the SMA (**106**) from the abdominal aorta (**89**). Enlarged lymph nodes may frequently be found in this vicinity. Branches of the portal vein (**102**) and the falciforme ligament (**124**) can be distinguished.

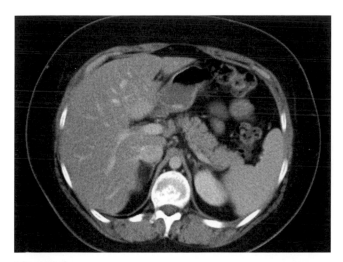

Fig. 105.1a

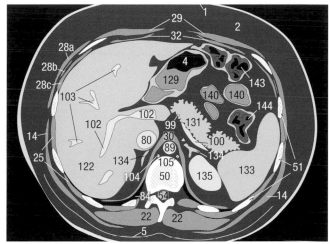

Fig. 105.1b

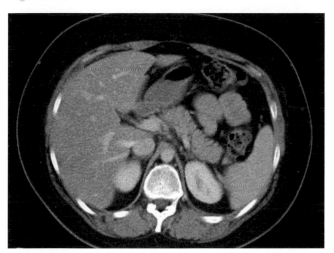

Fig. 105.2a

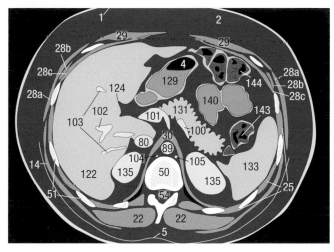

Fig. 105.2b

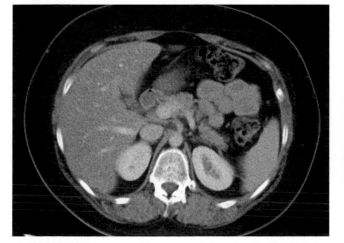

Fig. 105.3a

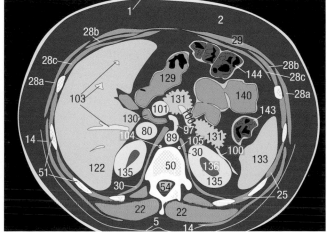

Fig. 105.3b

Look for arterial calcifications in the origins of the renal arteries (**110**) at the level of the renal veins (**111**). The left renal vein does not always pass between the aorta (**89**) and the SMA (**106**) to the inferior vena cava (**80**), as it does in Figure 106.1. Anatomic variations are not unusual (cf. p.116). Benign cysts frequently occur in the renal pelvis (**136**) next to the ureter (**137**) or in the renal parenchyma (**135**) (Figs. 106.2 and 106.3). Such cysts do <u>not</u> enhance after CM injection (cf. p.133).

In Fig. 106.2 the superior mesenteric artery (**106**) originates from the aorta (**89**) and can be followed down next to the SMV (**107**).

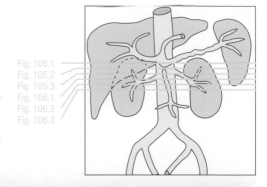

Fig. 105.1
Fig. 105.2
Fig. 105.3
Fig. 106.1
Fig. 106.2
Fig. 106.3

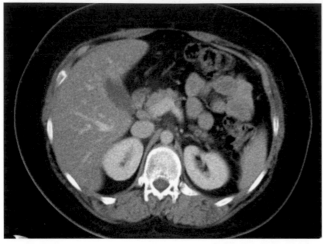

Fig. 106.1a

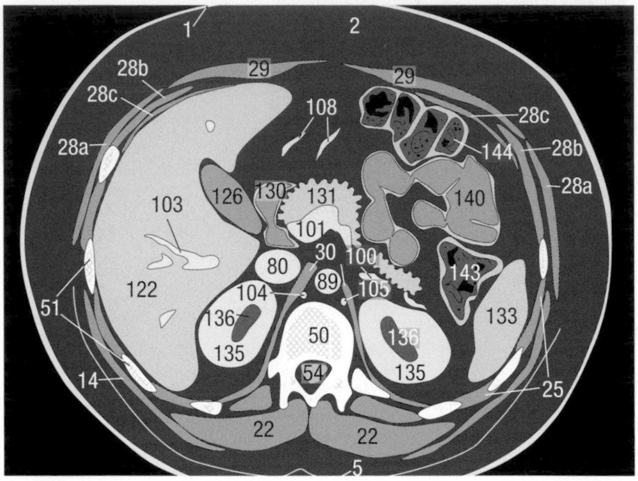

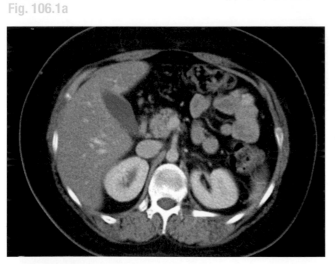

Fig. 106.1b

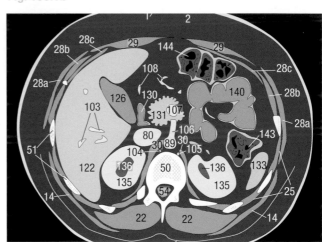

Fig. 106.2a

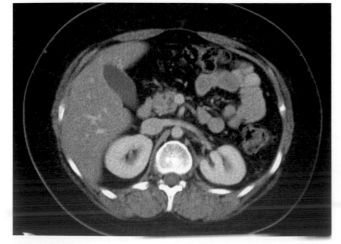

Fig. 106.2b

Fig. 106.3a

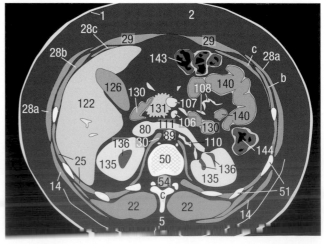

Fig. 106.3b

Close to the gallbladder (**126**), you can sometimes see partial volume effects (Fig. 107.1) of the adjacent colon (**143/144**), the walls of which (**152**) should normally be thin and well defined in contrast to the root of the small bowel mesentery (as in Fig. 107.3). The duodenum (**130**) can only be distinguished from the other intestinal loops (**140**) on the basis of its position. At this level, you should also check the kidneys (**135**) for smooth margins and possible parenchymal scarring. The presence of fat makes it easier to identify the rectus abdominis muscle (**29**) as well as the oblique muscles of the abdominal wall (**28a–c**).

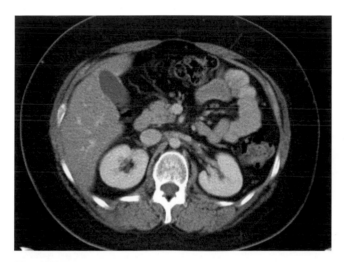

Fig. 107.1a

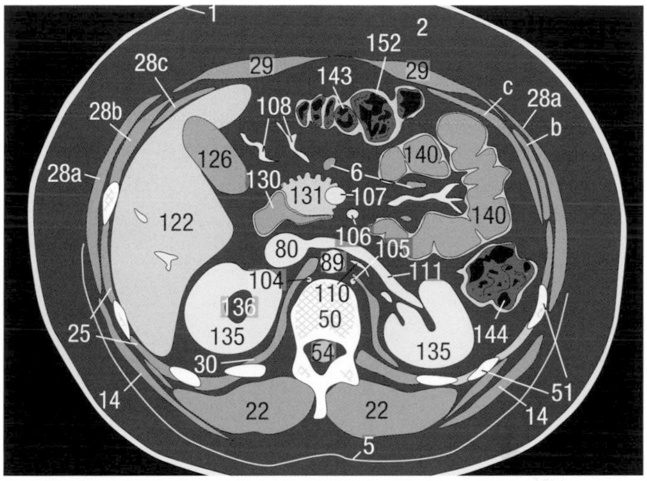

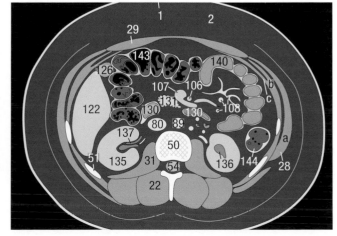

Fig. 107.1b

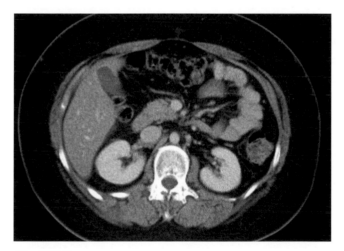

Fig. 107.2a

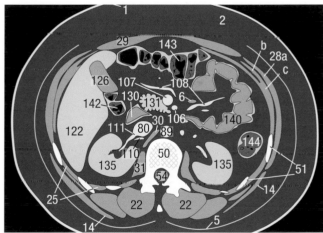

Fig. 107.2b

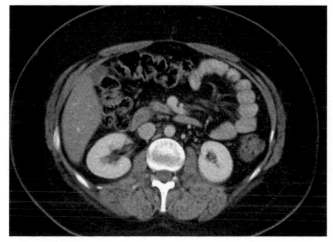

Fig. 107.3a

Fig. 107.3b

Note the typical position of the proximal parts of the ureters (**137**), medial to the inferior poles of the kidneys (**135**) and anterior to the psoas muscle (**31**).

In Figures 108.2 and 108.3, the lumina of both ureters could also appear hyperdense if CM is being excreted in the urine. Haustrations caused by the semilunar folds (haustral folds) (**149**) are typical of the colon (**142-144** in the figures below).

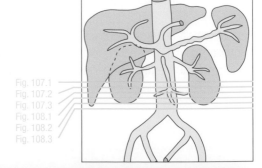

Fig. 107.1
Fig. 107.2
Fig. 107.3
Fig. 108.1
Fig. 108.2
Fig. 108.3

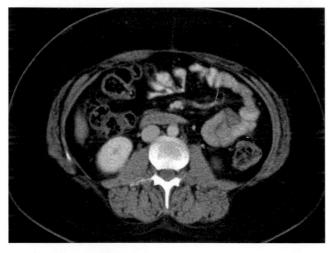

Fig. 108.1a

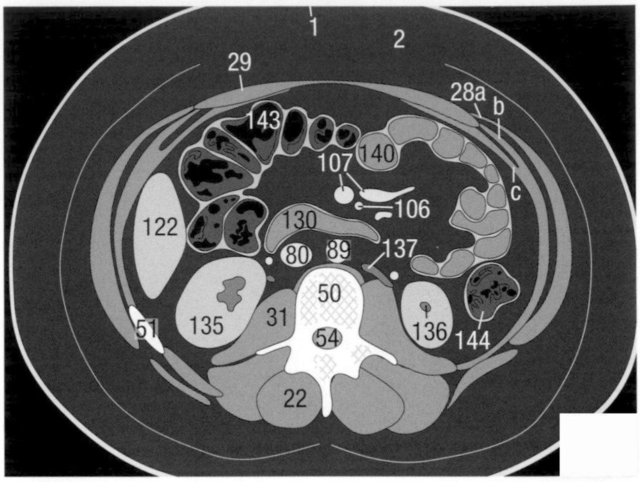

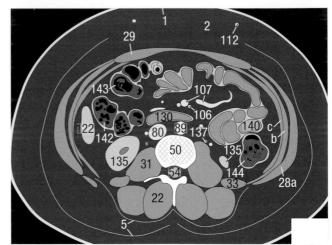

Fig. 108.1b

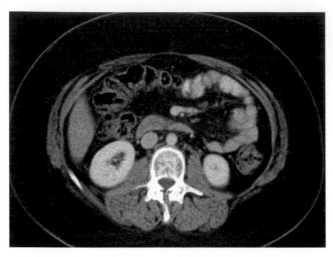

Fig. 108.2a

Fig. 108.2b

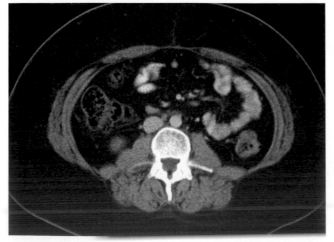

Fig. 108.3a

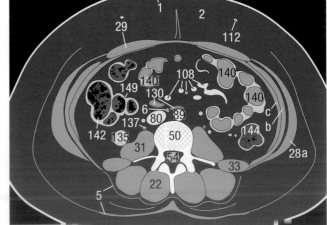

Fig. 108.3b

In Figure 109.1, the branching pattern of the superior mesenteric vessels (**108**) which supply the small bowel (**140**) can be seen. At the bifurcation of the aorta (**89**) (usually at L4 vertebral body, Fig. 109.1), the common iliac arteries (**113**) are anterior to the corresponding veins (**116**). The two ureters

(**137**) are located more laterally in front of the psoas muscles (**31**). Along with the iliac bones (**58**) the gluteus medius muscles (**35a**) appear (Fig. 110.2) and sometimes contain calcified intramuscular injections sites.

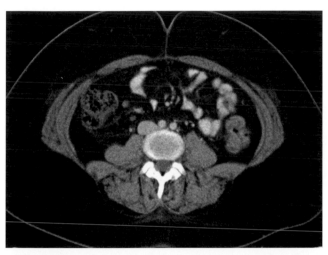

Fig. 109.1a

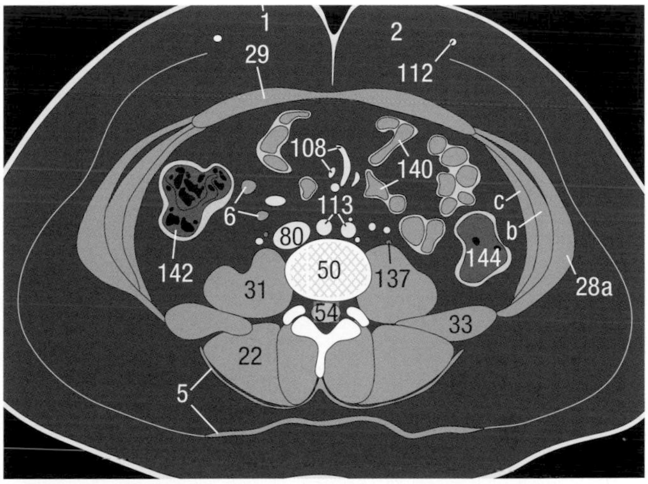

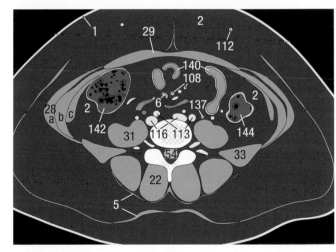

Fig. 109.1b

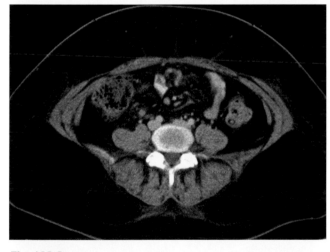

Fig. 109.2a

Fig. 109.2b

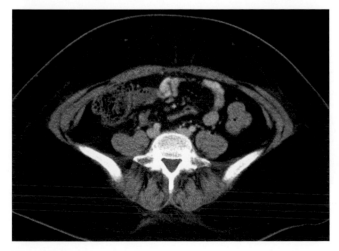

Fig. 109.3a

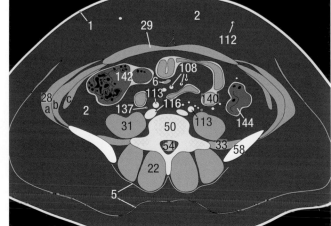

Fig. 109.3b

In order to exclude the presence of an abdominal hernia you should check for a normal width of the linea alba (**47**) between the rectus abdominis muscles (**29**). More caudally (Fig. 110.3) there is a site of predilection for enlarged LNs at the division of the iliac vessels into external artery/vein (**115/118**), which pass anteriorly, and internal artery/vein (**114/117**), which are located more posteriorly. The transition from the lumbar spine (**50**) to the sacrum (**62**) lies at this level.

Further down we find predominantly small bowel loops of jejunum and ileum (**140**) which can be distinguished from sigmoid colon (**145**) by its haustrations and semilunar folds (cf. p. 111).

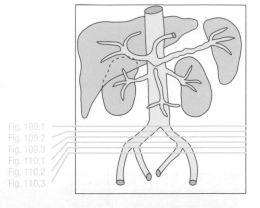

Fig. 109.1
Fig. 109.2
Fig. 109.3
Fig. 110.1
Fig. 110.2
Fig. 110.3

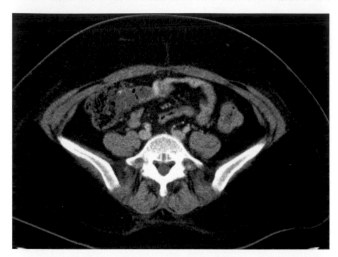

Fig. 110.1a

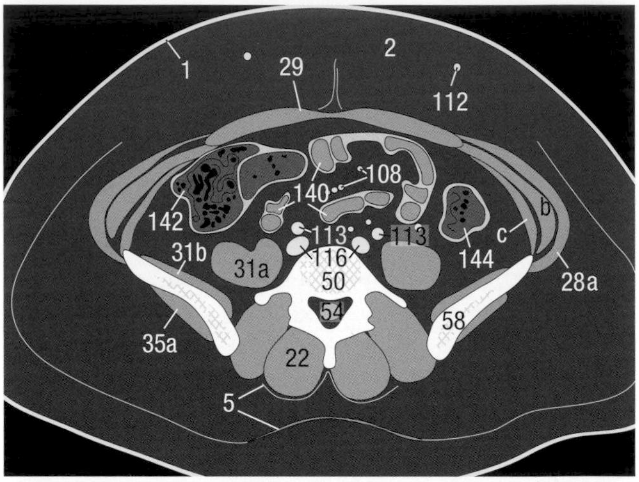

Fig. 110.1b

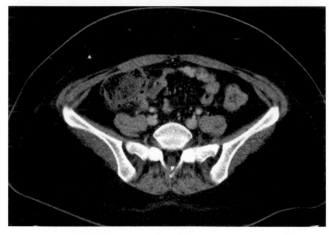

Fig. 110.2a

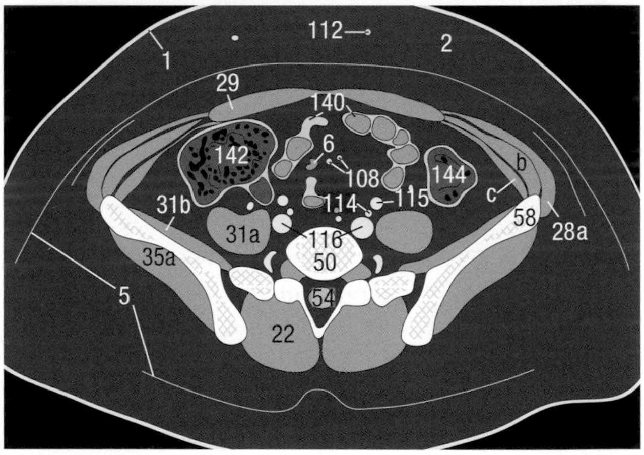

Fig. 110.2b

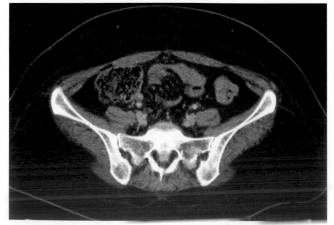

Fig. 110.3a

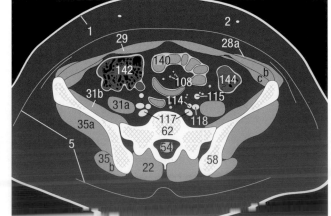

Fig. 110.3b

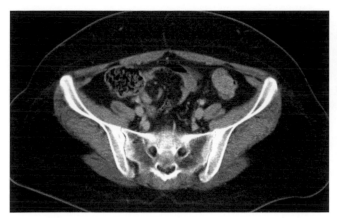

Fig. 111.1a

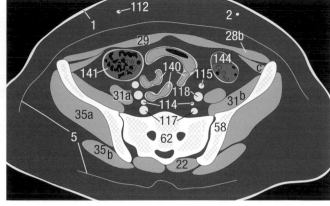

Fig. 111.1b

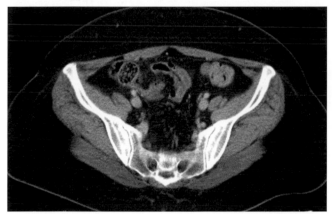

Fig. 111.2a

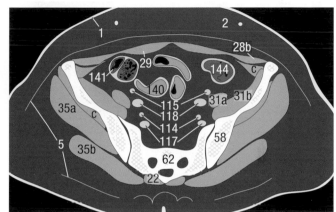

Fig. 111.2b

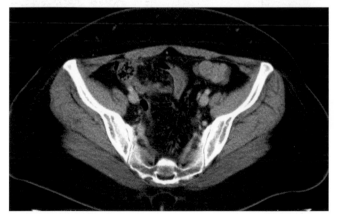

Fig. 111.3a

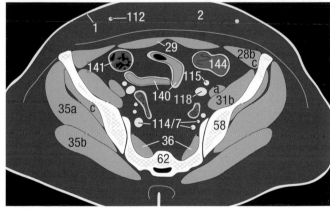

Fig. 111.3b

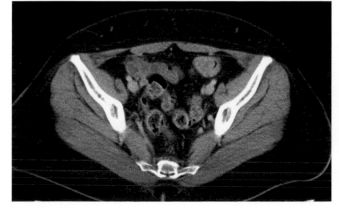

Fig. 111.4a

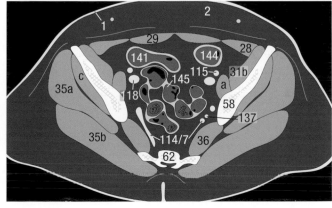

Fig. 111.4b

In the following images, the ureters (**137**) pass posteriorly to approach the lateral aspects of the base of the bladder (**138**). Within the bladder, differences in the concentration of excreted might be recognized as fluid–fluid levels of different densities without any clinical significance.

The ovaries (**159**) lie more laterally. Depending on age and the phase of the menstrual cycle, ovarian follicles (**169**) might be misinterpreted as cystic lesions (Fig. 112.3).

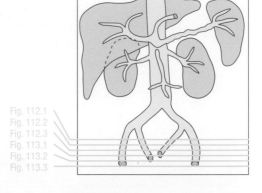

Fig. 112.1
Fig. 112.2
Fig. 112.3
Fig. 113.1
Fig. 113.2
Fig. 113.3

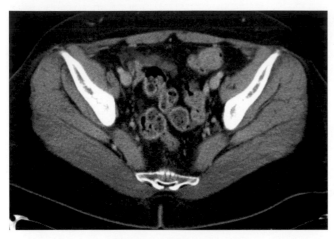

Fig. 112.1a

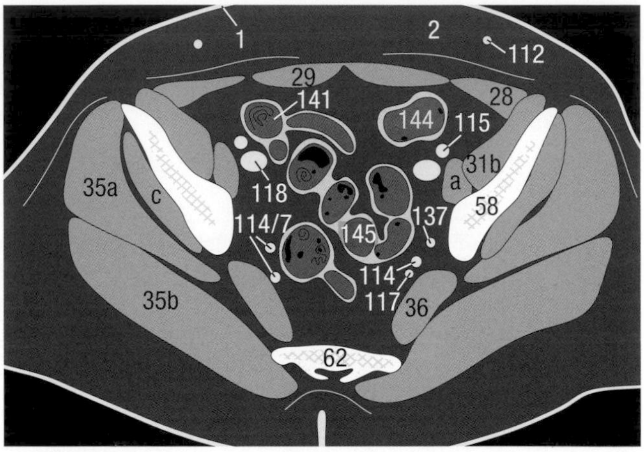

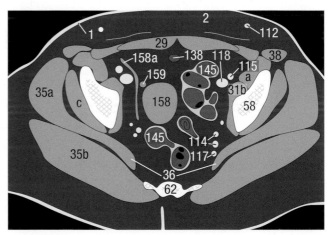

Fig. 112.1b

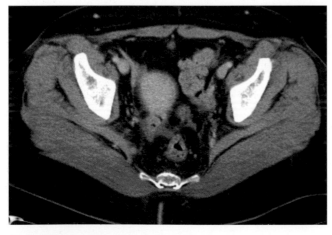

Fig. 112.2a

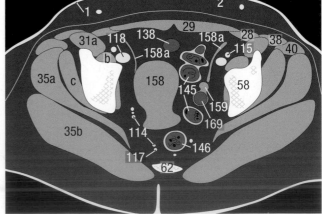

Fig. 112.2b

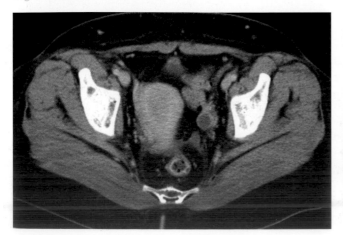

Fig. 112.3a

Fig. 112.3b

In the female pelvis, the size and position of the uterus (**158**) relative to the urinary bladder can vary considerably from patient to patient. The uterus may lie cranial or lateral to the bladder (Figs. 113.1–114.1). The cervix and the vagina (**160**) are situated between the bladder (**138**) and the rectum (**146**). Depending on age and the phase of the menstrual cycle, changing thicknesses of endometrium (★) can be seen within the uterus (**158** in Fig. 113.1).

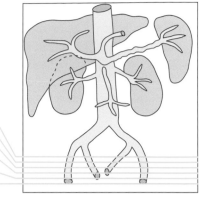

Fig. 113.1
Fig. 113.2
Fig. 113.3
Fig. 114.1
Fig. 114.2
Fig. 114.3

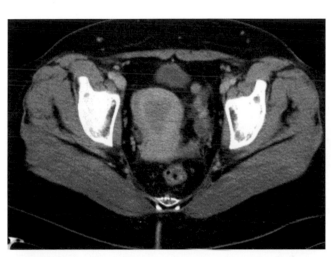

Fig. 113.1a

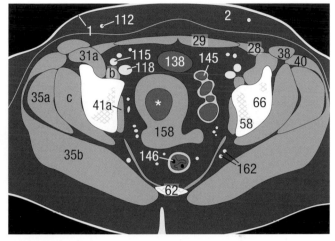

Fig. 113.1b

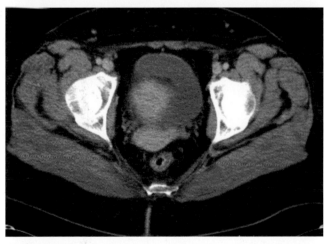

Fig. 113.2a

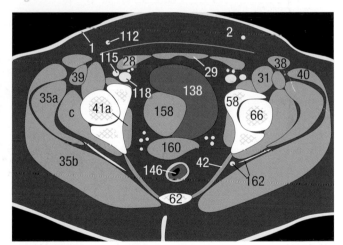

Fig. 113.2b

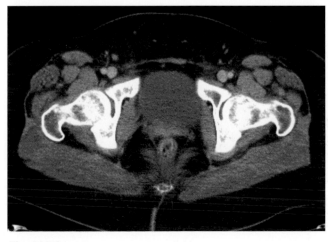

Fig. 113.3a

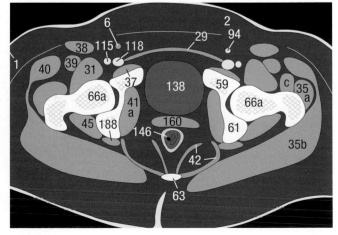

Fig. 113.3b

Free intra-abdominal fluid (ascites or hemorrhage) may occur in the rectouterine pouch between rectum and uterus, as well as in the vesicouterine space. In the inguinal region, lymph nodes (**6**) can be up to 2 cm in diameter and be normal (Figs. 114.2 and 114.3). The size of normal abdominal lymph nodes does not usually exceed 1 cm. It is not possible to examine the hip joints on soft-tissue windows (Fig. 114.3); the heads of the femurs (**66a**) in the acetabular fossae (**59/61**) can best be analyzed on bone windows (not shown here).

On the next pages, a male pelvis is shown, demonstrating the prostate (**153**), seminal vesicles (**154**), spermatic cord (**155**), and root of penis (**156**). Note in particular the internal obturator muscles (**41a**) and the levator ani muscles (**42**) lateral to the anal canal (**146a**). An assessment of bone windows completes the examination of the abdominal and pelvic images.

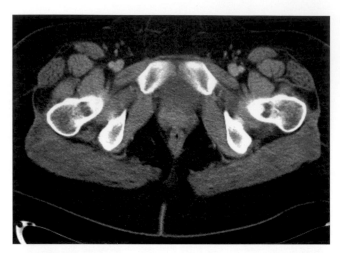

Fig. 114.1a

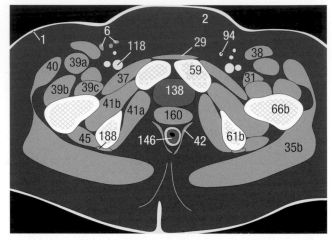

Fig. 114.1b

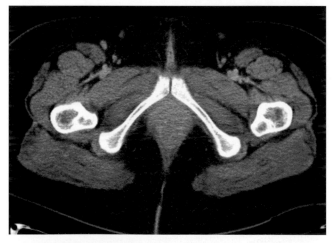

Fig. 114.2a

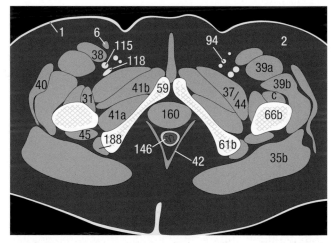

Fig. 114.2b

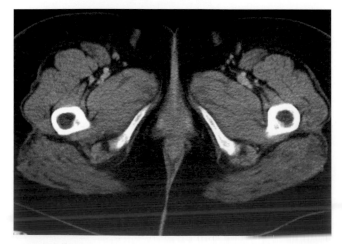

Fig. 114.3a

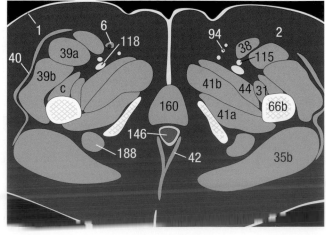

Fig. 115.3b

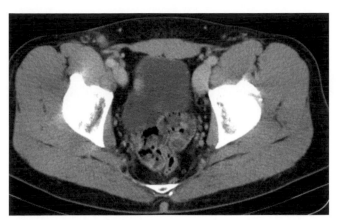

Fig. 115.1a

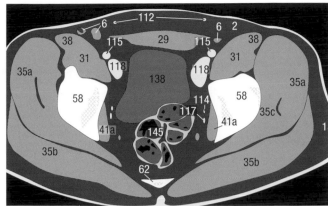

Fig. 115.1b

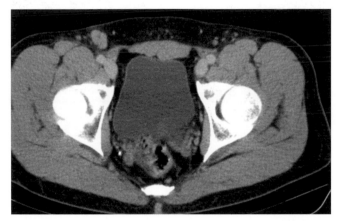

Fig. 115.2a

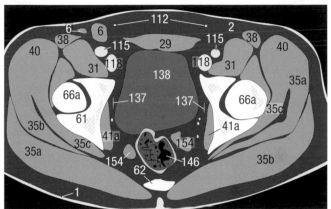

Fig. 115.2b

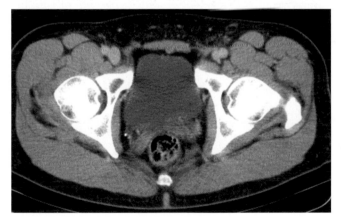

Fig. 115.3a

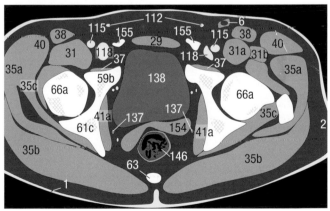

Fig. 115.3b

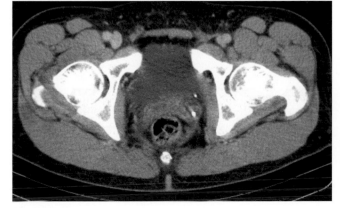

Fig. 115.4a

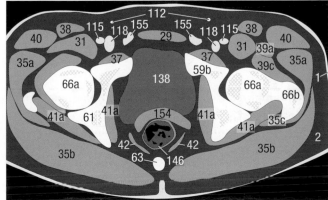

Fig. 115.4b

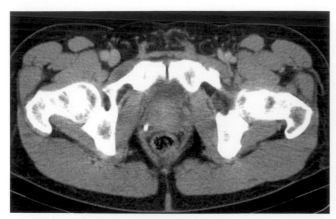

Fig. 116.1a

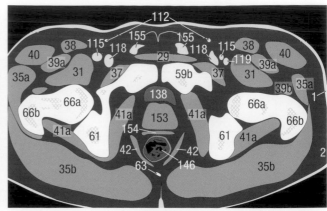

Fig. 116.1b

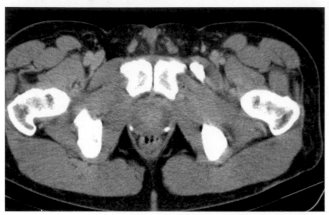

Fig. 116.2a

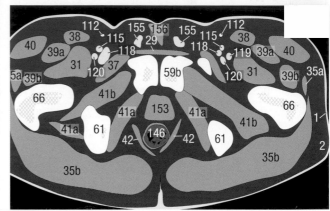

Fig. 116.2b

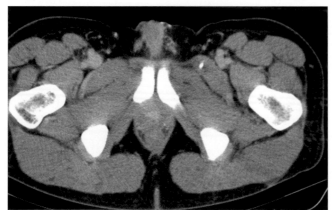

Fig. 116.3a

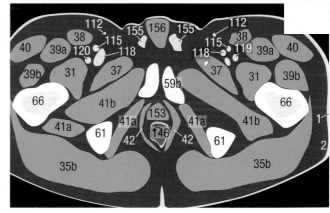

Fig. 116.3b

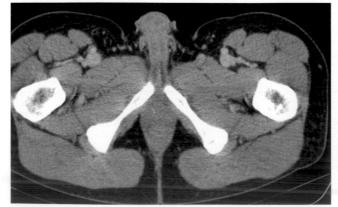

Fig. 116.4a

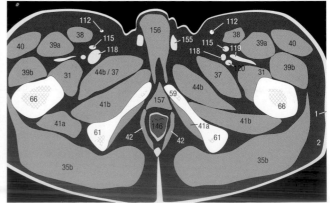

Fig. 116.4b

Anatomic Variations

For the beginner, it is important to be familiar with the most common anatomic variations which may lead to misinterpretations of CT images. In some patients, the contours of the right lobe of the liver (**122**) may appear scalloped by impressions of the diaphragm (**30**) which could be mistaken for liver lesions (Fig. 117.1). The walls of an empty stomach (**129**) are thick and may suggest a malignant lesion (**129a**).

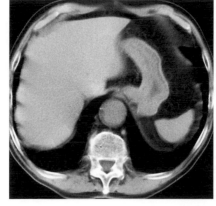

Fig. 117.1a

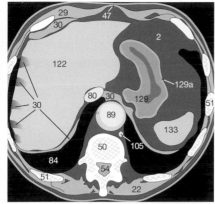

Fig. 117.1b

Ultrasound may mistake an anomalous left renal vein (**111**) for a retro-aortic LN. Usually the left renal vein passes between the SMA (**106**) and the aorta (**89**). However, the vein may be retroaortic and pass between the aorta and the spinal column (**50**) to the inferior vena cava (**80**) (Figs. 117.2 - 117.4). Duplication of the left renal vein with preaortic and retroaortic components can

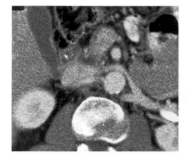

Fig. 117.2a

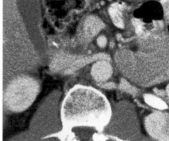

Fig. 117.3a

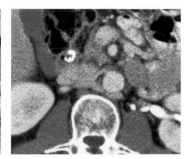

Fig. 117.4a

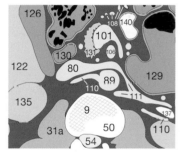

Fig. 117.2b

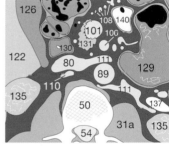

Fig. 117.3b

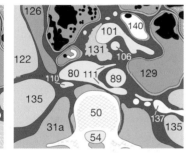

Fig. 117.4b

Characteristic Partial Volume Effects

If the wall of one organ indents that of another, cross-sectional images will make it look as if one organ were within the other. For example, the sigmoid colon (**145**) may appear "within" the urinary bladder (**138**) (Fig. 117.5a). By comparing adjacent sections (Figs. 117.5a and c), it is easy to recognize that only parts of both organs have been imaged. In a similar manner, the right colic flexure (**142**) may appear to be "within" the gallbladder (**126**) (Fig. 117.6).

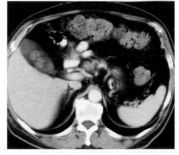

Fig. 117.6a

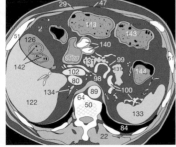

Fig. 117.6b

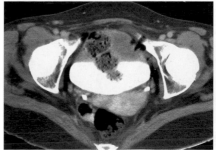

Fig. 117.5a

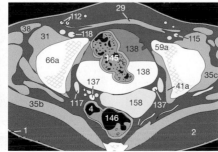

Fig. 117.5b

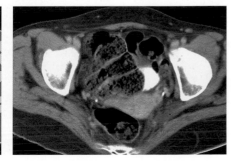

Fig. 117.5c

Lymph Node Hyperplasia

Pathologic lesions of the abdominal wall occur most frequently in the inguinal region. Lymph node hyperplasia with nodes up to 2 cm in dimension should not be considered abnormal. Large conglomerate masses of LNs (◄—) are found in non-Hodgkin's lymphoma (Fig. 118.1) and less frequently in Hodgkin's disease.

An inguinal hematoma (**173**) caused by hemorrhage from a femoral artery puncture site after coronary angiography should be considered (Fig. 118.2) in the DD.

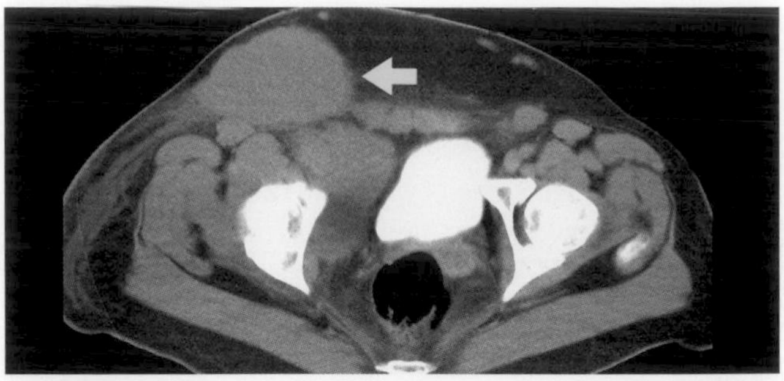

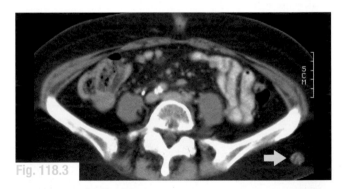

Fig. 118.1

Fig. 118.2b

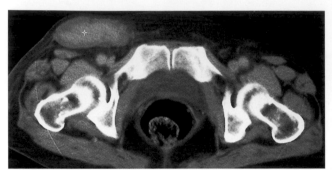

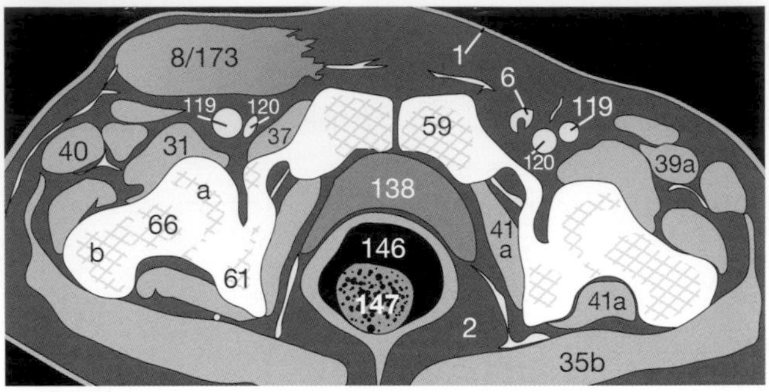

Fig. 118.2a

Abscesses

Intramuscular injection sites in the gluteal region resulting in subcutaneous fat (**2**) necrosis or postinflammatory residue (—►) typically are well-defined, hyperdense, partially calcified lesions (Fig. 118.3).

An abscess may spread from the gluteal muscles to the pelvis through the ischiorectal fossa. After diffuse infiltration (**178**) of the gluteal muscles (**35**) with surrounding edema (**185** in Fig. 118.4), liquefaction (**181**) may occur and, depending on the localization and size, the abscess can involve the sciatic nerve (Fig. 118.5).

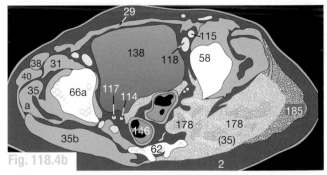

Fig. 118.3

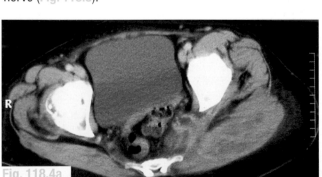

Fig. 118.4a

Fig. 118.4b

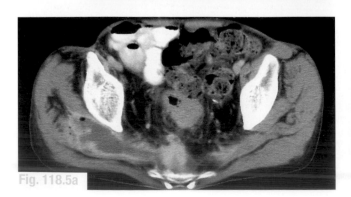

Fig. 118.5a

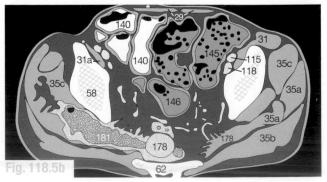

Fig. 118.5b

The CT in Figure 119.1 shows subcutaneous lesions, resulting from heparin injections (**173**) or small hematomas that may mimic cutaneous metastases (**7**) or malignant melanomas (Fig. 119.2). Larger metastases tend to invade the muscles of the abdominal wall (**29**) and often have hypodense, central

necrosis (**181**). Enhancement after intravenous CM may also point to malignancy or a florid inflammatory process. If the degree of CM enhancement is uncertain, a region of interest for densitometric analysis is placed in the lesion on a pre-CM and compared with a post-CM (Fig. 119.2).

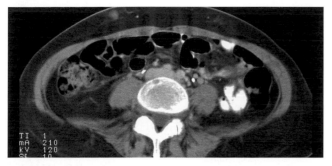

Fig. 119.1a

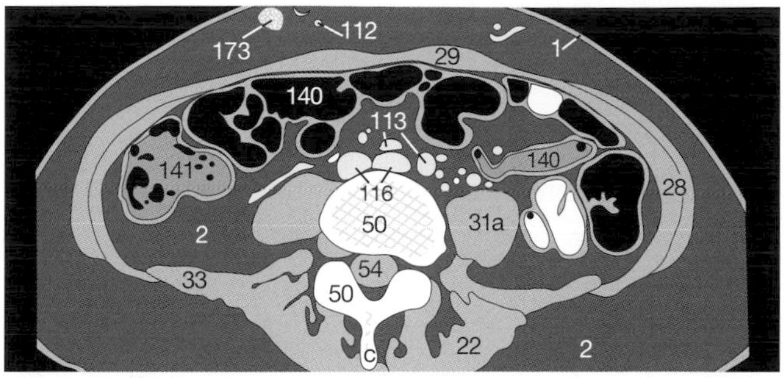

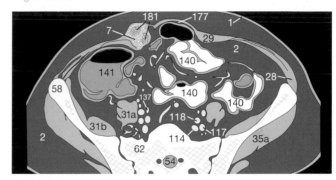

Fig. 119.1b

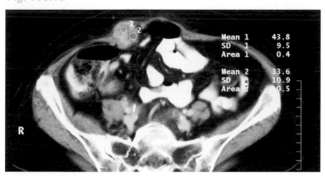

Fig. 119.2a

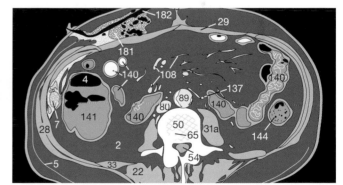

Fig. 119.2b

Metastases in the abdominal wall may not be evident until they become infected and develop into an abscess (**181**), which was catheterized and drained in the case illustrated (**182** in

Fig. 119.3). The second metastasis (**7**), just beneath the right abdominal wall (**28**), was not recognized at first because the patient's symptoms were attributed to the adjacent abscess.

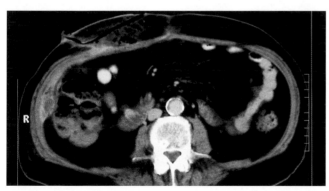

Fig. 119.3a

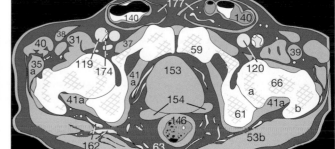

Fig. 119.3b

In elderly patients, an inguinal hernia containing small intestine, or even bilateral scrotal hernias containing loops of the

small bowel (**140**) may be diagnosed. In the case in Figure 119.4, the processus vaginalis (**177**) was open bilaterally.

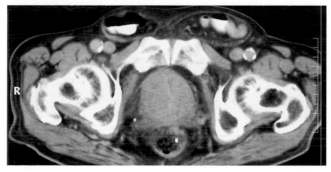

Fig. 119.4a

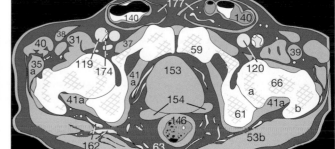

Fig. 119.4b

Segments of the Liver

If a liver biopsy or radiotherapy is planned, it is helpful to know in which segment a focal lesion is situated. The liver is horizontally subdivided (blue line in Fig. 120.1) by the main branches of the portal vein (**102**) into a cranial and caudal part. The main hepatic veins (**103**) mark the borders of the segments in the cranial part (Fig. 120.2). The border between the left and right lobes is <u>not</u> marked by the falciform ligament (**124**), but by the plane between the middle hepatic vein and gallbladder (**126**) fossa.

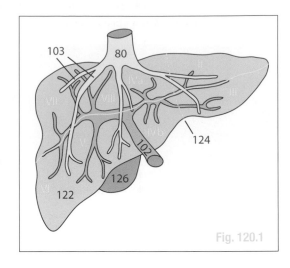

Fig. 120.1

Left lobe	I	caudate lobe
	II	lateral segment, cranial part
	III	lateral segment, caudal part
	IV	quadrate lobe (a: cranial, b: caudal)
Right lobe	V	anterior segment, caudal part
	VI	posterior segment, caudal part
	VII	posterior segment, cranial part
	VIII	anterior segment, cranial part

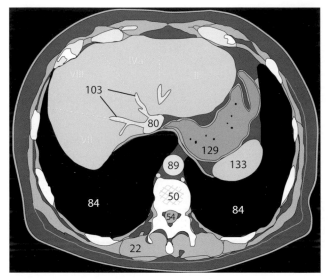

Fig. 120.2

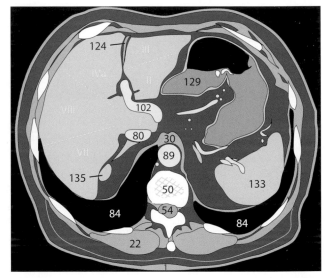

Fig. 120.3

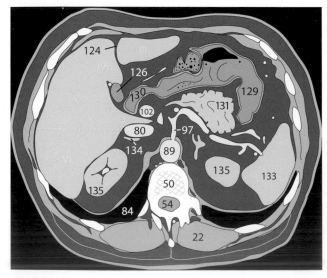

Fig. 120.4

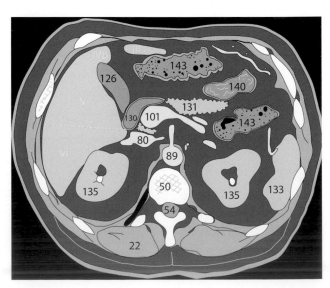

Fig. 120.5

Choice of Window

In conventional (nonhelical) CT, the unenhanced liver (**122**) is imaged on a special liver window width (Fig. 121.1a) set between 120 and 140 HU. Normal liver parenchyma can be more clearly distinguished from lesions on narrow window width images because they provide high image contrast. If there is no fatty infiltration of the liver (which would reduce attenuation), intrahepatic vessels (**103**) appear as hypodense structures. In cases of fatty infiltration, the veins may appear isodense or even hyperdense on unenhanced images. The post-contrast agents CT images are viewed using a window width of approximately 350 HU; this smoothes the gray scale contrast (Fig. 121.1c).

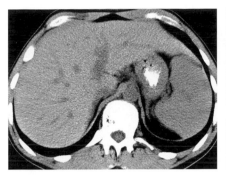
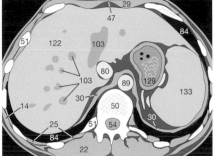
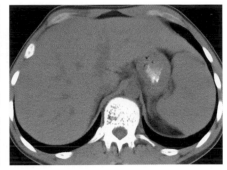

Fig. 121.1a | Fig. 121.1b | Fig. 121.1c

Passage of a Bolus of Contrast Agents

In a three-phase helical acquisition of early arterial, portal venous, and late venous phases of contrast agents enhancement, an unenhanced study is not necessary [17, 18]. Hypervascular lesions become much more clearly defined in the early arterial phase (Fig. 121.2a) than in the late venous phase. In the late venous (equilibrium) phase (Fig. 121.2b), the density levels of the arterial, portal venous, and venous systems are practically identical.

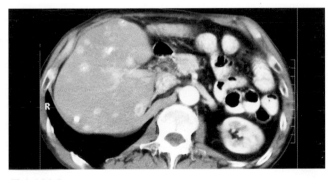
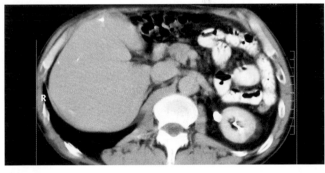

Fig. 121.2a | Fig. 121.2b

CT Portography

The chances of demonstrating the true extent of liver lesions (e.g. metastases) are greatly improved if contrast agents are injected directly into the SMA or the splenic artery and images are then acquired in the portal venous phase [17, 21]. Since the principal blood supply for most metastases and tumors comes from the hepatic artery, these lesions will appear hypodense within the hyperdense normal parenchyma that has enhanced with contrast agents (Fig. 121.3a). In the same patient, the early arterial phase image (Fig. 121.3b) shows that without contrast agents portography, the extent of the metastases would have been greatly underestimated.

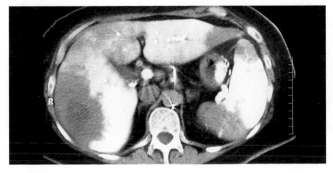
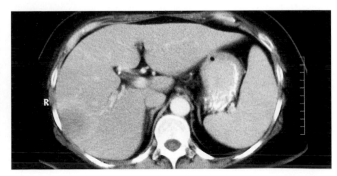

Fig. 121.3a | Fig. 121.3b

Hepatic Cysts

Hepatic cysts (**169**) containing serous fluid are sharply defined, thin-walled, homogeneous lesions with density values close to those of water (Fig. 122.1). Partial volume effects may cause poor delineation from adjacent hepatic parenchyma (**122**) if the cysts are small. If in doubt, a ROI should be positioned within the cyst for density measurement (Fig. 122.2a). It is important to ensure the ROI is correctly placed in the center of the cyst, well away from the cyst walls (cf. pp. 15 and 133). In small cysts, for example the poorly defined lesion in Figure 122.2b, the average density measurement was too high, because adjacent liver parenchyma was included in the calculation. Note that benign cysts do not show any significant enhancement after i.v. CM.

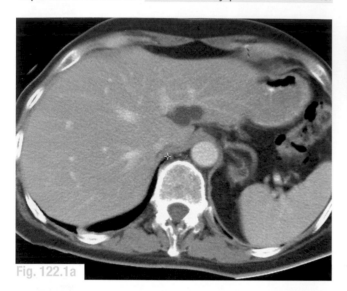

Fig. 122.1a

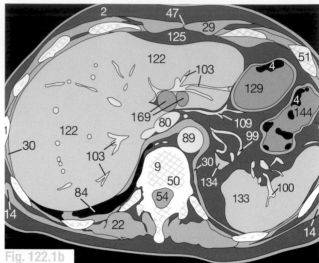

Fig. 122.1b

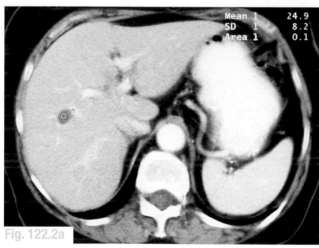

Fig. 122.2a

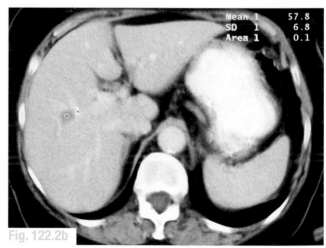

Fig. 122.2b

Echinococcus

Hydatid *(Echinococcus granulosus)* cysts have a very characteristic multiloculated appearance, often with radially arranged septations between different cysts (**169** in Fig. 122.3). It may prove difficult to differentiate between collapsed, dead cysts and other intrahepatic lesions. The right lobe of the liver is most frequently affected, sometimes the left lobe or the spleen (**133**) become involved, as shown in (Fig. 122.3). The density of the cyst fluid is usually between 10 and 40 HU on an unenhanced image. Partial or complete wall calcification is frequent and the outer membrane may enhance with CM. The DD includes infections with *E. alveolaris* (not shown) and occasionally hepatocellular carcinoma that is poorly defined with irregular satellite lesions.

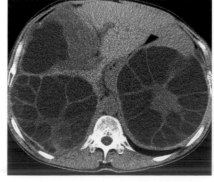

Fig. 122.3a

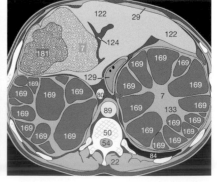

Fig. 122.3b

Liver Metastases

Multiple focal lesions within the liver suggest metastases. Common sites of origin are the colon, stomach, lung, breast, kidneys, and uterus. The morphology and vascularity differ between the types of liver metastases. An enhanced helical scan is therefore obtained in both the venous phase (Fig. 123.1a) and the early arterial phase (Fig. 123.1c). In this manner, smaller lesions (**7**) become well defined and hepatic veins (**103**) will not be mistaken for metastases.

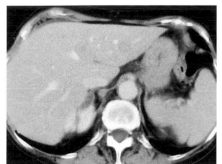

Fig. 123.1a

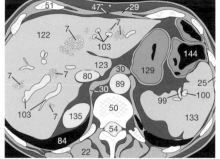

Fig. 123.1b

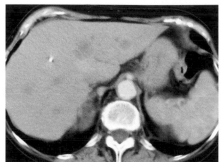

Fig. 123.1c

Hypo- and hypervascular metastases share the hypodense (dark) appearance in the venous phase because of rapid wash-out of contrast material. If spiral CT is not available, it is helpful to compare unenhanced images (Fig. 123.2) with enhanced images (Fig. 123.3). In the example on the right, number and size of the hepatic lesions (**7**) would have been underestimated on the enhanced images. It is easily comprehensible that individual small metastases can escape detection if unenhanced images are passed over. To increase the contrast in the hepatic parenchyma (**122**), a narrow window setting should always be used when viewing these unenhanced images (see page 117). This might even bring out small metastases (**7**) (Fig. 123.2). These small liver metastases (**7**) differ from small cysts by exhibiting an indistinct margin and a higher density after intravenous injection of contrast medium (Fig. 123.4) indicative of enhancement. The average density values were 55 and 71 HU, respectively (Fig. 123.4).

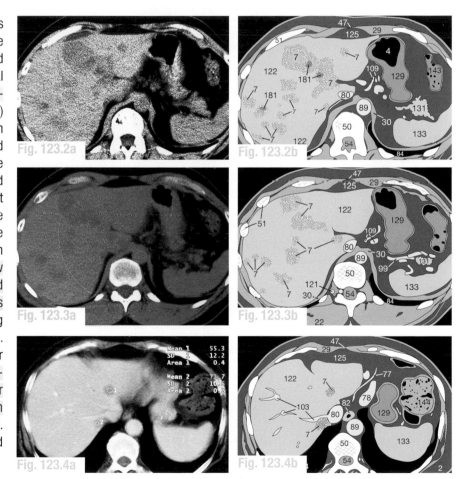

Fig. 123.2a

Fig. 123.2b

Fig. 123.3a

Fig. 123.3b

Fig. 123.4a

Fig. 123.4b

In case of diagnostic doubt and for reference at follow-up during therapy, it is useful to compare the CT images with ultrasound findings. Apart from the typical hypoechoic halo, metastases have varied ultrasound appearances, just as in CT images [23]. The ultrasound diagnosis may be difficult, especially when calcification in metastases leads to acoustic shadowing. Even though they are quite rare, slowly enlarging mucinous metastases (i.e. those from colon carcinomas) may become very calcified (✎ in Fig. 123.5).

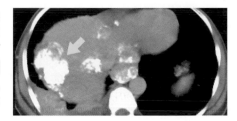

Fig. 123.5

Solid Hepatic Lesions

A hemangioma is the most common benign hepatic lesion. In unenhanced images small hemangioma are well-defined homogeneous areas of decreased attenuation. After injection of CM, enhancement typically begins in the periphery and progresses toward the center of the hemangioma (Fig. 124.1a), reminiscent of the closing of an optic diaphragm. In dynamic bolusenhanced CT sequences, enhancement progresses centripetally. Following administration of a CM bolus, a series of CT images is acquired every few seconds at the same location. Accumulation of CM within the cavities of the hemangioma ( ) leads to homogeneous enhancement in the late venous phase (Fig. 124.1b). In large hemangiomas, this might take several minutes or be inhomogeneous.

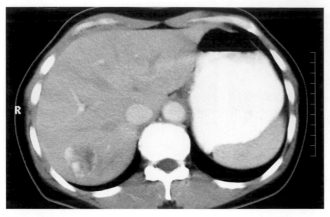

Fig. 124.1a

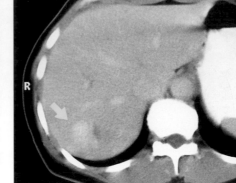

Fig. 124.1b

Hepatic adenoma ( ) occurs most frequently in women between the ages of 20 and 60 years who have a long history of taking oral contraceptives. An adenoma originates in hepatocytes and may be solitary or multiple. The adenoma is usually isodense, sometimes hypervascular (Fig. 124.2), and may be accompanied by hypodense infarction, central necrosis, and/or spontaneous hyperdense hemorrhage. Surgical excision is recommended due to the possibility of acute hemorrhage and malignant degeneration. By contrast, focal nodular hyperplasia (FNH) does not show any tendency of malignant degeneration, and lesions of this kind contain biliary ducts. On unenhanced images, FNH appears as hypodense, sometimes isodense, but well-defined lesions. After i.v. CM, FNH often demonstrates an irregularly shaped, hypodense central area (★) representing its central blood supply; however this feature is seen in only 50% of all FNH (Fig. 124.3).

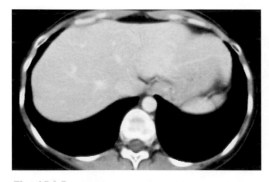

Fig. 124.2

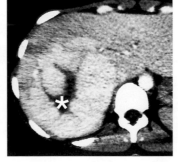

Fig. 124.3

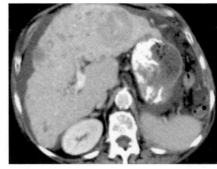

Fig. 124.4

Hepatocellular carcinoma (HCC) often occurs in patients who have a long history of hepatic cirrhosis and is seen most often in men over the age of 40 years. In one-third of all cases, HCC is solitary although multifocal lesions are not rare. Thromboses in the branches of the portal vein caused by tumor invasion into the lumen of the vessel may be seen in one-third of cases. The CT appearance of HCC (Fig. 123.4) is extremely variable. On unenhanced images, HCC usually appears hypodense or isodense; CM may show diffuse or rim enhancement and central necrosis. When there is also cirrhosis, it may be difficult to define the border of an HCC.

Secondary lymphoma should be considered in the DD because it may infiltrate the liver parenchyma and may be the cause of diffuse hepatomegaly. Of course, this does not mean that every case of hepatomegaly is due to a lymphoma. Non-Hodgkin's lymphomas resemble HCC because of their similarities in vascularity and nodular growth.

Diffuse Hepatic Lesions

In fatty changes of the liver, the density of the unenhanced parenchyma, which is normally about 65 HU, may reduce so that it is either isodense or even hypodense with regard to the blood vessels (Fig. 125.1; cf. also p. 120). In hemochromatosis (Fig. 125.2), the accumulation of iron leads to increased attenuation above 90 HU and may reach as much as 140 HU. In these cases, the natural contrast between parenchyma and vessels is even greater. Cirrhosis (Fig. 125.3), resulting from chronic liver damage, has a diffuse nodular appearance and usually gives the organ an irregular, lumpy contour.

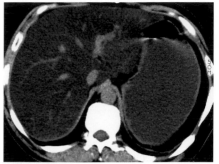
Fig. 125.1

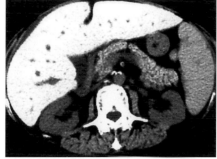
Fig. 125.2

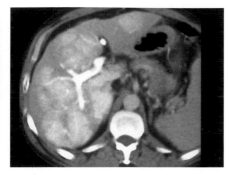
Fig. 125.3

Abdominal Pathology: Biliary Tract

Biliary Tract

After surgical choledochoenteric anastomosis, sphincterotomy, or endoscopic retrograde cholangiopancreatography (ERCP), hypodense gas (➡) is usually present within the intrahepatic bile ducts (Fig. 125.4). These causes of biliary gas must be differentiated from gas-forming anaerobic bacteria within an abscess.

Dilatation of the intrahepatic biliary tract (**128**) is called cholestasis (Fig. 125.5). It may result from gallstones, a malignant obstruction of the biliary tract, or from a pancreatic carcinoma at Vater's ampulla. In Figure 125.5, note the calcification (**174**) of the tortuous splenic artery (**99**) and the hepatic metastases (**7**). These poorly defined and only slightly hypodense metastases must be differentiated from artifacts (**3**) arising from the ribs adjacent to the liver (**122**) and spleen (**133**). These beam-hardening artifacts result from the abrupt changes in attenuation between the viscera and the rib (**51**).

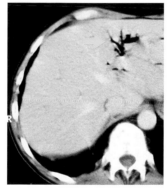
Fig. 125.4

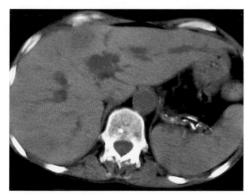
Fig. 125.5a

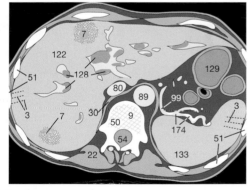
Fig. 125.5b

If it is not possible to treat the cause of cholestasis surgically, inserting a stent (**182** in Fig. 125.6) may decompress an obstructed biliary duct (**128**).

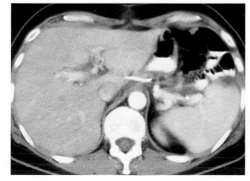
Fig. 125.6a

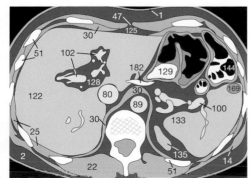
Fig. 125.6b

The size and shape of the gallbladder vary depending on when the patient last ate food. A hydrops of the gallbladder should only be diagnosed if there is very marked dilatation, that is if the diameter exceeds 5 cm in several transverse planes. The attenuation of bile is usually just greater than that of water (0 HU) but may increase to up to 25 HU if the bile is highly concentrated [4].

Cholecystolithiasis

Stones (**167**) within the gallbladder (**126**) may show different patterns of calcification (Fig. 126.1). Cup-shaped and ring-like calcifications can be seen in stones containing cholesterol and bilirubin (Fig. 126.2). If stones obstruct gallbladder drainage or inflammation has caused stenosis, sludge may form resulting in increased attenuation and sedimentation of bile (Fig. 126.3). Common duct stones should be diagnosed using thin-section CT because smaller stones might be missed in standard thickness sections.

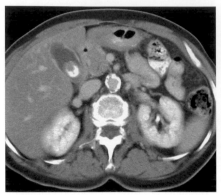

Fig. 126.1a

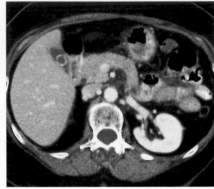

Fig. 126.2a

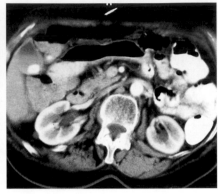

Fig. 126.3a

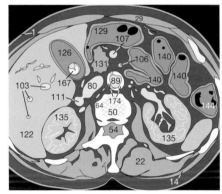

Fig. 126.1b

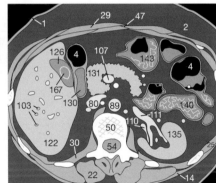

Fig. 126.2b

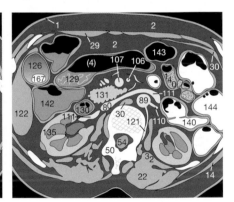

Fig. 126.3b

Chronic Inflammatory Lesions

Cholecystolithiasis can lead to chronic inflammation, resulting in a stone-filled, shrunken gallbladder, acute cholecystitis, or an empyema of the gallbladder (recognized by an irregularly thickened wall) (↖ ↗ in Fig. 126.4). There is an increased risk of malignant change with chronic inflammatory processes [24]. The development of a porcelain gallbladder (Fig. 126.5) with an egg-shell-like pattern of calcification (**174**) may be a premalignant lesion.

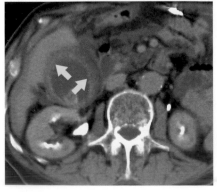

Fig. 126.4

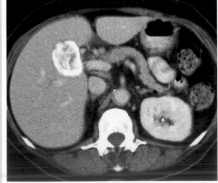

Fig. 126.5a

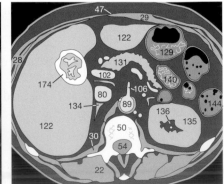

Fig. 126.6b

Contrast Enhancement

Before reading further, try to define a characteristic feature of the spleen by looking at Figure 127.1a. The normal splenic parenchyma (**133**) has an attenuation of approximately 45 HU on unenhanced images. The attenuation of the spleen will only appear homogeneous in an unenhanced image or in the late venous phase of an enhanced study (Fig. 127.1c). In the early arterial phase (Fig. 127.1a), it will enhance heterogeneously and appear patchy or marbled, a pattern representing its trabecular architecture. This pattern should not be misinterpreted as an abnormality. Note also the uneven distribution of CM within the inferior vena cava (**80**) and the three (!) hepatic metastases (**7**) in the same image (Fig. 127.1a). Did you spot the areas of near-water attenuation representing perisplenic/perihepatic ascites (**8**)?

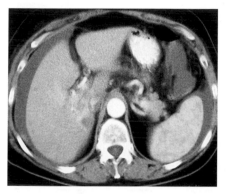
Fig. 127.1a

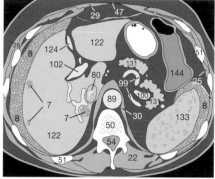
Fig. 127.1b

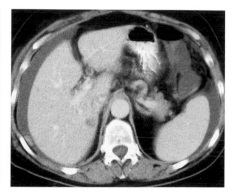
Fig. 127.1c

The splenic artery (**99**) is typically elongated and tortuous so that it may be imaged in several consecutive slices. In elderly patients, it is common to see atherosclerotic plaques (**174** in Fig. 127.2). Occasionally, a homogeneous splenunculus [accessory spleen ➚], well demonstrated in the surrounding fat, may be seen at the hilum or the inferior pole of the spleen (Fig. 127.3). Differentiating between a splenunculus and an abnormally enlarged LN may be difficult.

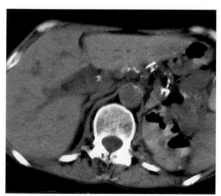
Fig. 127.2a

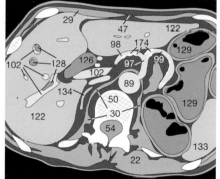
Fig. 127.2b

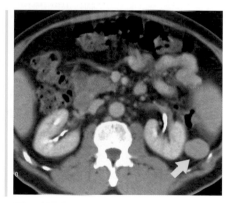
Fig. 127.3

Splenomegaly

Diffuse enlargement of the spleen (Fig. 128.1) may be caused by several conditions: portal hypertension, leukemia/lymphoma, myelofibrosis and hemolytic anemia, or by various storage diseases. Assessment of splenic size is made difficult by individual variations in shape. Marked splenomegaly is easily recognized, but in borderline cases of splenomegaly and for follow-up one should know the normal range of splenic size. In the transverse plane, the length of the spleen (l) should measure no more than 10 cm (dotted line) and its width (d, at right angle to the dotted line) should not exceed 5 cm (Fig. 127.4).

In ultrasound, the spleen is not measured in a transverse plane but in an oblique plane parallel to the intercostal space. In this plane, the upper limit of normal is 11 cm for the long axis [28].

The craniocaudal dimension of the spleen should not exceed 15 cm, so that at a slice thickness of 1 cm it should not be visible on more than 15 sections. Splenomegaly is diagnosed if at least two of these three parameters are exceeded.

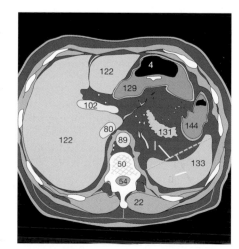
Fig. 127.4

As splenomegaly develops, the typical normal crescentic shape is lost (Fig. 128.1). Gross spleno-megaly, which may be caused by chronic lympho-cytic leukemia, acts as a space-occupying mass and displaces adjacent organs. In Figure 128.1, the left kidney is compressed (↓). If the blood supply cannot keep pace with splenic growth, infarctions (↙) may result. These appear as hypodense areas that do not enhance with CM (Fig. 128.2).

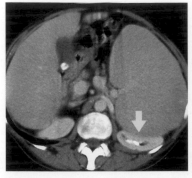 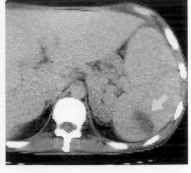

Fig. 128.1   Fig. 128.2

Focal Splenic Lesions

Splenic cysts share the same characteristics of hepatic cysts (cf. p.121). Metastases in the spleen (**7**) are rare and difficult to distinguish from cysts. In the case illustrated in Figure 128.3, the diagnosis of splenic metastases was relatively easy because there were hepatic lesions and malignant ascites (**8**). If there are multifocal lesions with inhomogeneous CM enhancement, a diagnosis of focal splenic lymphoma or splenic candidiasis should be considered.

Ascites (**8**) may accompany candidiasis, as shown in Figure 128.4. Splenic lymphoma is usually characterized by diffuse infiltration and the spleen may appear normal.

The examination of the spleen (**133**) after a blunt thoracic or abdominal trauma must be meticulous. Lacerations of the parenchyma (**181**) may lead to hematomas (**8**) beneath the capsule, and delayed rupture of the capsule may cause massive hemorrhage into the abdominal cavity (Fig. 128.5).

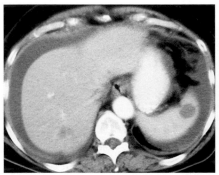 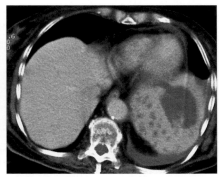 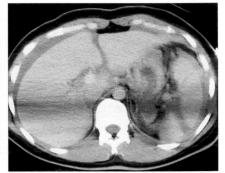

Fig. 128.3a   Fig. 128.4a   Fig. 128.5a

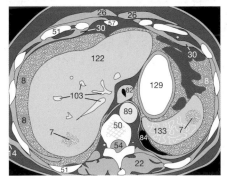 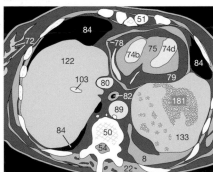 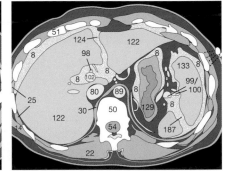

Fig. 128.3b   Fig. 128.4b   Fig. 128.5b

The remnants of smaller hematomas may present as subcapsular (↗) or paren-chymal (↑) calcifications (Fig. 128.6).

Septations within splenic cystic lesions (Fig. 128.7) are strongly suggestive of echinococcosis, and appear quite similar to those in the liver. In most cases the liver is also affected (cf. p.122).

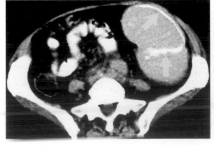 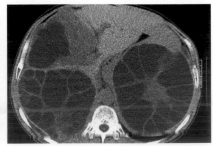

Fig. 128.6   Fig. 128.7

Acute and Chronic Pancreatitis

Acute pancreatitis may present as edematous interstitial pancreatitis (Fig. 129.1). Hypodense peripancreatic fluid (exudate) (**8**) and edema of the connective tissue (**185**) are frequent findings. CT shows blurring of the pancreatic contours; the normally lobular pattern of the pancreas is effaced (Figs. 129.1 and 129.2). In hemorrhagic necrotizing pancreatitis (Fig. 129.2), the extent of necrosis is a prognostic feature.

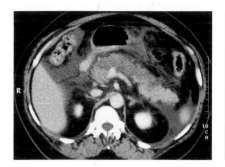

Fig. 129.1

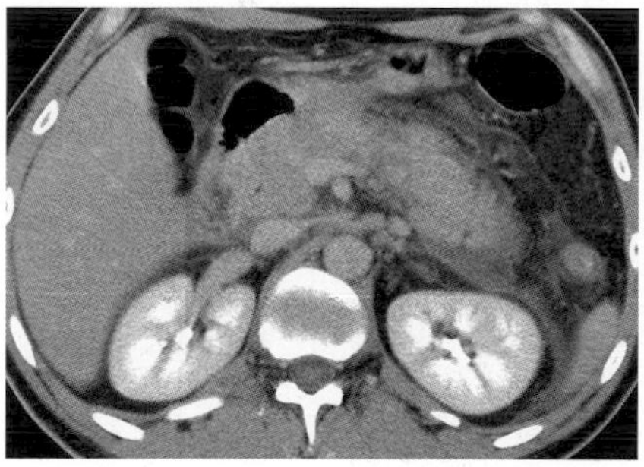

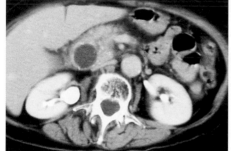

Fig. 129.2a

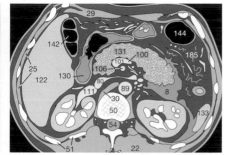

Fig. 129.2b

Chronic pancreatitis progresses either slowly and progressively or in recurrent episodes. The two most common causes of chronic pancreatitis are alcohol abuse and cholelithiasis.

Typical findings in chronic pancreatitis are fibrosis and multifocal calcifications (**174**), irregular dilatation of the pancreatic duct (**132**), and sometimes the formation of pseudocysts (**169**) within, or next to, the pancreas (**131**) (Figs. 129.3 and 129.4). The disease may lead to pancreatic atrophy as a late feature.

The possibility that pancreatic carcinoma develops in association with chronic calcific pancreatitis is presently being discussed.

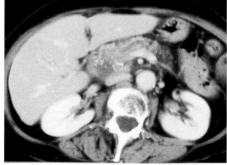

Fig. 129.3a

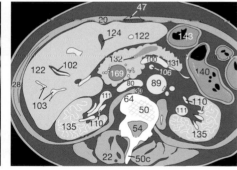

Fig. 129.3b

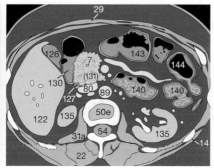

Fig. 129.4a

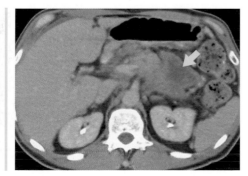

Fig. 129.4b

Pancreatic Neoplasms

Most pancreatic carcinomas (**7**) are located within the head of the pancreas (**131**). As a result, even small tumors may cause cholestasis by obstructing the common bile duct (**127**) (Fig. 129.5). Pancreatic carcinomas tend to metastasize very early to the liver and the regional LNs. In case of doubt, ERCP should be carried out to image the pancreatic and common bile ducts. Islet cell tumors, 75% of which are functional, are located within the body of the pancreas. The Zollinger-Ellison syndrome (Fig. 129.6) is caused by a gastrin-secreting tumor (✎). Other neoplasms associated with the pancreas are insulinomas, glucagonomas, and serotonin-producing masses.

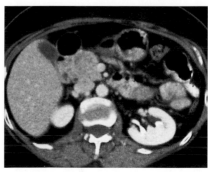

Fig. 129.5a

Fig. 129.5b

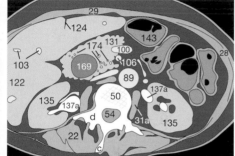

Fig. 129.6

The normal position and shape of the adrenal glands has been described on pages 104 to 105. The maximum lengths of the adrenal glands range between 2.1 and 2.7 cm, the right adrenal often being somewhat longer than the left. The thickness of the limbs should not exceed 5 to 8 mm in the transverse plane. A fusiform or nodular thickening (**7**) is likely to be abnormal in CT, and is usually indicative of hyperplasia or an adenoma of the adrenal gland (**134** in Fig. 130.1). Typically, the adrenals can be clearly differentiated from adjacent fat, the diaphragm (**30**), the kidney (**135**), the liver (**122**), and the inferior vena cava (**80**).

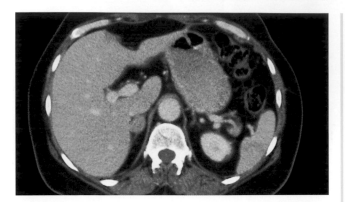

Fig. 130.1a

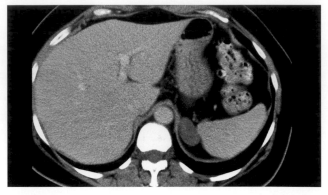

Fig. 130.2a

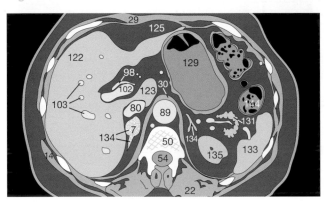

Fig. 130.1b

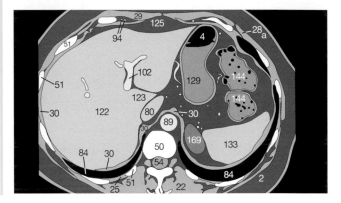

Fig. 130.2b

The following conditions may be dignosed according to the specific hormonal excess: congenital adrenal cortical hyperplasia (androgens), Conn's syndrome (aldosterone), and Cushing's syndrome (cortisone). An upper pole renal cyst (Fig. 130.2) or a renal angiomyolipoma (cf. Fig. 134.4) must be included in the DD. Attenuation values for benign cysts (**169**) should lie close to those for water (= −1 HU in the present case) (Fig. 130.2). (Compare with cysts on p. 133.)

In cases of heterogeneous enlargement of the adrenal gland or infiltration of adjacent organs, a metastasis or a carcinoma (Fig. 130.3) must be suspected. Since bronchogenic carcinomas often metastasize to the liver and the adrenals, staging chest CT studies for lung cancer should be extended to include the caudal margin of the liver and the adrenals. Tumors of the paravertebral sympathetic trunks, which are located close to the adrenal glands, may also be detected, but they are rare. The MRI images in Figures 130.4a and 130.4b show a neuroblastoma (→) in the sagittal (a) and coronal (b) planes.

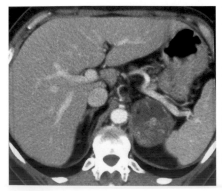

Fig. 130.3

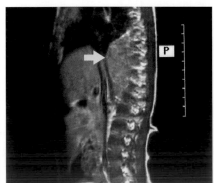

Fig. 130.4a

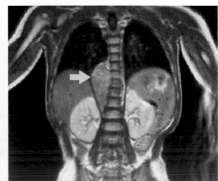

Fig. 130.4b

Whenever doubt exists whether an enlarged adrenal gland represents a benign process, densitometry (see pages 122 and 133) with determination of the enhancement pattern should be considered: benign adenomas of the adrenal gland show a tendency of a considerably more rapid wash-out of the contrast enhancement than malignant lesions, such as metastases and adrenal gland carcinomas (Fig. 131.1). This method requires an additional scan at the level of the adrenal glands after 3, 10, or 30 minutes.

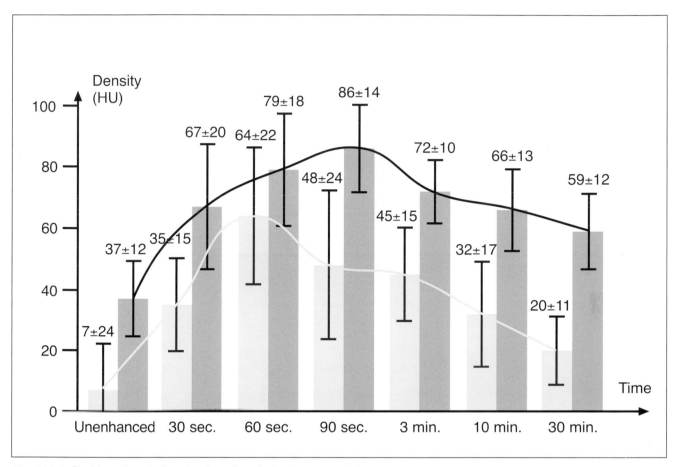

Fig. 131.1 Rapid wash-out of contrast medium in benign adrenal glands adenomas (blue) in comparison with non-adenomas (gray)

Malignant tumors of the adrenal gland tend to have a prolonged contrast enhancement. This difference can be applied to the differential diagnosis. The dynamic enhancement pattern in the adrenal glands has been extensively investigated in numerous studies, which revealed further differences in absolute and relative wash-out of the peak contrast enhancement. This wash-out pattern, however, shows a certain overlap between the tumor types, and therefore the assessment has been proven useful only when applying the following parameters [42]:

Densitometry in the DD of space-occupying lesions of the adrenal glands

Unenhanced:	< 11 HE	=>	Adenoma
10 min. after injection of contrast medium:	< 45 HE	=>	Adenoma
30 min. after injection of contrast medium:	< 35 HE	=>	Adenoma

For these three values, the range of the histograms or so-called box-whisker plots of Fig. 131.1 does not overlap for both tumor types, and a benign tumor of the adrenal glands can be safely assumed if the measured density values fall below these values. In all other cases, a benign adenoma cannot be assumed with acceptable degree of sensitivity and specificity and further evaluation is recommended.

Congenital Variations

The attenuation of the renal parenchyma (**135**) on unenhanced images is approximately 30 HU. The kidneys occasionally develop to different sizes. If the outlines are smooth and the parenchymal thickness is not irregular, it is likely to represent unilateral renal hypoplasia (Fig. 132.1). The smaller kidney need not be abnormal.

A kidney may have an atypical orientation as in Figure 132.2. However, if a kidney lies in the iliac fossa (Fig. 132.3), this does not indicate an ectopic location, but a renal transplant (**135**). The organ is connected to the iliac vessels (**113/116**) and the urinary bladder (**138**).

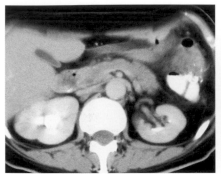

Fig. 132.1a

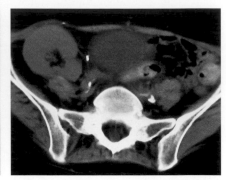

Fig. 132.2a

Fig. 132.3a

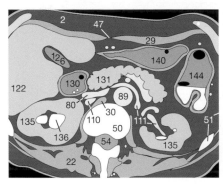

Fig. 132.1b

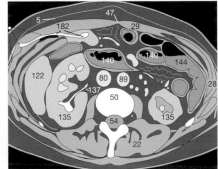

Fig. 132.2b

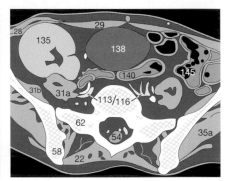

Fig. 132.3b

Marked differences in size, as in Figure 132.2, may indicate partial or complete renal duplication on one side. The positions and number of renal arteries may vary considerably (**110** in Fig. 132.1b). The renal arteries must be examined carefully for evidence of stenosis as a cause of renal hypertension. The ureter (**137** ➡) can be present as a partial or complete duplex ureter (Fig. 132.4). In complete renal duplication, the renal pelvis is also duplicated.

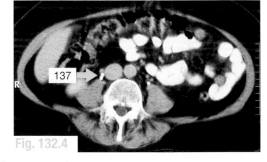

Fig. 132.4

Occasionally, the low-density fat in the hilum (✳ in Fig. 132.5b) is only poorly demarcated from the renal parenchyma (**135**) owing to a beam-hardening artifact or partial volume averaging (Fig. 132.5a). This gives the incorrect impression of a renal tumor. Comparison with an immediately adjacent section (Fig. 132.5c) demonstrates that only hilar fat was present. The actual tumor in this particular example (**7**) is situated at the posterior margin of the right lobe of the liver (**122**).

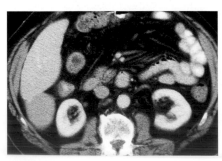

Fig. 132.5a

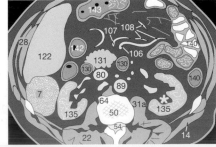

Fig. 132.5b

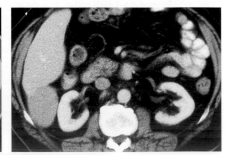

Fig. 132.5c

Cysts

Renal cysts are frequent incidental findings in adults and may be located anywhere in the parenchyma. They may be exophytic or parapelvic, in which case they can resemble a hydronephrosis. Benign cysts contain a serous, usually clear liquid with an attenuation of between −5 and +15 HU. They do not enhance with CM because they are avascular. The attenuation measurement may be inaccurate if there are partial volume averaging artifacts due to slice thickness (Fig. 133.1: ~ 25 HU) or to eccentric positioning of the ROI (Fig. 133.2: ~ 22 HU) (cf. pp. 15 and 121). Only the correct positioning of the ROI in the center of the cyst (⑯ in Fig. 133.3) will provide an accurate average of 10 HU. In rare cases, hemorrhage into benign cysts will result in hyperdense values on unenhanced images. The attenuation values will not change on post-contrast images.

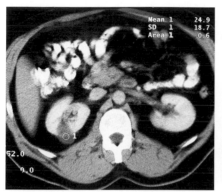
Fig. 133.1

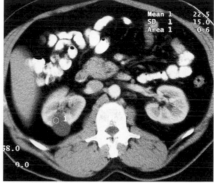
Fig. 133.2

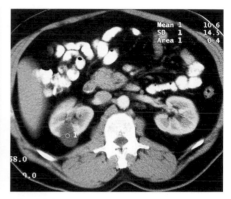
Fig. 133.3

Increased density or calcifications in a mass may indicate past renal tuberculosis, current Echinococcus infestation (hydatid disease), or a cystic renal cell carcinoma. The difference between pre- and post-contrast images also provides information on renal function: after approximately 30 seconds the well-perfused renal cortex is the first part of the kidney to accumulate the CM (cf. Figs. 133.2 and 133.3). After another 30 to 60 seconds the CM is excreted into the more distal tubules leading to enhancement of the medulla. The result is homogeneous enhancement of the renal parenchyma (cf. Fig. 133.1).

The appearances of multiple renal cysts in children with congenital autosomal recessive polycystic kidney disease are dramatically different from those of the occasional cysts found in adults, which are generally incidental findings. Polycystic kidney disease in the adult (**169** in Fig. 133.4) is autosomal dominant and associated with multiple cysts of the liver, the bile ducts and, more rarely, with cysts in the pancreas or with abdominal or cerebral aneurysms.

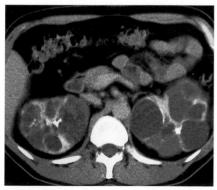
Fig. 133.4a

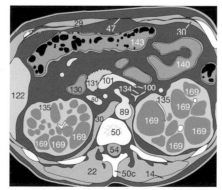
Fig. 133.4b

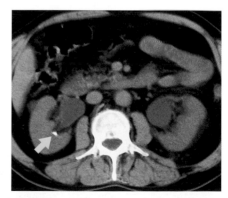
Fig. 133.5

Hydronephrosis

Parapelvic cysts may be confused with grade 1 hydronephrosis (Fig. 133.5), which is characterized in the unenhanced image by a dilated renal pelvis and ureter. In grade 2 hydronephrosis, the renal calyces become poorly defined. When parenchymal atrophy ensues, the hydronephrosis is categorized as grade 3 (see p. 134).

Since no CM had been given to the patient in Figure 133.5, the hyperdense lesion (↗) in the right kidney must be a renal calculus. For the diagnosis of nephrolithiasis alone, CT should be avoided because of undue radiation exposure (ref. p. 174ff.). Sonography is the method of choice for nephrolithiasis as well as hydronephrosis.

Hydronephrosis, which causes dilatation of the ureter (**137**) and the renal pelvis (**136**), impairs renal function (Fig. 134.1). In this image, the left renal parenchyma (**135**) shows delayed and reduced CM enhancement as compared with the normal right kidney.

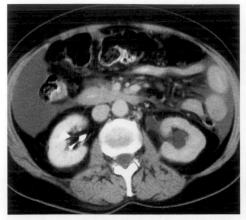

Fig. 134.1a

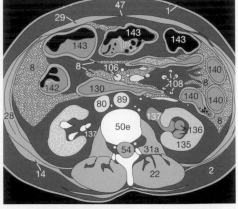

Fig. 134.1b

Chronic grade 3 hydronephrosis reduces the parenchyma to a narrow rim of tissue (Fig. 134.2), resulting finally in atrophy and a non-functioning kidney. In cases of doubt, identifying the dilated ureter (↘ in Fig. 134.2b) can resolve the DD between a parapelvic cyst and hydronephrosis. CM accumulates in a dilated renal pelvis, but not in a cyst.

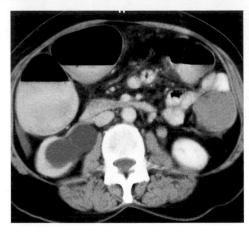

Fig. 134.2a

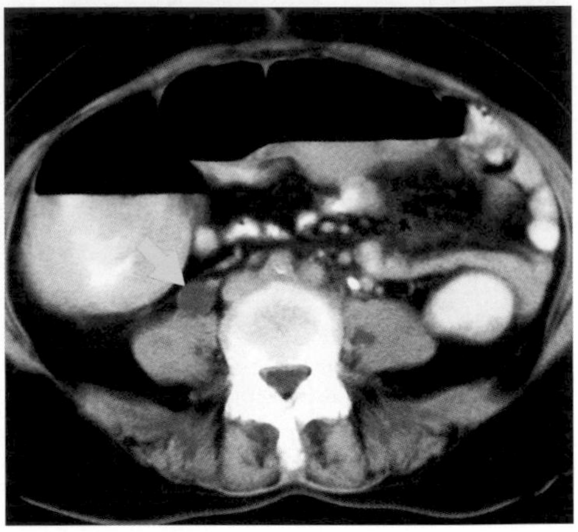

Fig. 134.2b

Solid Tumors

Enhancement with CM often helps to distinguish between partial volume averaging of benign renal cysts and hypodense renal tumors, since CT morphology alone does not provide sufficient information about the etiology of a lesion. This is especially so when a mass (✳) is poorly defined within the parenchyma (Fig. 134.3). Inhomogeneous enhancement, infiltration of adjacent structures, and invasion of the pelvis or the renal vein are criteria of malignancy.

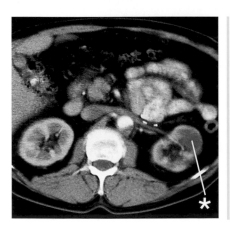

Fig. 134.3

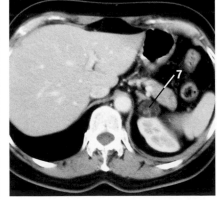

Fig. 134.4

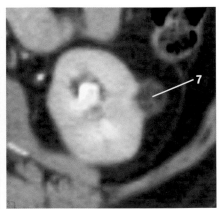

Fig. 134.5

However, when a mass consists not only of solid, inhomogeneous areas, but also contains fat, an angiomyolipoma (**7**) must be considered (Figs. 134.4 and 134.5). These benign hamartomas contain fat, atypical muscle fibers, and blood vessels. The vessel walls are abnormal, and the complication of intratumoral or retroperitoneal hemorrhage may occur (not depicted here).

Kidney Problems Related to Blood Vessels

If ultrasound shows fresh hemorrhage into the abdomen after penetration or blunt trauma, the source of bleeding must be located as soon as possible. The DD must include not only splenic rupture or major vessel disruption but also renal injury. On unenhanced images of a renal rupture (Figs. 135.1a and 135.1b), the contours of the kidney (**135**) appear blurred,

and depending on the extent of hemorrhage, hyperdense fresh hematoma (**8**) can be detected in the retroperitoneal spaces. In this case, enhanced images (Figs. 135.1c and 135.1b) show that the renal parenchyma (**135**) is still well perfused and function is maintained.

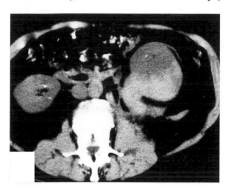

Fig. 135.1a

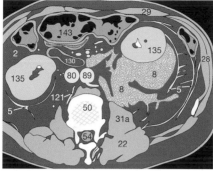

Fig. 135.1b

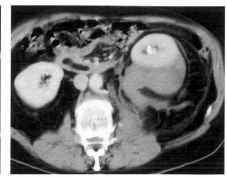

Fig. 135.1c

After extracorporeal shock-wave lithotripsy (ESWL), renal injuries may rarely occur that lead to small hematomas or extravasation of urine from the ureter. If there is hematuria or persisting pain after ESWL, it is essential to obtain delayed

images. Urine leaking into the retroperitoneal spaces (→ in Figs. 135.2a through 135.2c) would not be opacified in images obtained before the kidney has excreted CM.

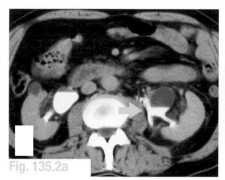

Fig. 135.2a

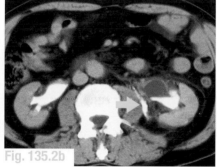

Fig. 135.2b

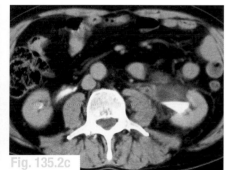

Fig. 135.2c

Renal infarctions (**180**) usually have a triangular shape on CT images corresponding to the vascular architecture of the kidney (Fig. 135.3). The broad base abuts the capsule and the triangle gradually tapers toward the pelvis (**136**). A typical feature is the lack of enhancement after i.v. CM in the early perfusion phase and in the late excretion phase. Embolisms usually originate in the left heart, or in the aorta in cases of atherosclerosis (**174** in Fig. 135.3) or aneurysms (cf. p. 142).

If there is a low attenuation filling defect (**173**) in the lumen of the renal vein (**111**) after a CM injection, the presence of bland thrombus (Fig. 135.4) or tumor thrombus from a renal carcinoma extending into the inferior vena cava (**80**) must be considered.

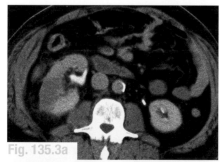

Fig. 135.3a

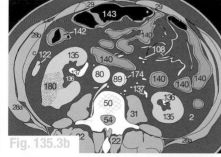

Fig. 135.3b

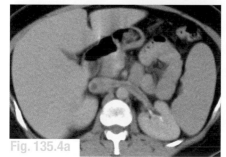

Fig. 135.4a

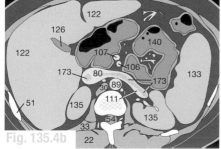

Fig. 135.4b

Catheters

The walls of the urinary bladder are best examined if the bladder is distended. If a urinary catheter (**182**) is in place at the time of CT (Fig. 136.1), sterile water can be instilled as a low-density CM. Focal or diffuse wall thickening of a trabeculated bladder, associated with prostatic hyperplasia, will be demonstrated clearly. If a ureter (**137**) has been stented (**182**) for strictures or retroperitoneal tumors, the distal end of the JJ stent may be visible in the bladder lumen (**138**) (bilateral JJ stents in Fig. 136.2).

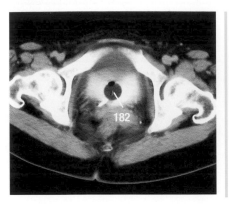

Fig. 136.1

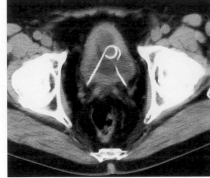

Fig. 136.2a

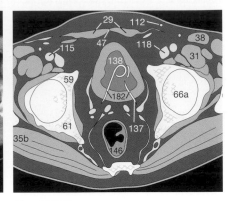

Fig. 136.2b

Diverticula

Diverticula situated at the periphery of the bladder can easily be distinguished from ovarian cysts by using CM (Fig. 136.3). The "jet phenomenon" is often seen in the posterior basal recess of the bladder and is caused by peristalsis in the ureters. They inject spurts of CM-opacified urine into the bladder, which is filled with hypodense urine (Fig. 136.4).

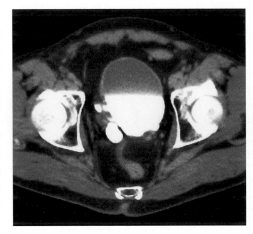

Fig. 136.3

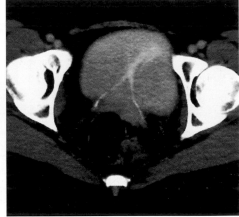

Fig. 136.4

Solid Tumors

Bladder wall tumors (**7**), which become visible after intravenous or intravesical CM, have characteristic, irregular margins that do not enhance with CM (Fig. 136.5). Tumors must not be confused with intravesicular blood clots that may occur following transurethral resection of the prostate. It is important to determine the precise size of the tumor and to what extent adjacent organs (e.g., cervix, uterus, or rectum) have been infiltrated (◀ in Fig. 136.6).

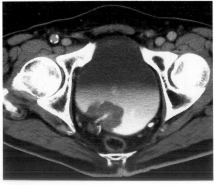

Fig. 136.5a

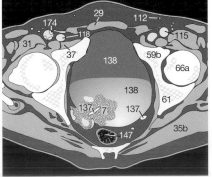

Fig. 136.5b

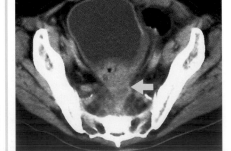

Fig. 136.6

If the bladder has been resected because of carcinoma, a urinary reservoir (∗) can be constructed using a loop of small bowel (ileum conduit) which has been isolated from the GIT. Urine is excreted from the reservoir into a urostomy bag (⬅ in Fig. 137.1b). In Figure 137.2 a colostomy (⬇) is also seen (cf. p. 140).

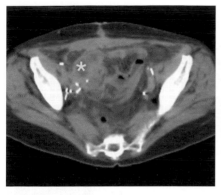

Fig. 137.1a

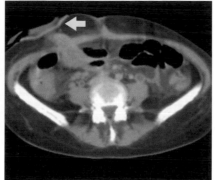

Fig. 137.1b

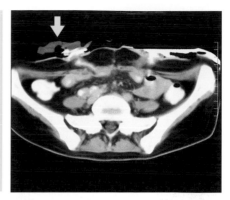

Fig. 137.2

Abdominal Pathology: Reproductive Organs

Uterus

Foreign bodies in the uterine cavity (158), e.g. an intrauterine contraceptive device (166), are not always as clearly visible in a transverse image as in Figure 137.3. Calcifications (174) are a characteristic feature of benign uterine myomas. Nevertheless it can be difficult to distinguish multiple myomas from a carcinoma of the uterus (7 in Fig. 137.4). If the adjacent walls of the bladder (138) or the rectum (146) are infiltrated, the tumor is most likely to be malignant (Fig. 137.5). Central necrosis (181) occurs in both kinds of tumors and is usually indicative of a rapidly growing, malignant tumor (Fig. 137.4).

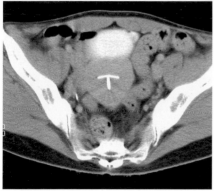

Fig. 137.3a

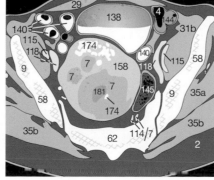

Fig. 137.4a

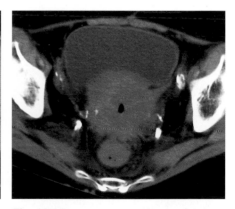

Fig. 137.5a

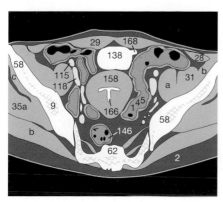

Fig. 137.3b

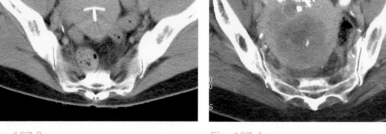

Fig. 137.4b

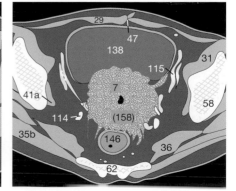

Fig. 137.5b

Ovaries

The most common ovarian lesions are thin-walled follicular cysts (**169**) that contain a clear fluid with a density equivalent to that of water, which is below 15 HU (Fig. 138.1). Density measurements, however, are unreliable in small cysts (cf. p. 133). These cannot be clearly differentiated from mucinous cysts or hemorrhagic cysts. This latter type of cyst may be caused by endometriosis. Sometimes cysts reach considerable sizes (Fig. 138.2) with consequent mass effect.

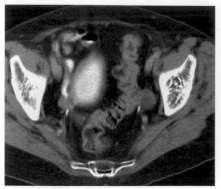

Fig. 138.1a

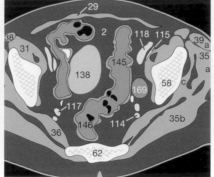

Fig. 138.1b

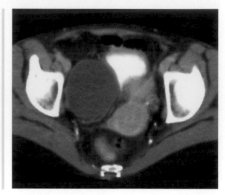

Fig. 138.2

The malignant nature of solid ovarian tumors can be suspected if there are the following general criteria used for other tumors:

1) ill-defined margins;
2) infiltration of adjacent structures;
3) enlarged regional LNs; and
4) inhomogeneous enhancement with CM.

Peritoneal carcinomatosis (Fig. 138.3) frequently occurs in advanced ovarian carcinoma, and is characterized by the appearance of multiple fine nodules and edema (**185**) in the greater omentum, the root of the mesenteric, and the abdominal wall, and by ascites (**8**).

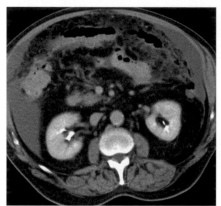

Fig. 138.3a

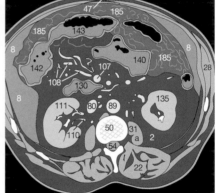

Fig. 138.3b

Prostate, Vas Deferens

High-density calcification representing postinflammatory residue is often encountered following prostatitis (Fig. 138.4). Calcifications are also occasionally seen in the vas deferens (Fig. 138.5). Carcinoma of the prostate is only detectable in advanced stages (Fig. 138.6) when the bladder wall or the adjacent ischiorectal fossa fat is infiltrated. If a prostate carcinoma is suspected, all images should be carefully viewed on bone windows for sclerotic metastases (see p. 145).

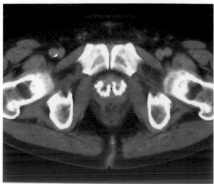

Fig. 138.4

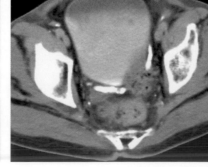

Fig. 138.5

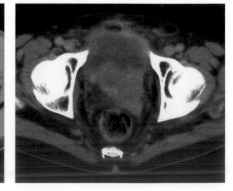

Fig. 138.6

Stomach

Despite the advantages of using water as a hypodense CM for imaging the stomach after intravenous Buscopan [15, 16], small tumors may escape detection during conventional CTs. Endoscopy and endosonography should be employed to complement CT. Marked focal wall thickening, which occurs in carcinoma of the stomach, is usually easily recognized (← in Fig. 139.1). In cases of diffuse wall thickening (Fig. 139.2), the DD should also include lymphoma, leiomyoma, or leiomyosarkoma of the stomach. It is vital to look for bubbles of intraperitoneal gas (← in Fig. 139.3), which is evidence of a small perforation possibly occuring with ulcers or advanced ulcerating carcinomas.

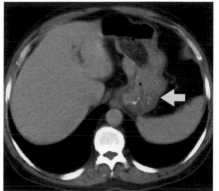

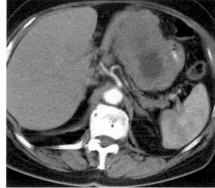

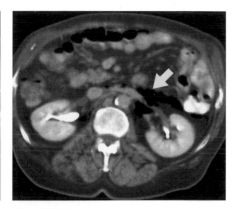

Fig. 139.1   Fig. 139.2   Fig. 139.3

Inflammation of the Intestines

The entire small and large bowel must be examined for wall thickening or infiltration of the surrounding fat as per the checklist on page 102. Both ulcerative colitis (Fig. 139.4) and Crohn's disease (Fig. 139.5) are characterized by thickening of the affected bowel wall (↑) so that several layers of the wall may become visible. Disseminated intravascular coagulopathy (DIC) or over-anticoagulation with warfarin may cause diffuse hemorrhage (8) in the bowel wall (140) and also lead to mural thickening (Fig. 139.6). The DD should include ischemia if the abnormality is limited to segments in the territory of the mesenteric vessels, e.g., in the walls of the colon (152), as a result of advanced atherosclerosis (174), or an embolus (Fig. 139.7). You should therefore check that the mesenteric vessels (108) and the walls of the intestine enhance homogeneously after i.v. CM.

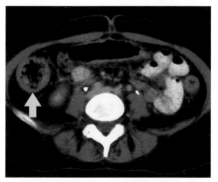

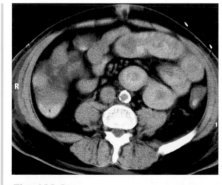

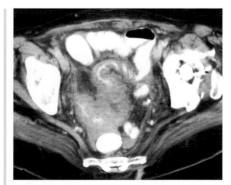

Fig. 139.4   Fig. 139.6a   Fig. 139.7a

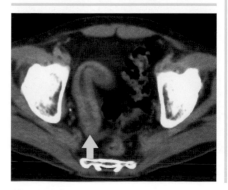

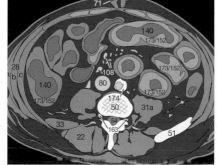

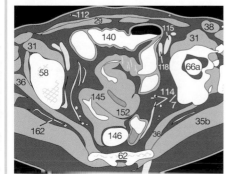

Fig. 139.5   Fig. 139.6b   Fig. 139.7b

Colon

Elderly patients frequently have diverticular disease (**168**) of the descending colon (**144**) and sigmoid colon (**145** in Fig. 140.1). The condition is more significant if acute diverticulitis

has developed (Fig. 140.2), which is characterized by ill-defined colonic walls and edematous infiltration of the surrounding mesenteric fat (⬊ in Fig. 140.2).

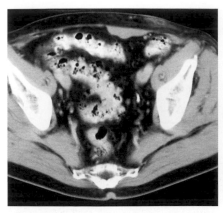

Fig. 140.1a

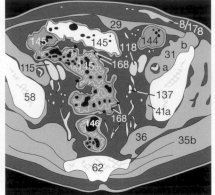

Fig. 140.1b

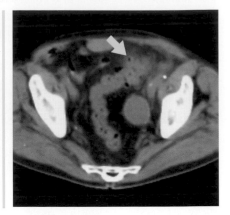

Fig. 140.2

Malignant thickening of the colonic wall (**152** in Fig. 140.3) is not always easily distinguished from that found in colitis (cf. p. 139): in both conditions there is stranding of the pericolic fat. The liver should always be checked for metastases if the cause of the colonic abnormality is uncertain.

A temporary colostomy (**170** in Fig. 140.4) may be necessary if a left hemicolectomy or sigmoid colectomy was performed

because of perforated diverticulitis or carcinoma. The colostomy is permanent if the rectum was excised. A potential complication of a colostomy can be seen in Figure 140.5: there is an abscess in the abdominal wall (**181**). A carcinoid lesion of the small bowel (⬈ in Fig. 140.6) may simulate a carcinoma of the colon.

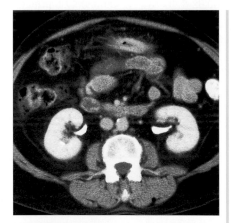

Fig. 140.3a

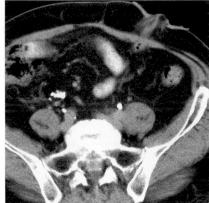

Fig. 140.4a

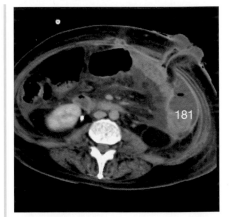

Fig. 140.5

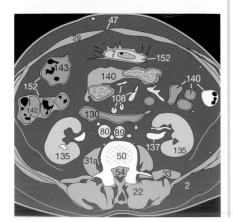

Fig. 140.3b

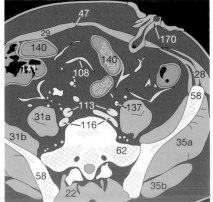

Fig. 140.4b

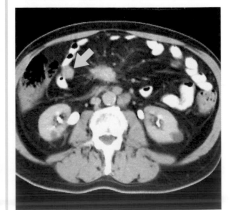

Fig. 140.6

Ileus

Horizontal air-fluid levels (↓ ↓) and atonic, dilated bowel loops (**140**) are typical features of ileus. If dilatation is recognized in the topogram (Fig. 141.1), or in an overview of the abdomen, an ileus must be suspected. If only the small intestine (Fig. 141.2) is involved, the most likely cause is a mechanical obstruction due to adhesions. A gallstone may cause obstruction of the small bowel (gallstone ileus). This follows cholecystitis with the formation of a cholecystoenteral fistula and the passage of a gallstone into the bowel. The gallstone may obstruct the narrower caliber of the distal ileum (**167** in Fig. 141.3).

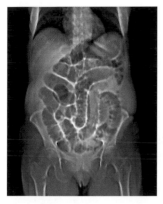

Fig. 141.1

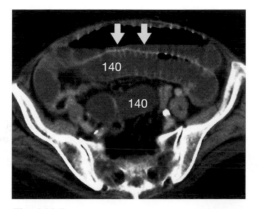

Fig. 141.2

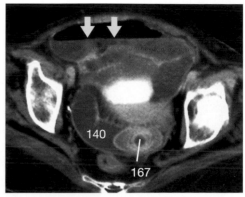

Fig. 141.3

Mechanical obstruction of the colon leads to similar air-fluid levels and dilatation (↓ ↓ in Fig. 141.4). When looking for the cause of an ileus, the entire colon must be examined for obstructing or constricting tumors or focal inflammation.

Test Yourself!   Exercise **29:**

Are there any suspicious findings other than the colic ileus in Figure 141.4? Does the image remind you of others in the manual? Make the most of the figures by returning to previous chapters, covering the text, and identifying as many structures as possible. You will improve your learning efficiency by reviewing the images and diagrams and using the legends to make sure you got it right.

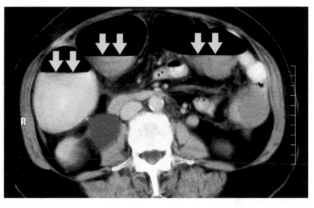

Fig. 141.4

Notes

Aneurysms

Ectasia or aneurysms of the abdominal aorta (**89**) are usually the result of atherosclerotic disease (**174**) which leads to mural thrombosis (**173** in Fig. 142.1). An aneurysm of the abdominal aorta is present if the diameter of the patent lumen has reached 3 cm or the outer diameter of the vessel measures more than 4 cm (Fig. 142.2). Surgical intervention in asymptomatic patients is usually considered when the dilatation has reached a diameter of 5 cm. The general condition of the patient and the rate at which dilatation is progressing must be considered. If the patent lumen is central and is surrounded by mural thrombosis (**173** in Fig. 142.2), the risk of rupture and consequent hemorrhage is reduced.

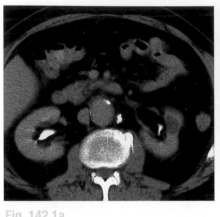

Fig. 142.1a

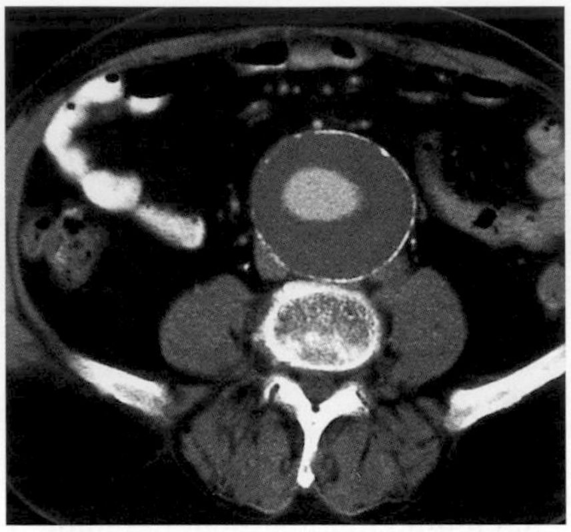

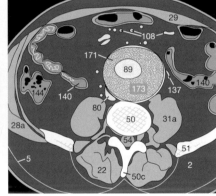

Fig. 142.2a

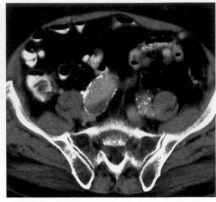

Fig. 142.3a

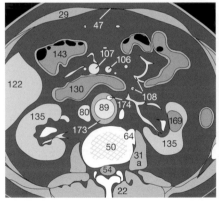

Fig. 142.1b

Fig. 142.2b

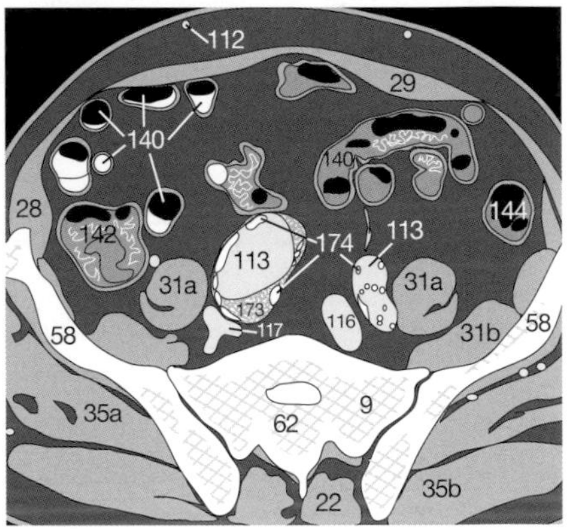

Fig. 142.3b

The risk of rupture is greater if the patent lumen is eccentric (↘ in Fig. 142.4) or if the cross-sectional shape of the vessel is very irregular. Dilatation in excess of 6 cm diameter also has a high risk of rupture. Surgical planning requires the determination of whether, and to what degree, the renal, mesenteric (**97**), and iliac (**113**) arteries are involved by the aneurysm (Fig. 142.3). Sudden pain may accompany rupture or dissection, which can extend from the thoracic to the abdominal aorta (cf. p. 93). Dynamic CM-enhanced CT will show the dissection flap (**172** in Fig. 142.5).

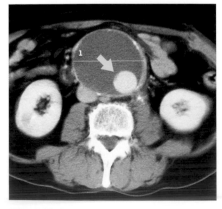

Fig. 142.4

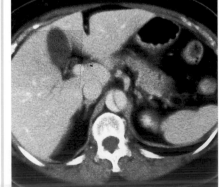

Fig. 142.5a

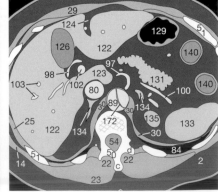

Fig. 142.5b

Venous Thromboses

In cases of thrombosis in a vein of the lower extremity (→), venography does not always clearly show whether or not the thrombus extends into pelvic veins (Figs. 143.1a and 143.1b). The CM, which is injected into a superficial vein of the foot, is often diluted to such a degree that it becomes difficult to assess the lumen of the femoral/iliac veins (↘ in Fig. 143.1c). In such cases, it is necessary to perform a CT with i.v. CM.

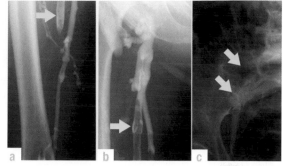

Fig. 143.1

The lumen of a vein containing a fresh thrombus (↘) is generally at least twice as large as normal (Fig. 143.2a). The segment containing the thrombus is either uniformly hypodense compared with the accompanying artery, or it shows a hypodense filling defect, representing the thrombus itself. In the case illustrated on the right, the thrombus extended through the left common iliac vein (↗) to the caudal segment of the inferior vena cava (Fig. 143.2b), where it can be seen as a hypodense area (↑) surrounded by contrast-enhanced, flowing blood (Fig. 143.2c). CT slices must be continued cranially until the inferior vena cava no longer shows any signs of thrombus (↓ in Fig. 143.2d).

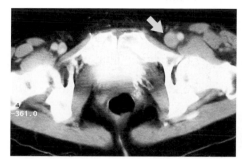

Fig. 143.2a

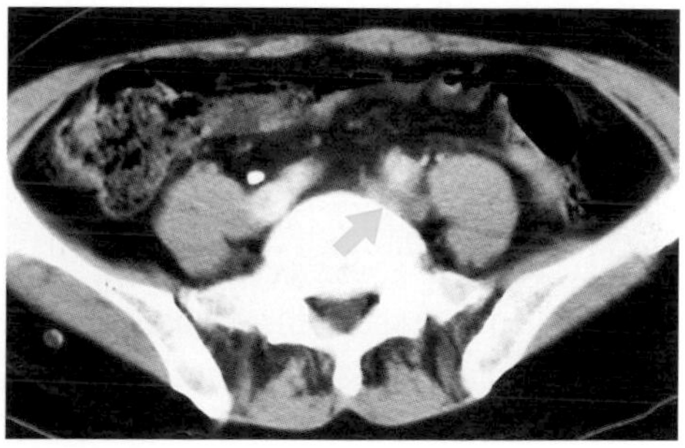

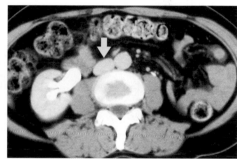

Fig. 143.2b

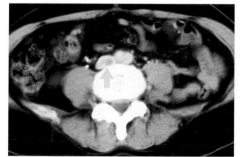

Fig. 143.2c

Fig. 143.2d

The injection of CM into a superficial foot vein opacifies satisfactorily only the ipsilateral leg, so it may be advisable to inject CM systemically through an arm vein in order to examine both sides of the pelvic venous system. If one side has become occluded, collaterals may develop (*) via the prepubic network of veins (Figs. 143.3a and 143.3b). Such collaterals are known as a "Palma shunt", and these can also be surgically created if a thrombus in a deeper vein resists dissolution.

You should be careful not to mistake an inguinal LN with physiologically hypodense hilar fat ("hilar fat sign" ✔ in Fig. 143.3c) for a partially thrombosed vein.

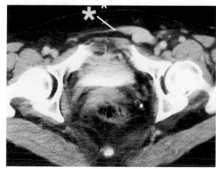

Fig. 143.3a

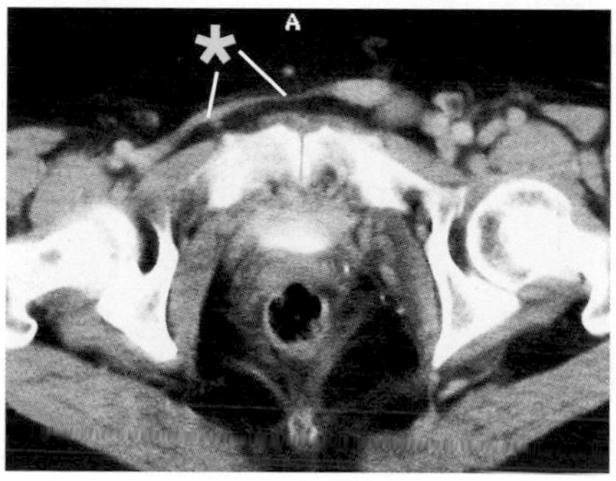

Fig. 143.3b

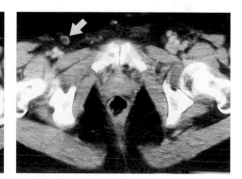

Fig. 143.3c

In order to avoid pulmonary embolism in cases of thrombosis (**173**) of the inferior vena cava (**80** in Fig. 144.1), the patient must be immobilized until the thrombus has either become endothelialized or has responded to therapy and dissolved (Figure 144.2). Occasionally, marked collateral circulation develops via the lumbar veins (**121**).

Depending upon the individual patient and the size of the thrombus, the vessel may be surgically explored and thrombectomy performed. If thromboses are recurrent, an arterio-venous shunt may be indicated in order to avoid relapse. The success of a particular therapy may also be checked with venography or color-Doppler ultrasound.

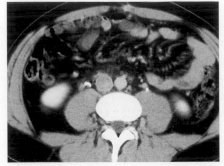
Fig. 144.1a

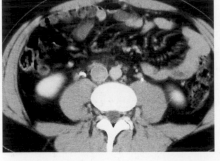
Fig. 144.1b

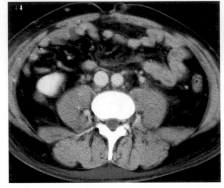
Fig. 144.2a

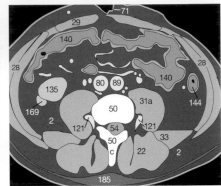
Fig. 144.2b

Enlarged Lymph Nodes

The density of LNs is approximately 50 HU, which corresponds to that of muscle. LNs with diameters below 1 cm are generally considered normal. Sizes between 1.0 and 1.5 cm are considered borderline, and those that exceed 1.5 cm are abnormally enlarged. Sites of predilection for enlarged LNs are the retrocrural, mesenteric ( ), interaortico-caval ( ), and para-aortic spaces (cf. p. 102).

Figure 144.3 illustrates the case of a patient with chronic lymphatic leukemia.

It is essential to be familiar with the major paths of lymphatic drainage. The drainage of the gonads, for example, is directly to LNs at renal hilar level. LN metastases (in Fig. 144.4) from a testicular tumor will be found in para-aortic nodes around the renal vessels but not in the iliac nodes, as would be expected with primary carcinomas of the urinary bladder, uterus, or prostate.

Conglomerate LN masses (**6/7**) surrounding the aorta (**89**) and its major branches such as the celiac trunk (**97**) are a typical finding in cases of non-Hodgkin lymphoma (Fig. 144.5).

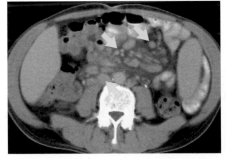
Fig. 144.3

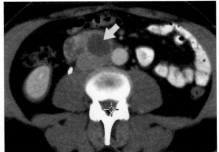
Fig. 144.4

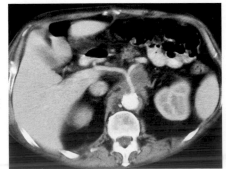
Fig. 144.5a

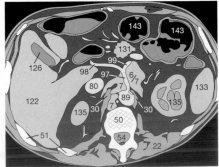
Fig. 144.5b

Normal Anatomy

The importance of examining bone windows during abdominal CTs has already been stressed on page 102. The marrow space of the iliac bones (**58**) and the sacrum (**62**) is normally homogeneous, and the surfaces of the sacroiliac joints should be smooth and regular (Fig. 145.1).

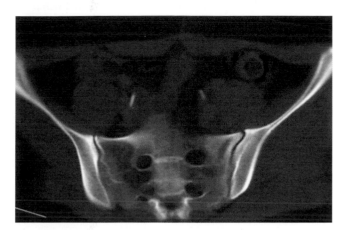

Fig. 145.1a

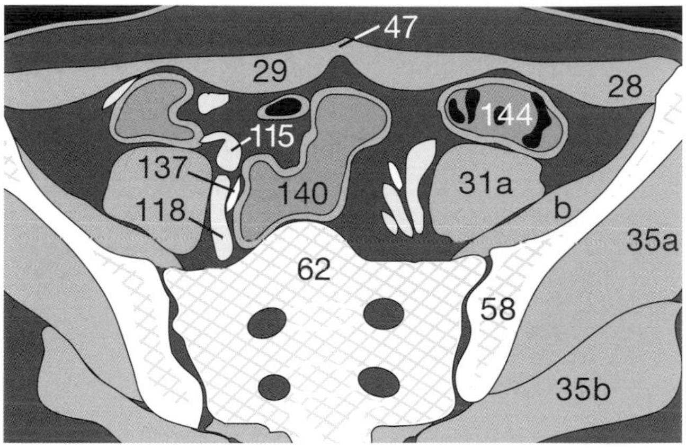

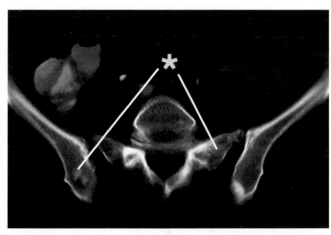

Fig. 145.1b

Metastases

Sclerotic bone metastases (**7**), for example from a carcinoma of the prostate, are not always as evident as in Figure 145.2a and may vary in size and degree of calcification. Even small and poorly defined metastases should not be overlooked (✳ in Fig. 145.2b). They cannot routinely be recognized on soft-tissue windows.

Lytic metastases (**7**), which can be seen on soft-tissue windows (Fig. 145.3a) only after they have reached considerable size, can be much more accurately detected on bone windows (Fig. 145.3c). This case shows a metastatic disease of the right ilium (**58**) that has destroyed the trabeculae and much of the cortex. The erosion extends to the sacroiliac joint. See the following pages for further images of this patient.

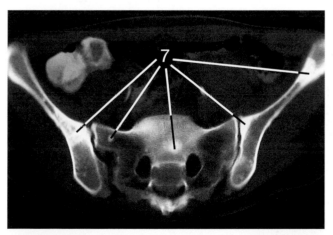

Fig. 145.2a

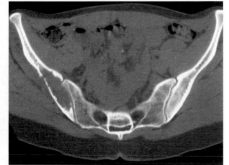

Fig. 145.2b

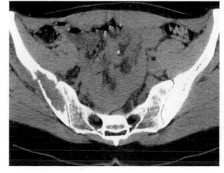

Fig. 145.3a

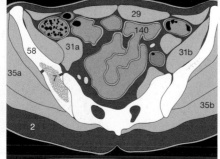

Fig. 145.3b

Fig. 145.3c

The mechanical integrity of a bone is suspect if any process involves its structure. Adjacent joint involvement must also be determined. MPRs (see p. 13) at various angles, for example sagittal or coronal, provide additional information. If necessary, 3D reconstructions can also be performed.

In the case shown on the previous page (see Fig. 145.3), the question of stability is easily answered: the coronal MPR (Fig. 146.1a) shows that the trabeculae of the right iliac bone have been completely destroyed for approximately 10 cm (➡). The lesion extends from the acetabulum to the mid-point of the sacroiliac joint and has also destroyed much of the cortex. In several areas, the cortex is disrupted (⬅). If you compare the bilateral sagittal reconstructions (Figs. 146.1b and 1c), it is easy to see that there is acute risk of fracture.

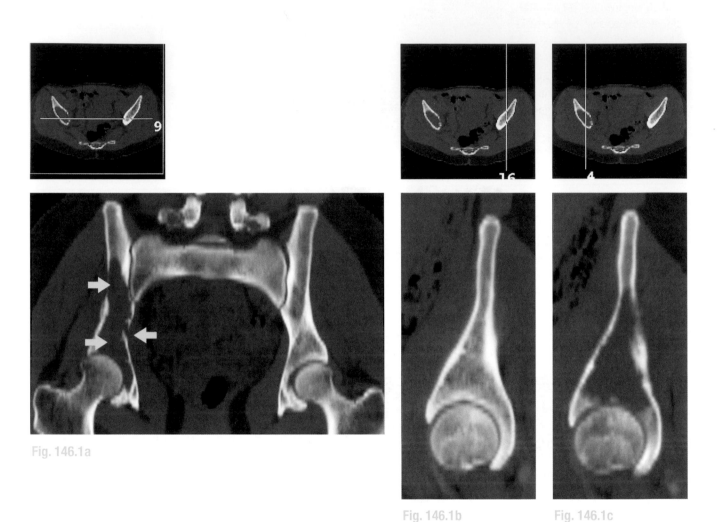

Fig. 146.1a

Fig. 146.1b   Fig. 146.1c

The 3D reconstruction of this pelvis (Fig. 146.2) does not add any more information, because it shows only the cortical disruption ( ) as seen from the lateral perspective.

The degree to which the trabeculae and marrow have been destroyed cannot be seen in this reconstruction because the attenuation level was set to detect the cortical bone, and the deeper trabeculae are therefore covered.

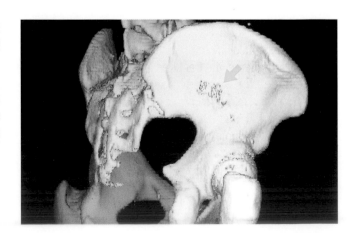

Fig. 146.2

Fractures

Bone windows should of course be used for the detection of fractures: hairline fractures and minimal dislocations cannot usually be recognized on soft-tissue windows.

It is also essential to give information on the precise fracture site and position of possible fragments for preoperative planning. In the case on the right, the fracture **(187)** of the femoral head **(66a)** is seen both in the axial plane (Fig. 147.1) and in the sagittal reconstruction (Fig. 147.2) (cf. p. 13).

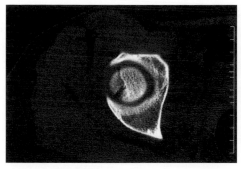

Fig. 147.1a

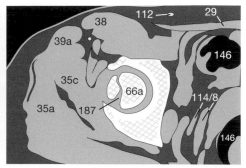

Fig. 147.1b

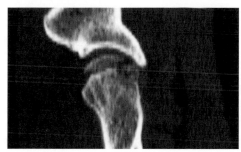

Fig. 147.2a

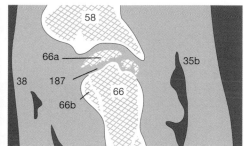

Fig. 147.2b

For joints such as the hip joint, it may be helpful to make an MPR in the oblique plane (Figs. 147.3). The angle of reconstruction is shown in Fig. 147.3a. Be careful not to mistake the acetabular suture ( ) with the real ischial fracture ( )!

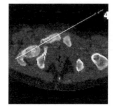

Fig. 147.3a

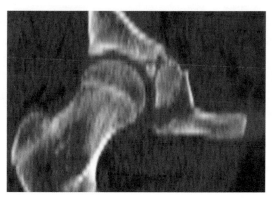

Fig. 147.3b

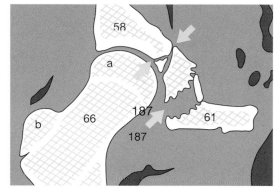

Fig. 147.3c

Another example of a fracture that may be mistaken for a suture is illustrated in Figure 147.4. The sutures ( ) are bilaterally symmetric, the fractures are not.

In this case, several fragments of bone (←——→) are seen at the right iliopubic junction, but the right acetabulum is intact. Note also the asymmetry in the image which is caused by differences in the levels of the femoral heads. The patient had left acetabular dysplasia (cf. figures on p. 148).

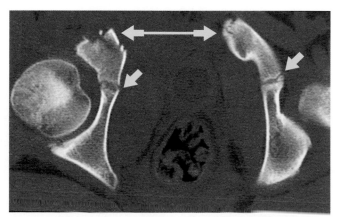

Fig. 147.4

Fragments are not always as obviously displaced nor is the fracture gap ( ) as wide as in the case illustrated in Figure 148.1. Look for fine breaks ( ) and discrete irregularities ( ) in the cortical outline in order not to miss a fracture or a small fragment (Fig. 148.2).

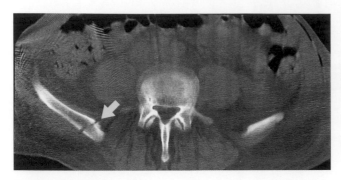

Fig. 148.1

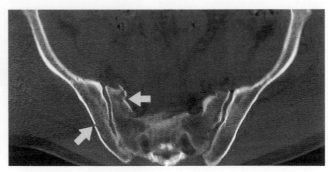

Fig. 148.2

Femoral Head Necrosis and Dysplasia of the Hip Joint

A fracture through the femoral head or even direct trauma to the hip joint may interrupt the blood supply to the head via the acetabular artery (see also Figures 147.1 and 147.2). Necrosis of the head makes it appear poorly defined ( ) as seen in Figure 148.3a and causes shortening of the leg. An image obtained 2 cm more cranially shows that a pseudoarthosis has developed in association with the right acetabular dysplasia (Fig. 148.3b). A 3D reconstruction gives an overview, but does not provide as much detail as a series of coronal MPRs (Fig. 148.5b with orientation in Fig. 148.5a).

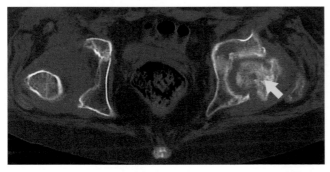

Fig. 148.3a

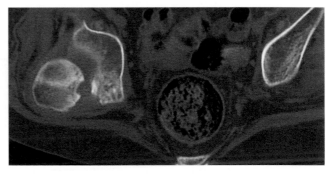

Fig. 148.3b

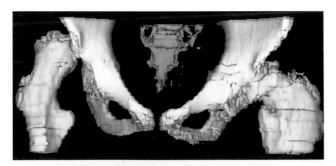

Fig. 148.4

MPRs are often used for diagnostic purposes and in planning surgery of complex fractures. They contribute valuable additional information to the conventional axial images. SCT produces particularly accurate MPR images because disruptive step artifacts can be avoided if the patient is able to cooperate by holding his or her breath.

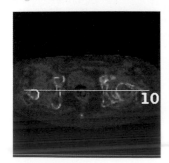

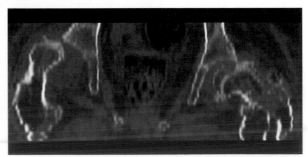

Fig. 148.5a   Fig. 148.5b

3D reconstructions, such as the one in Figure 142.4, yield impressive images, but are helpful only for specific problems such as plastic surgery. The amount of time and cost necessary to acquire and reconstruct 3D images are in most cases also very high.

The images and questions on this page will again help you to check on how much you have understood; the questions become contin-ually more difficult to answer. If you always remember the basic rules of CT reading, you will avoid jumping to the wrong conclusions. Don't look up the answers too soon!

Exercise 30:

What abnormality can you identify in Figure 149.1? Name as many blood vessels as you can!

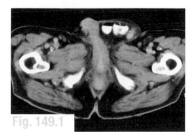

Fig. 149.1

Exercise 31:

Identify as many organs and blood vessels as possible in Figure 149.2. Look for any abnormalities.

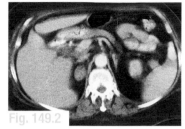

Fig. 149.2

Exercise 32:

What anatomic variation or abnormality do you recognize in Figure 149.3? Be sure you haven't missed anything.

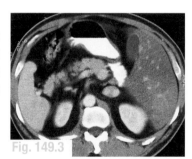

Fig. 149.3

Exercise 33:

"Do you smoke?" What abnormalities did you find in Figure 149.4?

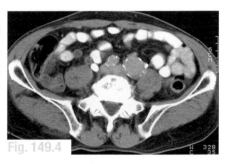

Fig. 149.4

Exercise 34:

It is easy to recognize the hepatic lesion in Figure 149.5. What is your DD?

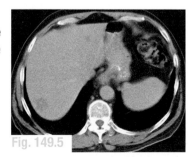

Fig. 149.5

Exercise 35:

Often abnormalities are not limited to one organ. What do your recognize in Figure 149.6?

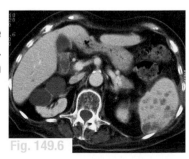

Fig. 149.6

The following questions may seem tricky, but you should be able to answer most of them if you go by the "rules of the book."

Describe the hepatic lesion in Figure 150.1. What steps did you take to arrive at your differential diagnosis? How would you proceed to verify it?

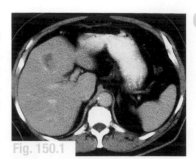

Fig. 150.1

Are the changes in Figure 150.2 "normal," or do you suspect that they are pathologic findings?

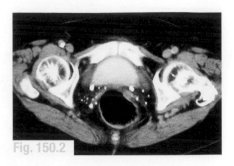

Fig. 150.2

Which of the two image levels on the right would you select for performing densitometric measurements of the kidney lesion? Why?

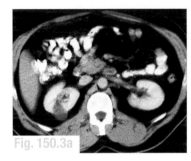

Fig. 150.3a

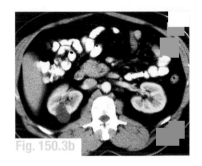

Fig. 150.3b

A patient is admitted for staging of a malignant melanoma (Figure 150.4). How far advanced is the lesion? What else would you do to obtain more information?

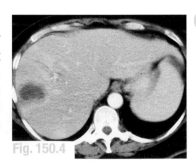

Fig. 150.4

A trauma patient could not be scanned in the prone position. What do you suspect in Figure 150.5, and what would you do to obtain more information?

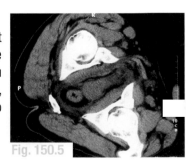

Fig. 150.5

Exercise 41:

A problem for those who already have some routine (Figure 151.1). How long did it take you to find two pathologic alterations and diagnose them accurately?

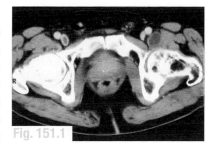

Fig. 151.1

Exercise 42:

Do you see anything abnormal in Figure 151.2? If so, what would you call it (the small figure indicates a structure filled with liquid)?

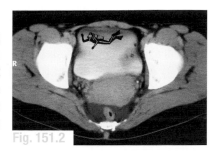

Fig. 151.2

Exercise 43:

At least three differential diagnoses should be considered for Figure 151.3. Which one is the most likely?

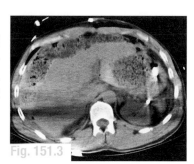

Fig. 151.3

Exercise 44:

In Figure 151.4, there are also several possibilities to explain the obvious alteration. Are you able to find **all** possible lesions in an image of this kind?

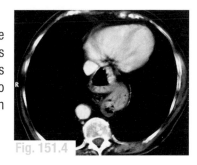

Fig. 151.4

Exercise 45:

What do you suspect is the case in Figure 151.5? What additional information do you need?

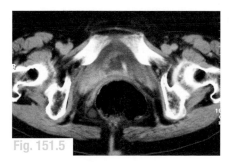

Fig. 151.5

Exercise 46:

This image (Figure 151.6) may contain several puzzles. Again, list the most likely diagnoses and then ask yourself what further information you need.

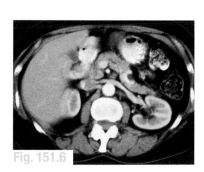

Fig. 151.6

The occipital condyles at the base of the skull articulate with the first vertebra, the atlas (**50a**), which is the only vertebra to lack a body. The dens (**50b**) of the axis protrudes upward into the atlas and is held in place by the transverse ligament (✳) (Figs. 152.1 and 152.2). This ligament may be torn by a whiplash injury during road traffic accidents.

The width of the space (⟷) between the anterior arch of the atlas (✳✳ in Figs. 152.1 and 152.2) and the dens is also measured, as in conventional x-ray images (Fig. 152.3). In adults it should not exceed 2 mm; in children, 4 mm. The vertebral artery passes through the transverse foramen (**88**).

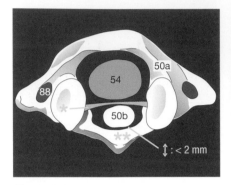

Fig. 152.1

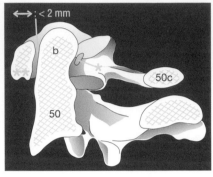

Fig. 152.2

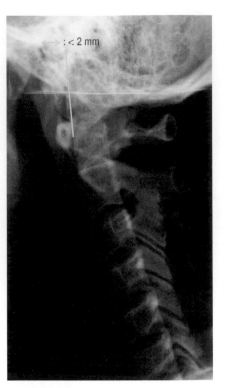

Fig. 152.3

The images below show normal anatomy at the level of the atlas (Fig. 152.4) and the body of the axis (Fig. 152.5). The cartilage of an intervertebral disc (**50e** in Fig. 152.6) will appear more homogeneous and hypodense than the typical pattern of trabeculae.

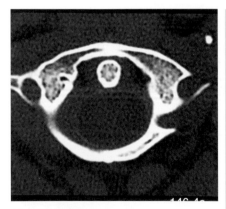

Fig. 152.4a

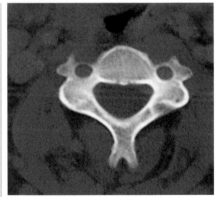

Fig. 152.5a

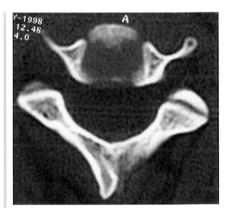

Fig. 152.6a

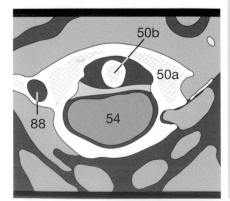

Fig. 152.4b

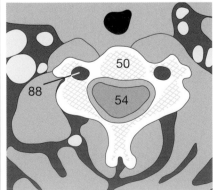

Fig. 152.5b

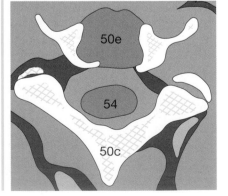

Fig. 152.6b

Cervical Disc Protrusion

A disc protrusion (prolaps of the nucleus pulposus) is demonstrated optimally in CT sections after myelography (CM in the SAS). The spinal cord is virtually isodense to CSF in unenhanced images, making it difficult to define the contours of the cord. After a myelogram, the CSF (132) will appear hyperdense to the cord (54) as well as to a disc. Normally, the CSF uniformly surrounds the cervical cord (Fig. 153.1). A disc prolapse (7), protruding into the CSF space can be seen because it is hypodense to the opacified CSF (Fig. 153.2). The gap between the cord (54) and vertebral body (50) is filled in. Did you recognize the pyriform fossa (172), the hyoid bone (159), the thyroid cartilage (169), and the cricoid cartilage (167)?

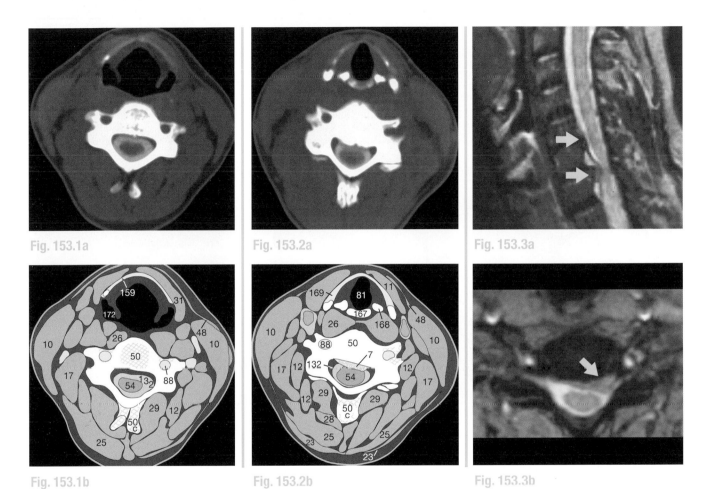

Fig. 153.1a   Fig. 153.2a   Fig. 153.3a

Fig. 153.1b   Fig. 153.2b   Fig. 153.3b

A disc prolapse will be seen even more clearly in an MR image. The sagittal T$_2$-weighted image in Figure 153.3a shows the extent of protrusions at two disk spaces. The disk protrudes into the hyperintense CSF space (→) in front of the cord. The axial T$_2$-weighted image (Fig. 153.3b) shows that the prolapse extends to the left and has caused stenosis of the intervertebral foramen (↘).

Cervical Spine Fractures

It is especially important to look for fractures of the cervical spine or for torn ligaments after trauma (ref. p. 152) so that damage to the cord is avoided if the patient needs to be moved or transported. Figures 153.4a through c show a coronal MPR in which the right occipital condyle (160) is fractured (188) but the dens (50b) is still in normal position.

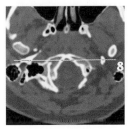
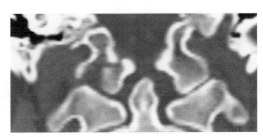
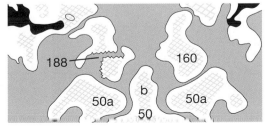

Fig. 153.4a   Fig. 153.4b   Fig. 153.4c

The thoracic vertebrae articulate with each other at their superior and inferior articular facets (**50d**) and with the ribs (**51**) at the inferior and superior costal facets and the transverse processes (**50f**). Figure 154.1 shows a normal thoracic image: the contours of the cortical bone are smooth and the trabeculae have a homogeneous pattern.

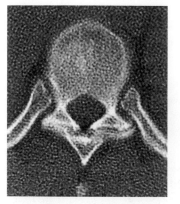

Fig. 154.1a

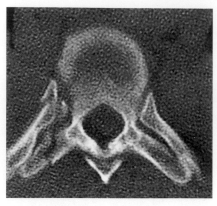

Fig. 154.2a

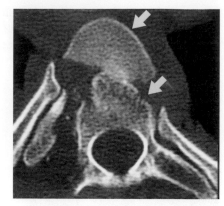

Fig. 154.3a

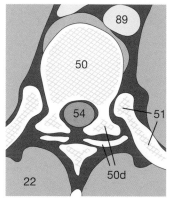

Fig. 154.1b

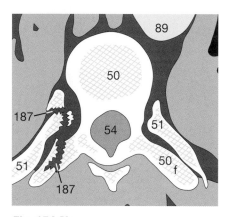

Fig. 154.2b

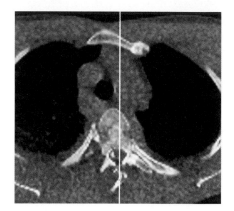

Fig. 154.3b

Fractures of the Thoracic Spine

Displaced fragments are identified by virtue of the fracture lines (**187**) and are best seen on bone windows. In Figure 154.2, both the transverse process (**50f**) and the corresponding rib (**51**) are fractured. In complex fracture dislocations (Figs. 154.3), torsion or shearing may cause compression or complete dislocation of the spine as a whole (Figs. 154.3a, e).

The axial image in Figure 154.3a shows two vertebrae ( ) at one level; the topogram in 154.3b indicates the position of the sagittal MPR shown in Figure 154.3e. The MPR gives a more precise picture of the fracture and the fragments than the oblique anterior and oblique posterior 3D views in Figures 154.3c and d.

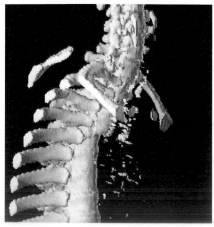

Fig. 154.3c

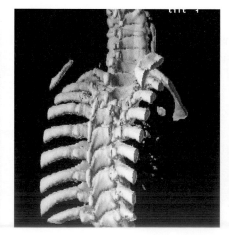

Fig. 154.3d

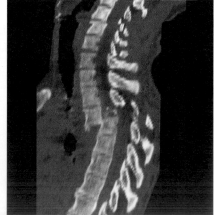

Fig. 154.3e

The transverse processes (**50f**) of the lumbar vertebrae are occasionally called costal processes. Lumbar vertebrae have much larger bodies (**50**) than thoracic vertebrae, and the angle of their intervertebral joints (**50d**) is smaller. Lumbar spinous processes do not extend as far caudally as the thoracic ones. Images of the normal lumbar spine usually show well-defined cortical bone and homogeneous trabeculae. At the level of a disk (Fig. 155.2), the hypodense cartilage (**50e**) may seem irregularly surrounded by bone: this is an oblique partial volume effect in which parts of an adjacent body (**50**) are included with the disk. The ligamenta flava (*) extend from one lamina to the next and can sometimes be seen behind the cord (Fig. 155.1a).

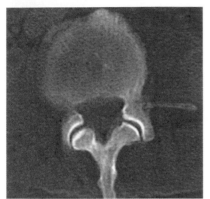

Fig. 155.1a

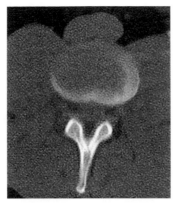

Fig. 155.2a

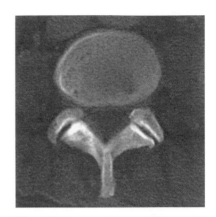

Fig. 155.3a

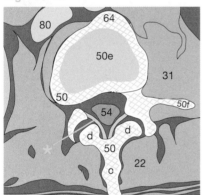

Fig. 155.1b

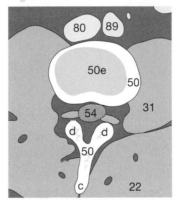

Fig. 155.2b

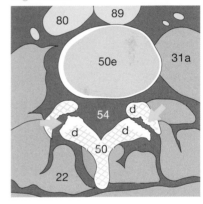

Fig. 155.3b

Degenerative change of the vertebrae can be seen in the facet joints (**50d**) (Fig. 155.3). There is increased subchondral sclerosis (→, ⬈) indicative of arthrosis of the joint.

Lumbar Disk Prolapse

As with cervical disk protrusions (see p. 153), it is important to establish whether the nucleus pulposus has protruded through the posterior longitudinal ligament. This ligament is applied to the posterior borders of the vertebral bodies and disks. Disk material that has penetrated the posterior longitudinal ligament and become detached from the disk is referred to as a sequestration (**). This can narrow the spinal canal or a lateral recess (Fig. 155.4). These structures are not well demonstrated on soft-tissue windows (Fig. 155.4a) because of their high density, but are clearly seen on bone windows (Fig. 155.4b). A T$_2$-weighted MR image (Fig. 155.5) shows the extent of the prolapse: the abnormal disk ( ) is thinner, is desiccated (shows a lower signal level [darker]), and the extruded material (⬈) impinges on the theca.

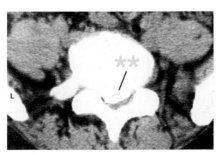

Fig. 155.4a

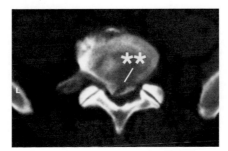

Fig. 155.4b

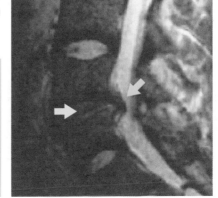

Fig. 155.5

Fractures

In conventional x-rays, it is often difficult to see the fracture of a lumbar transverse process (**50f**) if the fragment is not or only minimally dislocated (**187**). In CT sections, however, a fracture can be clearly demonstrated (Fig. 156.1). Figure 156.2 illustrates a case in which the spinous process (**50c**) was fractured. An arthrosis may develop if a fracture has involved a joint (Fig. 156.3). There are fractures of both the superior and the inferior articular processes (**50d**).

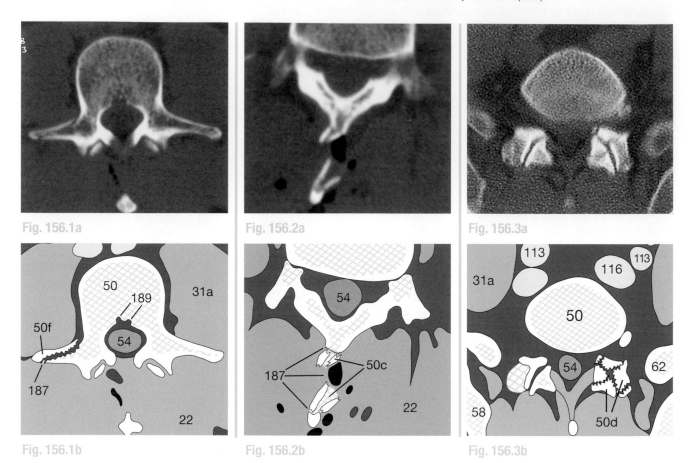

Fig. 156.1a　　　Fig. 156.2a　　　Fig. 156.3a

Fig. 156.1b　　　Fig. 156.2b　　　Fig. 156.3b

Do not confuse the vessels that supply the lumbar vertebra (**189**) and enter it posteriorly in the midline with a pathologic lesion or fracture (Fig. 156.1). Chronic fractures no longer show a definable fracture line (**187**) whose width varies with the degree of displacement. Sclerosis and bone remodeling adjacent to the fracture line will also be present. These pro-cesses can bridge the fracture line in bony union or can lead to pseudarthrosis (Fig. 156.4), as is seen here in a chronic pedicle fracture. On conventional radiographs these increased sclerotic processes can occasionally be very difficult to distinguish from purely degenerative osteophytes.

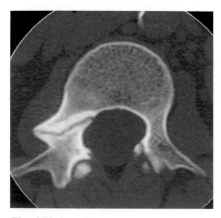

Fig. 156.4a

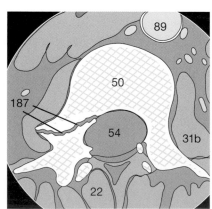

Fig. 156.4b

Stability Criteria

Lumbar fractures involving the posterior margin of the vertebral body and those with kyphotic angulation exceeding 30° are regarded as potentially unstable. Denis described three columns in the cervical spine: the anterior longitudinal ligament with the anterior two-thirds of the vertebral body; its posterior third with the posterior longitudinal ligament; and the vertebral arches with the ligamenta flava, interspinous ligament, and the capsules of the facet joints. Cervical fractures involving at least two of these columns are considered unstable.

Tumors and Metastases

Not all bone lesions originate within the bone. Malignant tumors of paravertebral tissues can also invade the bones.

Figure 157.1 shows an osteolytic lesion (⬀) in the body of a lumbar vertebra in a patient with carcinoma of the cervix. On soft-tissue windows (Fig. 157.2), there is a paravertebral metastasis (**7**) which has surrounded the bifurcation of the common iliac artery (**114/5**) and has infiltrated the right anterolateral aspect of the vertebral body.

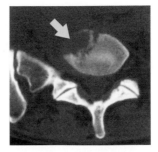

Fig. 157.1

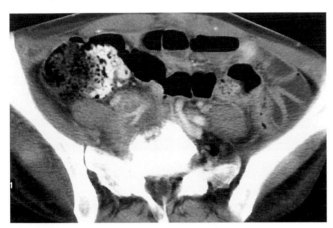

Fig. 157.2a

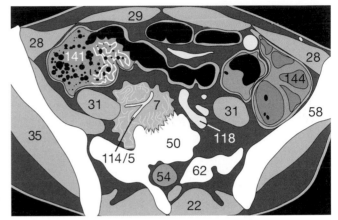

Fig. 157.2b

MPRs in the coronal (Figs. 157.3a and b) and sagittal (Figs. 157.4a and b) planes show the extent to which the bone has been eroded and that there is risk of fracture. As in Figure 146.2, the 3D reconstructions (Figs. 157.5a and b) clearly show the lesion from anterior and lateral perspectives, but not the degree to which the interior trabeculae have been destroyed.

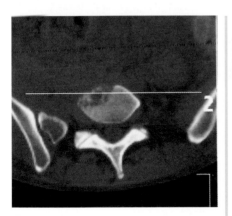

Fig. 157.3a

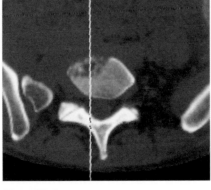

Fig. 157.4a

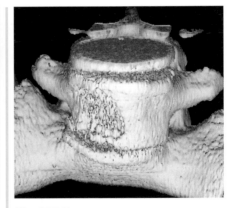

Fig. 157.5a

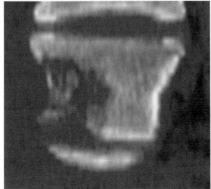

Fig. 157.3b

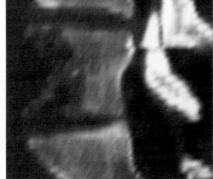

Fig 157.4b

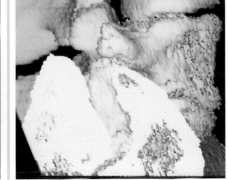

Fig. 157.5b

Infection

Abscesses in the paravertebral soft tissues or infective or inflammatory arthritides (**181**) in the small joints of the spine may lead to diskitis which ultimately destroys the intervertebral disk (Fig. 158.1). An advanced abscess can be detected on softtissue windows (Fig. 158.1a) as an area of heterogeneous density surrounded by a hyperdense enhancing rim representing reactive hyperperfusion. On bone windows (Fig. 158.1c), only small remnants of bone belonging to the vertebral body are present and some are displaced.

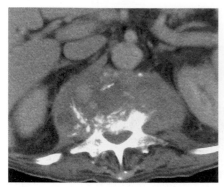

Fig. 158.1a

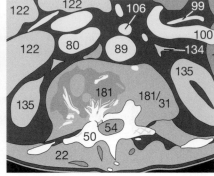

Fig. 158.1b

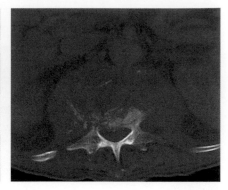

Fig. 158.1c

Methods of Stabilization

If therapeutic measures such as chemotherapy, antibiotics, and / or surgery have been effective in the treatment of a metastasis or infection, it is possible to stabilize the spine by inserting bone prosthetic material (Fig. 158.2a, b).

The choice of material depends upon the size of the defect and upon other individual factors. In follow-up examinations, these materials may cause considerable image artifacts because of their high relative density.

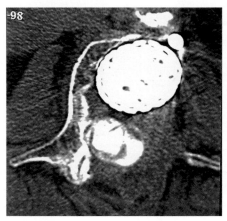

Fig. 158.2a

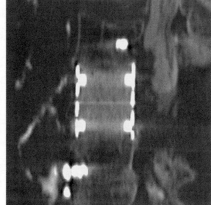

Fig. 158.2b

Notes

The anterior muscles of the thigh include the sartorius muscle (38), and the four components of the quadriceps muscle (39). The most anterior is the rectus femoris (39a), and lateral to this is the vastus lateralis (39b). The vastus intermedius (39c) and vastus medialis (39d) form the anterolateral borders of the adductor canal. This contains the superficial femoral artery and vein (119/120).

The adductor muscles comprise the superficially located gracilis muscle (38a) and the adductor longus (44a), brevis (44b), and magnus (44c) muscles. The pectineus muscle (37) is only seen in the most caudal images of the pelvis.

The posterior muscles of the thigh extend the hip joint and flex the knee joint. The group consists of the long and short heads of the biceps femoris muscle (188) and the semi-tendinosus (38b) and semimembranosus muscles (38c). In the proximal third of the thigh (Fig. 159.1), the hypointense tendon of the biceps muscle is adjacent to the sciatic nerve (162). In the distal third of the thigh (Fig. 159.3), the medial popliteal nerve (162a), which supplies the dorsal muscles, can be seen separate from the lateral popliteal nerve (162b). Note the close relationship of the profunda femoris artery and vein (119a/120a) to the femur (66) and the superficial position of the long saphenous vein (211a).

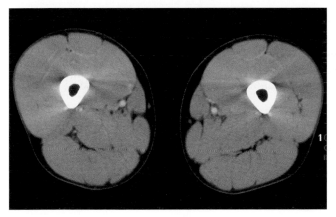

Fig. 159.1a

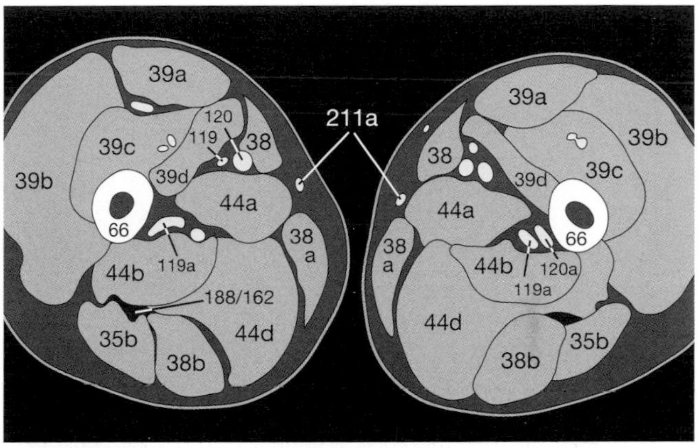

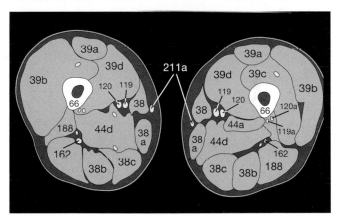

Fig. 159.1b

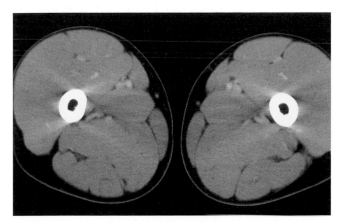

Fig. 159.2a

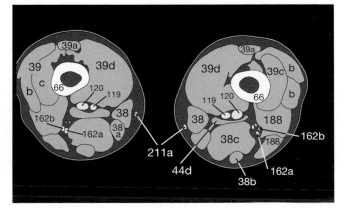

Fig. 159.2b

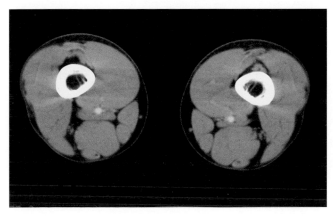

Fig. 159.3a

Fig. 159.3b

The popliteal artery (**209**) and vein (**210**), formed cranial to the joint line, are demonstrated at the level of the patella (**191**) in the fossa between the femoral condyles (**66d**) (Fig. 160.1). The tibial nerve (**162a**) lies directly posterior to the vein, whereas the fibular (peroneal) nerve (**162b**) lies more laterally. The medial (**202a**) and lateral (**202b**) heads of the gastrocnemius muscle and the plantaris muscle (**203a**) can be seen posterior to the femoral condyles. The long saphenous vein (**211a**) lies medially in the subcutaneous fat covering the sartorius muscle (**38**), and the biceps femoris muscle (**188**) lies laterally.

On the section just caudal to the patella (Fig. 160.2), the patellar tendon (**191c**) can be identified, posterior to which is the infrapatellar fat pad (**2**). Between the femoral condyles lie the cruciate ligaments (**191b**).Transverse sections such as these are frequently combined with coronal and sagittal MPRs (see also the images of a fracture on p. 167).

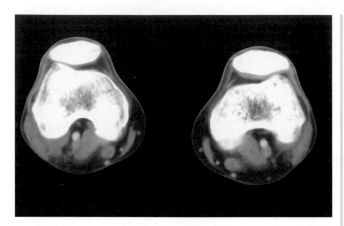

Fig. 160.1a

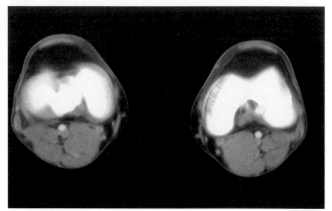

Fig. 160.2a

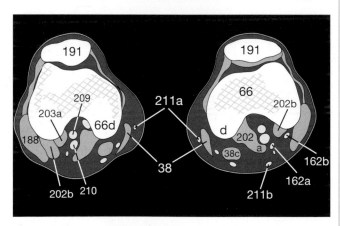

Fig. 160.1b

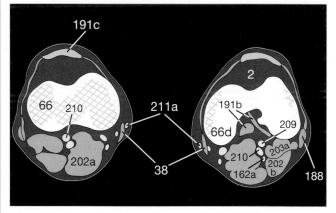

Fig. 160.2b

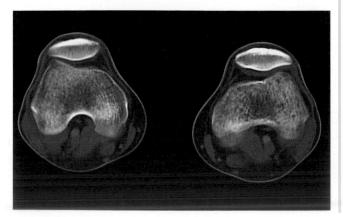

Fig. 160.1c

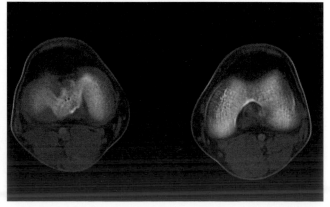

Fig. 160.2c

The muscles of the lower leg are separated into four compartments by the interosseus membrane between the tibia (**189**) and the fibula (**190**) and by the lateral and posterior intermuscular septa (Figs. 161.1 to 161.3). The anterior compartment contains the tibialis anterior muscle (**199**), the extensor hallucis longus muscle (**200a**) and the digitorum longus muscle (**200b**) next to the anterior tibial vessels (**212**). The lateral compartment contains the peroneus longus (**201a**) and brevis (**201b**) muscles next to the peroneal vessels (**214**). In slender individuals who have no fat between the muscles, these vessels and the peroneal nerve are only poorly defined (Fig. 161.2). The flexor muscles can be separated into a superficial and a deep group. The superficial group encompasses the gastrocnemius muscle with medial (**202a**) and lateral (**202b**) heads, the soleus muscle (**203**), and the plantaris muscle (**203a**). The deep group includes the tibialis posterior (**205**), the flexor hallucis longus (**206a**), and the flexor digitorum longus muscles (**206b**). These muscles are particularly well defined in the distal third of the lower leg (Fig. 161.3). The tibil alis posterior vessels (**213**) and the tibial nerve (**162a**) pass between the two flexor groups.

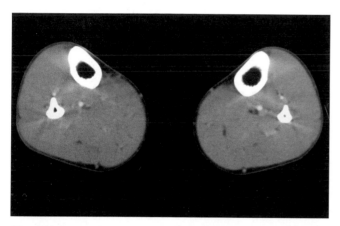

Fig. 161.1a

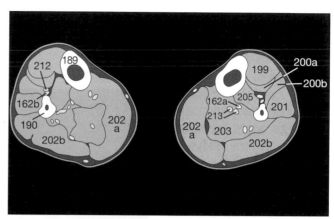

Fig. 161.1b

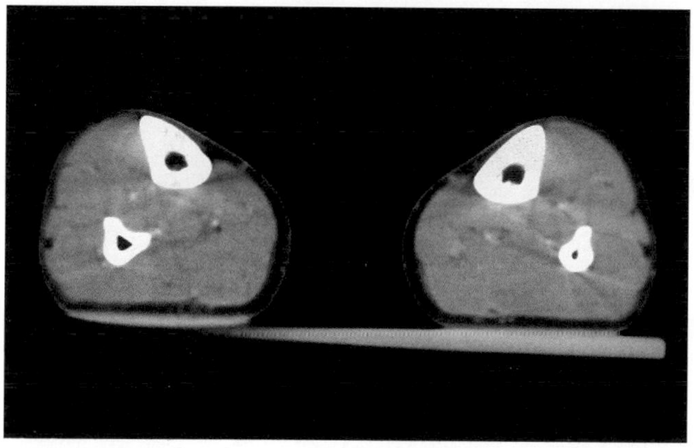

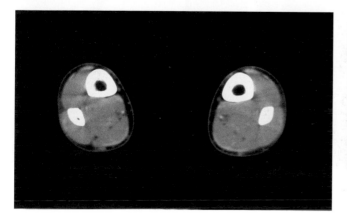

Fig. 161.2a

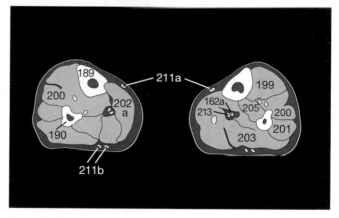

Fig. 161.2b

Fig. 161.3a

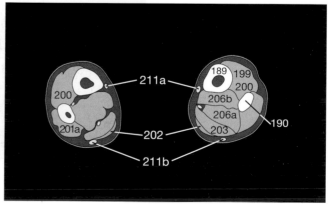

Fig. 161.3b

Multiplanar reconstructions are very valuable for visualizing fractures of the foot. The lateral digital radiograph in Figure 164.1a indicates the angle of the image plane, parallel to the long axis of the

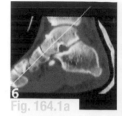

Fig. 164.1a

foot, seen in Figure 164.1b. This reconstructed image extends from the lateral (**190a**) and medial (**189a**) malleoli (at the lower edge of the image) through the talus (**192**) and the navicular (**194**) to the three cuneiform bones (**196a-c**). Two of the metatarsal bones (**197**) are included in the section. Note that the surfaces of the joints are smooth and evenly spaced. The sagittal image in Figure 164.2b was reconstructed slightly more laterally (see position in Fig. 164.2a) so that the cuboid bone (**195**) is included. The short flexor muscles (**208**) and the plantar ligaments are seen below the arch of the foot. The Achilles tendon (**215**) is seen posteriorly.

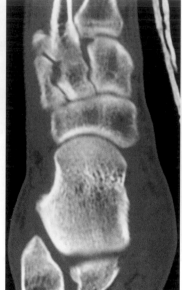

Fig. 164.1b

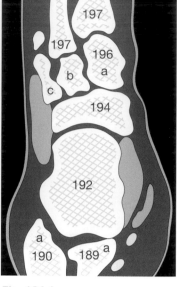

Fig. 164.1c

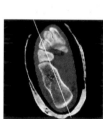

Fig. 164.2a

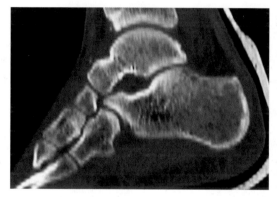

Fig. 164.2b

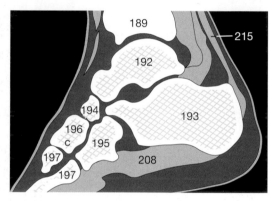

Fig. 164.2c

Diagnosis of Fractures

Typical signs of a fracture can be seen in the original axial plane (Fig. 164.3a): irregularities in the cortical outline (↓), displaced fragments (↗) and a fracture line (←) in the calcaneous. The MPR in the coronal plane (indicated in Fig.

164.3b) shows that not only is the calcaneous (↖) fractured, but there is a hairline fracture of the talus (→) involving the ankle joint (Fig. 164.3c).

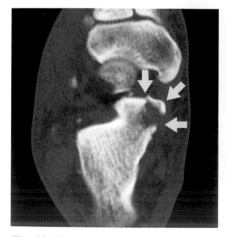

Fig. 164.3a

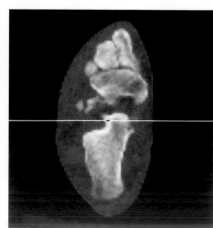

Fig. 164.3b

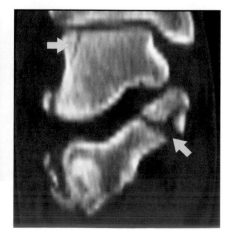

Fig. 164.3c

Fractures of the foot may initially escape detection in conventional x-rays if there is no major displacement of bone fragments. If the foot remains painful, a follow-up x-ray may show the fracture because fine hairline fractures can be seen when filled with hemorrhage. As an alternative, CT would show discrete fracture lines (**187**), as for example of the talus (**192**) in Figure 165.1.

In chronic fractures, the displaced fragment (✻) has usually become rounded off (Fig. 165.2). In this example, it is obvious that there were actually two fragments because a second fracture line (⬇) is seen next to the main one (**187**).

It is often difficult to treat comminuted fractures of the calcaneus (**193**), incurred for example during a fall (Fig. 165.3), because there are many small displaced fragments. A stable reconstruction of the arch of the foot may not be possible, resulting in a long period of sick leave.

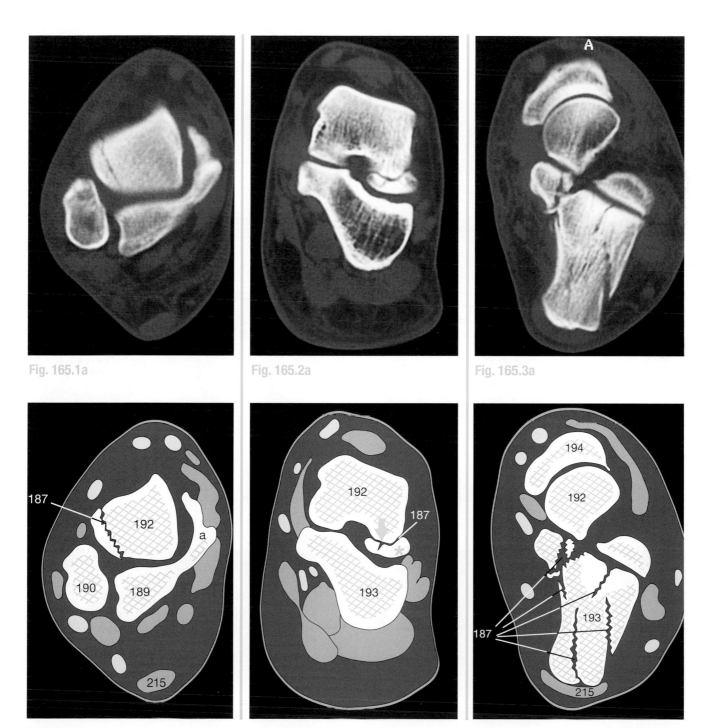

Fig. 165.1a   Fig. 165.2a   Fig. 165.3a

Fig. 165.1b   Fig. 165.2b   Fig. 165.3b

The assessment of fractures of long bones is generally the domain of conventional radiology. But CT examinations are helpful for locating displaced fragments and in the preoperative planning of comminuted fractures. Infections, however, are more accurately imaged by CT than by conventional radiographs because bone destruction is more readily seen on bone windows (Fig. 166. 1c) and soft-tissue involvement (**178**) is documented on soft-tissue windows (Fig. 166.1a). This patient had septic arthritis of the left hip joint with involvement of the acetabulum (**60**) and femoral head (**66a**).

The abscess appears more clearly after contrast enhancement (cf. Figs. 166.2a and 166.2c). The increased vascularity of the wall and the fluid within the abscess (**181**) are well demarcated from surrounding fat (**2**). Adjacent muscles (**38, 39, 44**) are no longer individually defined because of edema (compare with the right leg). Gas (**4**) has been produced and is loculated in the adjacent tissues.

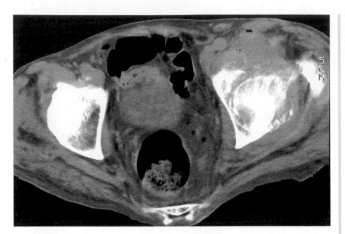

Fig. 166.1a

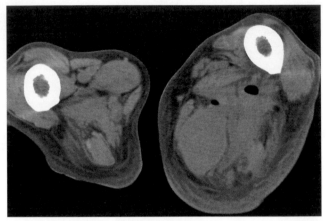

Fig. 166.2a

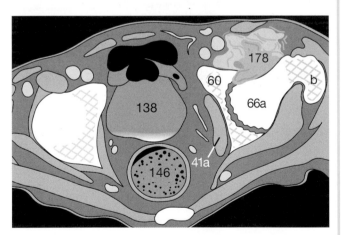

Fig. 166.1b

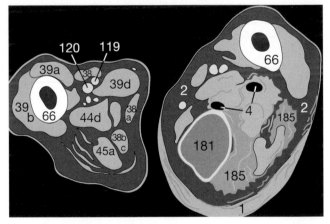

Fig. 166.2b

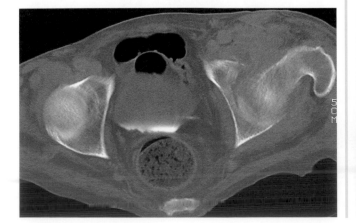

Fig. 166.1c

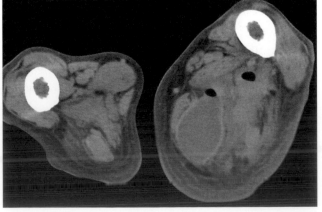

Fig. 166.2c

Fractures

If a fracture involves the knee joint, it is particularly important to reduce the fragments accurately to avoid joint surface incongruities that might lead to arthosis. In the case below, axial sections clearly show the lateral displacement of a large fragment ( ) of the tibia (Figs. 167.1a and 167.1b). The coronal MPR (Fig. 167.2b, with level shown in 167.2a) illustrates how much of the tibial plateau is affected.

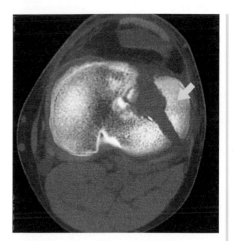

Fig. 167.1a

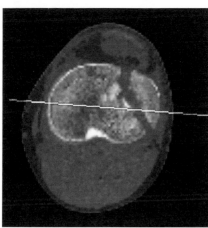

Fig. 167.2a

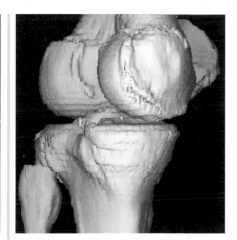

Fig. 167.3a

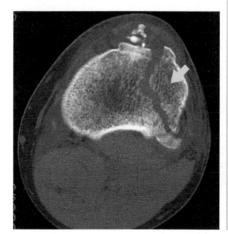

Fig. 167.1b

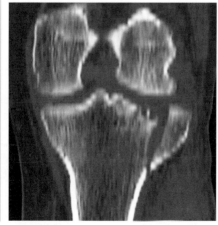

Fig. 167.2b

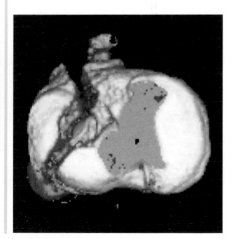

Fig. 167.3b

The 3D reconstruction seen from a posterolateral projection (Fig. 167.3a) is not very helpful, but the view from cranial (Fig. 167.3b) gives a good impression of the tibial plateau and fracture line because the femoral condyles have been excluded.

Checklist Skeletal System: Fracture Diagnosis

➡ Step-off or discontinuity of the cortex (evidence of fracture)?

➡ Articular involvement of a fracture (risk of secondary degenerative changes)?

➡ Stability on weight-bearing?

   Spine: e.g., 3-column model according to Denis (C-spine); A-B-C classification according to Magerl (T-spine)

➡ Simple fracture or comminuted fracture, extent of displacement of the fracture fragments (surgical planning)?

➡ Age of the fracture?

   • Acute => ragged and sharply demarcated fracture clefts

   • Old => sclerotic rim, callus formation

      Risk of pseudoarthrosis with persistent fracture cleft?

➡ Traumatic or pathologic fracture (underlying bone tumor)?

It is not always possible to determine the nature of a lesion from CT appearance and densitometry alone. In these cases, needle biopsies may be carried out under ultrasound or CT guidance. The patient's platelet count and coagulation status must be checked and informed consent obtained.

In Figure 161.1, a mass in the caudate lobe (✳) of the liver (**122**) is being biopsied. The close proximity of the hepatic artery and portal vein (**98/102**) and inferior vena cava (**80**) leave only a narrow path for the needle to approach from the right side (Fig. 168.1a).
Firstly the section on which the lesion appears largest is determined. The skin is cleaned and anesthetized with local anaestheic.

The needle is then inserted through the liver parenchyma toward the lesion. Slight changes in angle may be necessary (Figs. 168.1b, 168.1c, and 168.1d). Distances can also be calculated during the procedure, as seen in Figure 168.1b. After biopsy has been completed, an image is acquired to detect any hemorrhage. If a pneumothorax occurred following lung biopsy, expiratory images of the thorax are acquired to check for a tension pneumothorax.

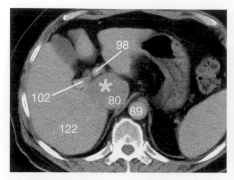

Fig. 168.1a

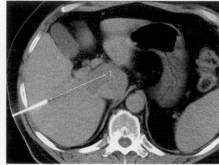

Fig. 168.1b

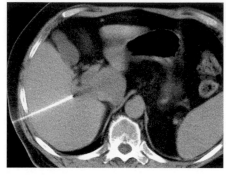

Fig. 168.1c

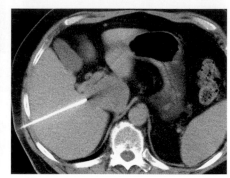

Fig. 168.1d

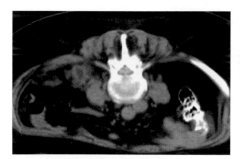

Fig. 168.2a

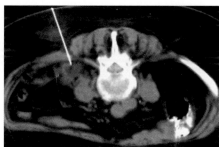

Fig. 168.2b

If there is a retroperitoneal lesion close to the spinal column, a biopsy may be carried out in the prone position. The orientation in Figure 168.2 is therefore unusual and one must be careful not to confuse left with right, but the procedure is identical.

After selection of the optimal level (largest diameter of the lesion), and after skin cleaning and local anesthesia, the needle is inserted (Fig. 168.2b) and the biopsy taken. The material should be promptly prepared for cytology and histology.

The size and extent of a cutaneous fistula can often be more clearly assessed if CM is instilled through a tube (Fig. 168.3). In this example, the hip had become infected and an abscess filled the joint after prosthetic surgery.

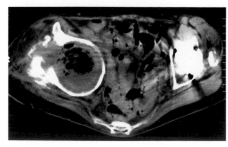

Fig. 168.3a

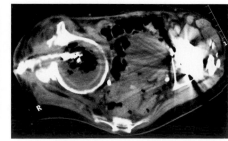

Fig. 168.3b

Occasionally, the beginner faces the question to decide whether a finding represents a true lesion or just an artifact. A contralateral comparison or a comparison with adjacent cranial or cauda sections can often be helpful. Furthermore, uncertainty arises when describing a lesion without familiarity with the appropriate vocabulary. This primer aims to remedy these problems.

A   General Approach to an Abnormality of the CT Morphology:

Where ?	Location, lateralization, relative position to other organs/vessels
Size ?	Size (diameter in [mm, cm]; important, e.g., monitoring of therapy)
Density ?	Relative to its surrounding: isodense (equal density); hyperdense (denser); or hypodense (less dense)
Structure ?	Homogenous (e.g., fluids) or heterogenous / septate / geographic
Shape ?	Tubular (vessels, muscles, …) or nodular (tumor, lymph nodes)? Reticular (resembling a net), striate or diffuse?
Demarcation ?	Sharply marginated (more likely benign) or indistinctly marginated (infiltration into the surrounding, e.g., inflammation, malignancy) Caution: Partial volume effect can mimic an indistinct margin!
Perfusion ?	No, peripheral, homogenous or heterogenous contrast enhancement
Expansion ?	Space-occupying effect not invariably a sign of malignancy: e.g., large benign cysts can displace adjacent vessels

B   Useful Terms, in Alphabetic Order   (⇨ Application, Possible Significance)

Air inclusions	⇨ Infection with gas-forming bacteria ⇨ compound fracture
Ampullary	Dilatation of the renal pelvis (⇨ physiologic variant or obstructive uropathy)
Articular involvement	Evaluation of fractures (⇨ risk of degenerative osteoarthritis)
Bolus CT	Dynamic examination, often without table movement to assess the contrast enhancement pattern
Bullae	Lung (⇨ pulmonary emphysema)
Capping	Periventricular abnormality in the white matter (⇨ transependymal diffusion of CNS; sign of SAE)
Cavity	Intrapulmonary hollow space (⇨ tuberculosis)
Central	In the center of a lesion or close to the hilum of parenchymatous organs
Clubbing	e.g., of a limb of the adrenal gland (⇨ adenoma, metastases)
CM	Contrast medium, given orally, rectally or intravenously
Concentric	Location of intravascular thrombi (⇨ aortic aneurysm)
Course of fracture lines	Evaluation with additional MPR (⇨ surgical planning)
Crescentic	Typical configuration, e.g., subdural hematoma or perihepatic effusion / ascites
Defect	Pathologic phenomenon in opacified vessels / urinary collecting system
Defect	In opacified vessels (⇨ thrombus), in urinary bladder (⇨ tumor, blood clot)

Demarcation	Depending on the vascularization, lesions become visible only after administration of contrast medium
Dense band	Band-like density (⇨ lung, connective tissue: post-inflammatory, scar)
Densitometry	Measuring of density (⇨ differential diagnosis)
Diffuse	Uniform, neither focal nor nodular; e.g., liver: hypodense ⇨ hepatic steatosis (fatty liver) hyperdense ⇨ hemochromatosis
Dumbbell-like	Typical calcification pattern of benign hamartomas (⇨ lung)
Eggshell-shaped	Calcification pattern of perihilar lymph nodes (lung ⇨ silicosis; porcelain gallbladder)
Enhancement	Increased density due to accumulation of contrast medium
Enhancement pattern	Perfusion pattern (homogenous, timely or delayed)
Excentric	Intravascular location of thrombi (⇨ aortic aneurysm)
Fluid Levels	Phenomenon (⇨ sedimented hematoma) or air-fluid levels (⇨ paralytic ileus or intestinal obstruction)
Fractures	Cortical step deformity, displacement, number of fragments, stability, articular surface?
Ground glass density	Diffuse, slight increase density seen in perifocal edema (⇨ fat, lung)
Halo	Confined perifocal edema (⇨ around inflammatory foci and metastases)
Hemorrhagic	Blood-containing (⇨ large infarcts, e.g., cerebral)
Hilar fat	Benign criterion for lymph nodes (⇨ nodal index)
Honeycombing	Typical for vascular rarefaction in the lung (⇨ emphysema)

HRCT	High resolution computed tomography (thin sections) (⇨ lung; also for MPR and 3D)	**Patchy**	Parenchymal perfusion pattern in the spleen during the early arterial phase
Hyperdense	Denser than the surrounding tissue (bright ⇨ fresh cerebral bleeding or calcification)	**Perifocal**	Circular around a lesion (edematous zone)
		Perihilar	Topographic description of an intrapulmonary lesion
Hyperperfusion	Enhancement (⇨ inflammation, hypervascular tumor)	**Peripheral**	Along the periphery, in contrast to central
Hypodense	Less dense than the surrounding (dark ⇨ fluid, fat, air)	**Pitch**	Ratio of table feed per rotation and section thickness (⇨ spiral technique, see p. 8 / 9)
		Pixel	Picture element (image formation, see p. 14)
Imbibition	Striate to diffuse enhancement (⇨ fatty tissue: scar, inflammation)	**Plaque**	Intravascular (⇨ arteriosclerosis), pleura-based (⇨ asbestosis)
Indentation	Blunt convex bulging / displacement of adjacent structures (⇨ tumors)	**Polycyclic**	= scalloped, cauliflower-like (⇨ hilar lymph nodes of the lung, e.g., Boeck's disease)
Indistinct	Outline of a lesion (see marginal indistinctness)	**Popcorn**	Typical pattern of benign calcifications (⇨ lung)
Indistinct margin	Caused by inflammatory and tumorous infiltration of the surrounding tissue (caution: DD partial volume effect)	**Process**	Favored term for "I don't know what is means"
		Pseudocysts	⇨ chronic pancreatitis
Induration	Thickened fibrous tissue (⇨ scar, pulmonary fibrosis)	**Pulsation**	Can induce artifacts along vessels (⇨ aortic aneurysm)
Infiltration	Perifocal extension of an inflammatory or malignant process	**Rarefaction**	Less vessels per pulmonary volume (⇨ emphysema, S/P lobectomy)
Inflow effect	Incomplete mixing of contrast medium, can mimic intravascular thrombi	**Respecting soft-tissue planes**	Lacking in malignant tumors or advanced inflammations (no longer respecting natural borders => infiltration)
Intramural	Located in the wall of a hollow viscus (⇨ gas, tumor)	**Retention cyst**	Convex projection into the paranasal sinus, homogenous
Iris effect	Centripetal enhancement (⇨ hepatic hemangiomas)	**Reticular**	Net-like pattern (⇨ fibrosis of the pulmonary interstitium)
Isodense	As dense as … (= isointense)	**Retrocrural**	Preferred posterior paravertebral lymph node station
Jet effect	Inflow of opacified urine from the ureter into the urinary bladder	**Risk of herniation**	Internal herniation of brain stem due to increased intracranial pressure (⇨ quadrigeminal and ambient cisterns)
Lacuna	Lacunar defect (⇨ late stage after cerebral infarct, isointense with CSF)		
LN	Lymph node (for size see checklists, ⇨ hilar fat)	**ROI**	Region of interest (⇨ densitometry)
Lymphangiomatosis	Ground glass-density (⇨ pulmonary parenchyma, breast carcinoma)	**Round lesion**	Focal space-occupying lesion (only intrapulmonic)
		Scalloped enhancement	Peripheral contrast enhancement (⇨ glioblastoma)
MPR	Multiplanar reconstruction of various image planes (sagittal, coronal ⇨ diagnostic evaluation of e.g. fractures)	**Site of predilection**	Preferred site for certain changes (⇨ lymph nodes, metastases)
Multiphase technique	Data acquisition during early arterial, portovenous or late venous passage of the contrast medium bolus (⇨ spiral CT of the liver)	**Sludge**	Thickened bile (⇨ cholestasis, cholecystitis)
		Space-occupying process	Tumor of unknown nature (ubiquitously applicable)
Multislice	New multislice technique consisting of simultaneous acquisitions of several sections in spiral mode	**Spindle-shaped**	Biconvex configuration (⇨ aortic aneurysm; epidural hematoma)
Mural thickness	Single or multiple layers (wall of a hollow viscus: ⇨ ischemia, inflammation)	**Spiral CT**	Acquisition of a 3D data set with continuous table feed and any section reconstruction, see p. 7
Narrowed parenchymal rim	⇨ Renal atrophy (degenerative, hydronephrosis)	**Stellar**	Hypodense star-like figure (⇨ FNH of the liver)
		Stellate	Septation (⇨ echinococcal cyst)
Necrosis	Central, hypodense or homogenous liquefaction	**Stent**	Short tube of various materials to stent vessels, ureter or common bile duct
Nodal index	Longitudinal-transverse diameter ratio (characterization of lymph nodes)	**Step deformity**	bony cortex (⇨ fracture diagnosis)
Nodular	Nodular configuration (⇨ lymph nodes, tumors, adenomas), miliary < granular < fine-nodular < large-nodular < confluent (⇨ pulmonary interstitium)	**Structure**	Non-descriptive term of a lesion, try to use more precise term
		Subcarinal	Preferred lymph node station
		Timely	Symmetric and timely renal enhancement and excretion of contrast medium = normal
Obliterated	Surface of cerebral gyri (⇨ cerebral edema, DD: child) or pancreas outline (⇨ acute pancreatitis)	**Triangular**	Wedge-shaped (⇨ typical infarct pattern, scar residue)
Osteolytic	Destruction of bony matrix (⇨ metastases, multiple myeloma)	**Tumor extension**	Renal vein or vena cava (⇨ renal tumor)
Osteoproliferative	Osseous apposition (⇨ degenerative), less frequent due to sclerotic metastases	**Vascular configuration**	Normal configuration of the pulmonary hila
		Voxel	Volume element (image formation, see page 14)
Partial volume effect	Effect of partial volume (causes apparent indistinctness)	**Wedge-shaped**	Triangular configuration (⇨ typical infarct pattern, scar residue)

B **Practical Terms,** Organ-related

The following list contains helpful terms, which are used for interpreting CT examinations of a particular organ. Terms locating the findings are followed by terms describing typical morphologic changes, which are incorporated with possible conclusions and subsequent organ-related peculiarities.

The list does not claim to be complete (this would make it far too convoluted), but should help the reader to look up some of the most frequent organ-related terms quickly.

Skull, intracranial

Locational descriptions

- Supra- / infratentorial
- Frontal / temporal / parietal / occipital
- Singular / multiple
- White matter / cortical

Typical morphology ⇨ possible diagnoses

- Midline displacement, obliterated cisterns, effaced sulci, narrow subarachnoid space or small ventricles;
  Obliterated white matter / cortex interface
  ⇨ increased intracranial pressure; possible herniation
- Capping
  ⇨ Transependymal diffusion of advanced increased ventricular CSF pressure
- Intracranial air inclusions
  ⇨ Compound fracture of the cranial vault or cranial base
- Cystic homogeneous hypodense
  ⇨ Hygroma / arachnoidal cyst
- Hyperdense, biconvex / crescentic space-occupying process along the internal table of cranial vault
  ⇨ epidural / subdural hematoma
- Hyperdense extracerebral CSF space
  ⇨ Subarachnoidal hemorrhage
- Hypodense white matter lesions
  ⇨ Infarcts, embolic residues
- CSF-isodense lacunar defect
  ⇨ Infarct residue
- Peripheral scalloped enhancement
  ⇨ Typical for glioblastoma
- Subtle rounding of the temporal horn
  Early increase in CSF pressure
- Ventricular enlargement
  ⇨ Internal hydrocephalus
  ⇨ increased CSF pressure !

Notable findings

- Immediate therapeutic intervention with pending herniation !

Paranasal sinuses

Locational descriptions

- Frontal sinus, ethmoid sinus, sphenoid sinus, maxillary sinus
- Semilunar canal (important drainage duct)

Typical morphology ⇨ possible diagnoses

- Round, broad-based, convex homogeneous space-occupying lesion ⇨ retention cyst

Notable findings

- Normal variants: Haller's cells, pneumatic nasal conchae or uncinate process
- Risk of visual loss with orbital fracture
- Fracture classification of facial bones according to Le Fort [33] (see p. 63)

Orbit

Locational descriptions

- Orbital floor, orbital roof, medial and lateral orbital wall, retrobulbar

Typical morphology ⇨ possible diagnoses

- Thickened extraocular muscles
  ⇨ Endocrine ophthalmopathy, Myositis

Notable findings

- Risk of vision loss with fractures of the orbital floor solely through cicatricial pull on the orbital fatty tissue

Neck

Locational descriptions

- Nuchal, submandibular, prevertebral, paratracheal, parapharyngeal, epiglottic, subglottic, neurovascular bundle, intra- / suprahyoidal

Typical morphology ⇨ possible diagnoses

- Heterogenous internal structure, possibly with intrathyroidal calcifications ⇨ nodular struma
- Multiple ovoid lesions along the neurovascular bundle ⇨ lymph nodes

Chest

Locational descriptions

- Peripheral = subpleural / central = perihilar;
- Basal / apical, segmental / lobular;
  Name segment !

Typical morphology ⇨ possible diagnoses

- Polycyclic bulky hila
  ⇨ Boeck's disease; hilar nodal metastases
- Multiple, only indistinctly outlined nodules
  ⇨ pulmonary metastases / granulomas
- Sharply outlined, striate density without perifocal edema ⇨ fibrotic edema
- Perifocal ground glass-like density in HRCT
  ⇨ Acute inflammatory process

- Irregular nodular thickened interlobar septae with fine-reticular thickening
  ⇨ Lymphangiomatosis
- Bullae with vascular rarefication, honey combing ⇨ emphysema
- Cavity with layered ground glass density below air pocket ⇨ aspergilloma
- Fusiform thickening along interlobar space
  ⇨ encapsulated pleural effusion
- Apical pleural thickening, cavities, hilar lymph nodes ⇨ tuberculosis
- Popcorn-like or club-like calcifications
  ⇨ benign hamartomas, post-inflammatory residues

Notable findings

- Normal variant of the azygous lobe
- HRCT with thinner sections (do you remember the rational? Refer to pp. 86-87)
- Don't forget the pulmonary window

Liver

Locational descriptions

- Subdiaphragmatic, subcapsular, perihilar, name the segment (not only the lobe), periportal, diffuse / focal / multifocal, parahepatic

Typical morphology ⇨ possible diagnoses

- Diffuse hypodensity with resultant hyperdense vessels (unenhanced)
  ⇨ fatty liver (hepatic steatosis)
- Diffuse hyperintensity ⇨ hemochromatosis
- Homogeneous-hypodense, round sharply marginated round lesion without enhancement ⇨ benign cysts
- Focal round lesion with enhancement
  ⇨ metastases; abscess
- Round lesion with central hypodense stellar figure ⇨ FNH
- Cameral cysts with stellate septations
  ⇨ echinococcus (splenic involvement?)
- Hypodense cannulated, but irregularly branching ⇨ cholestasis
- "intraparenchymal" hypodense air pockets
  ⇨ pneumobilia; S/P biliointestinal anastomosis

Notable findings

- Multiphase spiral CT: early arterial, portal and late venous for improved detection of focal lesions
- Dynamic bolus CT without table feed
  ⇨ iris effect in hemangiomas
- Portography CT after preceding catheter-placement into splenic or mesenteric artery

Gallbladder

Typical morphology ⇨ possible diagnoses

- Multi-layered edematous wall thickening with perifocal "ascites" ⇨ acute cholecystitis
- Intraluminal wall-based thickening with calcification ⇨ polyp
- Intraluminal sedimentation phenomenon ⇨ sludge
- Eggshell-like peripheral calcification ⇨ Porcelain gallbladder, precancerosis

Spleen

Locational descriptions

- Subdiaphragmatic, subcapsular, perihilar, perisplenic

Typical morphology ⇨ possible diagnoses

- Leopard-like marble pattern during the early arterial phase of enhancement ⇨ physiologic
- Wedge-shaped perfusion defect ⇨ infarct
- Perisplenic round lesion, isodense with splenic parenchyma ⇨ accessory spleen; LN

Pancreas

Locational descriptions

- Head, body, tail, peripancreatic fatty tissue, uncinate process

Typical morphology ⇨ possible diagnoses

- Diffuse enlargement with obliterated outline and exudate pathways ⇨ acute pancreatitis
- Atrophic organ, dilated ducts, calcifications and pseudocysts ⇨ chronic pancreatitis

Kidneys

Locational descriptions

- Parapelvic, medullary, parenchymal, cortical, subcapsular, arising, polar, perirenal, uni-/ bilateral, lateralization

Typical morphology ⇨ possible diagnoses

- Homogenous-hypodense, round, sharply demarcated space-occupying lesion without contrast enhancement ⇨ benign cyst
- Hypodense clubbing of the collecting system ⇨ obstruction; ampullary renal pelvis, parapelvic cyst
- Irregular wall thickening of the cyst with contrast enhancement ⇨ suspicious for malignancy
- Thinning of the parenchymal rim, generalized decrease in size ⇨ renal atrophy
- Heterogenous space-occupying lesion extending beyond the organ outline ⇨ renal cell carcinoma
- Hypodense wedge-shaped perfusion defect crenal infarct

Notable findings

- Densitometry of cystic changes for comparison with unenhanced sections
- Evaluation of excretion: symmetric, timely? Dilated ureteral lumen?

Urinary Bladder

Locational descriptions

- Intra-, extra-, paravesical, bladder floor, bladder roof, trigonum

Typical morphology ⇨ possible diagnoses

- Diffuse wall thickening ⇨ cystitis, trabeculated bladder; edema following radiation
- Focal wall thickening, polypoid projecting into the lumen ⇨ suspicious for malignancy

Notable findings

- Jet effect, diverticulum, catheter balloon; indwelling catheter to be clamped before examination!

Genital Organs

Locational descriptions

- Parametrial, intramural, submucosal, endometrial, ischial fossa, pelvic wall, periprostatic

Typical morphology ⇨ possible diagnoses

- Hypodense, water-isodense space-occupying lesion in the scrotum ⇨ hydrocele, varicocele
- Nodular thickening of the myometrium ⇨ benign myomas, but also small uterine cancers
- Growth beyond organ outline, infiltration of rectal and bladder wall ⇨ suspicious for malignancy

Notable findings

- Thin sections through the lesser pelvis, rectal administration of contrast medium

Gastrointestinal Tract

Typical morphology ⇨ possible diagnoses

- Generalized diffuse wall thickening ⇨ lymphoma; ischemia; ulcerative colitis
- Segmental wall thickening ⇨ Crohn's disease
- Air-fluid levels within lumen and dilatation ⇨ intestinal atony to ileus
- Free air in the abdomen ⇨ perforation
- Intramural air ⇨ suspicious for necrotic intestinal wall (ischemic or inflammatory); caution: DD diverticulum!

Notable findings

- Selection of suitable oral contrast medium (refer to p. 19)

Vessels / retroperitoneum

Locational descriptions

- Para-aortal, paracaval, interaortocaval, prevertebral, retrocrural, mesenteric, para-iliac, inguinal, cervical

Typical morphology ⇨ possible diagnoses

- Dilated aortic lumen with different times of opacification and detection of a septum ⇨ dissected aneurysm
- Reticulonodular thickening of the peritoneum with nodular projections and ascites ⇨ peritoneal carcinomatosis
- Endoluminal hypodense defects c thrombi; caution: DD inflow effect (refer to pp. 21-23, 73)

Bone / Skeleton

Locational descriptions

- Cortical, subchondral, juxta-articular, metaphyseal, diaphyseal, epiphyseal, intra- and extraspinal

Typical morphology ⇨ possible diagnoses

- Step-deformity of the cortex, cortical break, fracture line ⇨ fracture
- Articular involvement ⇨ risk of secondary degenerative osteoarthritis
- Focal hypodensity of the spongiosa with absent trabeculae ⇨ pathologic bone marrow infiltration

Notable findings

- Evaluation of stability, MPR, 3D reconstruction, myelo-CT of the spine

C   Checklists

The checklists represent the third part of this primer. They are not repeated here. They can be found as inserts or on the following pages:

The **physical radiation dose D** (energy absorbed per unit mass) is expressed in Gray (Gy), used for any type of radiation and also in the radiation therapy of malignant tumors. It has to be distinguished from the **equivalence dose H** expressed in Sievert (Sv), which represents the physical radiation dose multiplied by a proportionality factor that considers the unique radiation sensitivity of a particular tissue: Epithelium, mucosa of the respiratory and gastrointestinal tract and other tissues with a high rate of cell division (e.g., blood forming cells of the bone marrow) are more sensitive to ionizing radiation than tissue with dormant cell division.

An even better comparison of the biologic effect can be achieved with the **effective dose E**, which is the sum of the doses delivered to the individual organ. This effective dose, which weighs the relative inherent sensitivities, is also expressed in Sievert (Sv) or Millisievert (mSv). Furthermore, the patient's age at the time of radiation exposure must be included in a rational assessment of the radiation risk since the latency period of a radiation-induced tumor can be rather long (decades). Table 174.1 lists the risk coefficients of different organs following a low-dose exposure to the entire body.

Age-dependency of cancer mortality caused by ionizing radiation Estimated risk factors in (% / Sv) for men / women						
Age at exposure	Total	Leukemia	Lung / Respiratory	MDT	Chest	Others
5 years	12.8 / 15.3	1.1 / 0.8	0.2 / 0.5	3.6 / 6.6	1.3	7.8 / 6.3
15 years	11.4 / 15.7	1.1 / 0.7	0.5 / 0.7	3.7 / 6.5	3.0	6.1 / 4.8
25 years	9.2 / 11.8	0.4 / 0.3	1.2 / 1.3	3.9 / 6.8	0.5	3.7 / 2.9
45 years	6.0 / 5.4	1.1 / 0.7	3.5 / 2.8	0.2 / 0.7	0.2	1.2 / 1.0
65 years	4.8 / 3.9	1.9 / 1.5	2.7 / 1.7	0.1 / 0.5	-	0.1 / 0.2
85 years	1.1 / 0.9	1.0 / 0.7	0.2 / 0.1	- / 0.04	-	- / -
Mean	7.7 / 8.1	1.1 / 0.8	1.9 / 1.5	1.7 / 2.9	0.7	3.0 / 2.2

Table 174.1

This implies that the risk of radiation-induced malignancies markedly decreases with increasing age at the time of exposure. But not only the patient's age, but also the amount of the individual dose and the length of the time intervals play a decisive role. As a rule of thumb, the lower the individual dose and the longer the intervals between several radiation exposures, the lower the risk of a subsequently induced neoplasm. Among other factors, this depends on the capability of the cellular nuclei to repair DNA breaks with the help of repair enzymes as long as the reparative capacity is not exceeded

by high individual doses. Evidence even exists that protective effects predominate in the low-dose range through activation of protective cell factors (DNA reparase and others). For a better assessment of the risk associated with the medical application of ionizing radiation, it is revealing to consider the daily exposure from natural background radiation: The major component of the natural radiation exposure comes from radon, a noble gas, which gets into the air through the building materials of houses and apartments. Using a strictly theoretical calculation, radon and its decay products may induce 5 to 10% of all bronchial carcinomas. In contrast, medical application of ionizing radiation "only" induces less than 1.5% of all malignancies.

The average annual radiation exposure of about 2.4 mSv has to be put in perspective with the manmade radiation exposure of 1.8 mSv (Table 174.2).

Radiation Source	effektive annual dose	% of annual exposure
Inhalation of radon in aparments	~1.4	33.3 %
Terrestric radiation	~ 0.4	9.5 %
Cosmic radiation	~ 0.3	7.1 %
Incorporation of radioactive isotopes	~ 0.3	7.1 %
Subtotal of natural radiation exposure	**~ 2.4 mSv**	**57.0 %**
Application of ionizing radiation in medicine	~ 1.5	35.7 %
Accident of the Chernobyl nuclear reactor (Europe)	~ 0.02	0.5 %
Fall-out from nuclear weapon tests	~ 0.01	0.2 %
Operation of nuclear reactors	~ 0.01	0.2 %
Occupational radiation exposure	~ 0.01	0.2 %
Subtotal of man-made radiation exposure	**~ 1.8 mSv**	**43.0 %**
Total annual radiation exposure in Germany	**~ 4.2 mSv**	**100.0 %**

Table 174.2 Relative contribution of several radiation sources to the total annual exposure (Europe)

In general, "hard" X-rays used for conventional radiography of the chest are scattered and absorbed less in human tissue than "soft" X-rays used for mammography. The scatter radiation also contributes to the absorption and consequently to the risk associated with a particular examination. Because of the tissue-dependent variability of the risk factors and the different characteristics of the various modalities used in diagnostic radiology, the organ doses are quite diverse.

Examination	Organ / tissue	Organ dose	Effektive dose E
Conventional radiology, chest	Lung, breast	0.3 mSv	0.2 mSv
Conventional radiology, skull	Red bone marrow	4.0 mSv	0.2 mSv
Radiology, C-spine	Thyroid gland	4.5 mSv	2.0 mSv
Radiology, T-spine	Breast, lung	14.0 mSv	5.0 mSv
Radiology, L-spine	Red bone marrow	1.0 mSv	0.4 mSv
DSA of the heart	Lung	20.0 mSv	10.0 mSv
DSA of the kidneys	Red bone marrow	30.0 mSv	10.0 mSv
Fluoroscopy, UGI series	Red bone marrow	17.0 mSv	6.0 mSv
Fluoroscopy, BE	Red bone marrow	3.0 mSv	3.0 mSv
Cranial CT	Red bone marrow	5.0 mSv	2.0 mSv
Chest CT	Lung, chest	20.0 mSv	10.0 mSv
Abdomen CT	Red bone marrow	10.0 mSv	7.0 mSv

Table 175.1 Radiation dose of different radiographic examinations

Type of Spiral CT	Head	Chest	Abdome	Pelvis
16-rows scanner	1,6	2,8	5,4	4,3
32-rows scanner	1,5	2,5	4,8	3,9
64-rows scanner	1,4	2,4	4,7	3,9
128-rows scanner	1,6	2,7	5,3	4,3
Dual Source 128-rows scanner	1,1	2,0	3,0	3,2
Dual Source 192-rows scanner	1,4	1,3	3,2	3,4

Table 175.2

Together with arteriography and fluoroscopy, CT is responsible for a rather high radiation exposure in diagnostic radiology. Multiplying the individual values with the number of the different examinations performed annually reveals that CT is responsible for about a third of the collective total dose.

The different CT examinations deliver the following average radiation doses (Table 175.2). All scan protocols should be used with automatic dose- and kV modulation and with iterative recon with a mean strenght, if possible.

A comparison with air travel is often used in public health discussions: On a long, high altitude transatlantic flight, cosmic rays cause a not irrelevant additional exposure. On a flight from Europe to the West Coast of the U.S.A., this can easily be in the range of certain CT examinations. Other calculations of the cancer risk compare conventional chest radiography with cigarette smoking: A single chest radiograph is believed to have the same cancer risk as smoking seven cigarettes. It should be kept in mind, however, that all mathematical models include several aspects and cofactors that are elusive to exact statistic calculations.

While these comparisons put into perspective an excessive concern of the potential risk of medical radiographic exami-nations, they should not be misused to belittle the radiation risk. To avoid unnecessary risks to the general population, it has become established policy to avoid dispensable radiation exposure in conventional radiology and CT, and to take advantage of any possible reduction of radiation exposure to patients.

It is for the same reason that pulsed fluoroscopy has replaced continuous fluoroscopy for upper GI series, enteroclysis and barium enema: The examiner selects between several pulse sequences with 1, 2, 4, and 8 images per second. The resultant dose reduction is considerable. The next pages describe solutions suitable for dose reduction that are especially applicable for CT.

Automatic Bolus Tracking (BT)

For CT, several techniques are available for reducing the radiation dose to the patient. Especially CT requiring optimal contrast enhancement in the vessels, e.g., above all CT angiography, should be performed with automatic bolus tracking to avoid unnecessary duplications because of inadequate intravascular contrast enhancement. This software solution offers the examiner the possibility to place a region of interest (ROI) (✐) just before or at the beginning of the target region, e.g., the lumen of the descending aorta (Fig. 176.1a). After selecting a certain threshold value for the density of the aorta, e.g., 100 HU, the unit measures the density automatically at the preselected site every second after the beginning of the intravenous injection of contrast medium, usually through the cubital vein.

Data acquisition (the actual scanning process) begins as soon as the density in the aortic lumen exceeds the threshold value, i.e., exactly when the bolus of the contrast medium has reached the selected target region after passage through the pulmonary circulation (Fig. 176.1b).

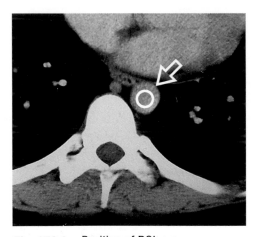

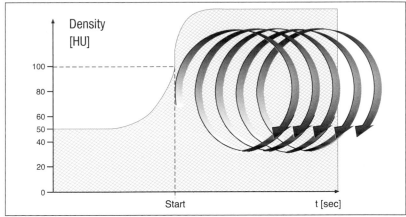

Fig. 176.1a   Position of ROI, e.g., over the descending aorta.

Fig. 176.1b   Automatic delay of data acquisition until arrival of the CM bolus at the target region.

In addition, the amount of contrast medium needed to achieve the same contrast enhancement can be reduced: sterile physiologic NaCl solution is injected from a second syringe of the injection pump (see front cover flap) at the same flow rate immediately following the injection of contrast medium in order to push the contrast medium faster and at a higher concentration through the brachial veins toward the heart and through the pulmonary circulation.

Taking Advantage of the Pitch

By using a faster table feed to increase the pitch, a few singleslice CT units can reduce the effective patient dose by spreading the spiral of data acquisition (see Fig. 8.4).

The software of the multislice technology uses a compensatory mechanism that automatically increases the tube current when-ever the examiner increases the pitch – effectively delivering the same total dose for the examination. For a 16-slice CT, the examiner can select the craniocaudal span of the z-axis, the collimation and scan time for the desired volume – and the software determines the optimal table feed or, respectively, pitch, and the tube current.

Reduced Tube Current for Thin Patients and Children

As a rule of thumb, the noise doubles for each 8-cm increase in the patient's diameter. Dose and noise are exponentially related: Doubling the dose reduces the noise only by a factor of 1.4. To penetrate thin patients and children for a satisfactory image, a markedly lower radiation dose is adequate. In older units lacking instant radiation measurements at the level of the detectors and modulation of the tube current (see below), the dose can be reduced by lowering the preselected tube current (mAs).

Automatic Tube Current Modulation

The idea underlying this feature of the combined applications to reduce exposure (CARE) is as simple as it is effective: it is based on the assumption that the cross-sections of most body regions are oval rather than circular. With the patient supine, the AP diameter (↕) of the chest, abdomen, and pelvis is definitely shorter than the transverse diameter (↔). Consequently, the tube current is higher in lateral angulation than in anterior or posterior angulation (Fig. 177.1). After each semi-circulation, e.g., every 180 degrees, the same dosis is needed since the additive attenuation of the x-rays is directionally neutral (Fig. 177.2). It is the essence of the automated modulation that the tube current measures the attenuation profile for each tube angulation and calculates the corresponding minimal dose still adequate to achieve an optimal image after an additional 180-degree angulation. As a result, the tube current is modulated

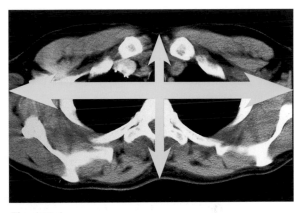

Fig. 177.1

with a 180-degree delay. Plotting the tube current along the time axis displays a curve reminiscent of a sinus curve with the amplitudes tending to decrease from the shoulder to the legs (Fig. 177.3) and with maxima at the level of the shoulder and pelvis.

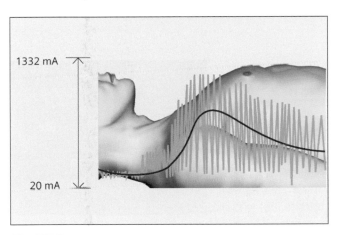

Fig. 177.2

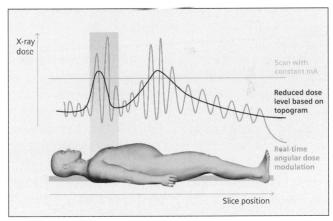

Fig. 177.3

Compared with units delivering the same image quality without tube current modulation, the dose-reducing potential of this technique is impressive, with the highest reduction coinciding with areas of considerable radiation absorption, e.g., at the shoulder and pelvis (Table 177.4).

In addition, the life expectancy of the x-ray tube is extended and image artifacts induced by the arms placed along the patient's body, as frequently found in trauma and ICU patients, are reduced.

Effects of automatic tube current modulation	
Body region	**Dose reduction**
Skull	14 – 26 %
Shoulder region	22 – 56 %
Chest	19 – 27 %
Abdomen	11 – 24 %
Pelvis	21 – 30 %
Extremities	33 – 41 %

Tab. 177.4

Bringing out the information contained in images of CT angiography requires a review using different perspectives (MIP = maximum intensity projection), different reconstruction planes (MPR = multiplanar reconstruction) or a three-dimensional visualization (VRT = volume rendering technique). All these reconstruction images used to be degraded by the resolution of 0.5 mm per pixel length in the transverse plane (xy-plane) and a markedly higher resolution along the body axis (z-axis), resulting in an anisotropic voxel (see page 8) with different lengths. The advances of the multidetector CT (MDCT) with the introduction of the 16-slice technology in the year 2001 permit the inclusion of an adequately large body volume with almost isotropic voxels in the sub-millimeter range with justifiable scan times. The following pages present recommended examination protocols for different vascular regions including several representative images.

Intracranial Arteries

The individual axial sections are usually supplemented with displays using MIP and, e.g., sagittal MPR as well as VRT (see above). A good diagnostic evaluation of the cerebral arteries can be achieved with thin overlapping section reconstructions using a section thickness of 0.6 to 1.25 mm and a reconstruction interval (RI) of 0.4 to 0.8 mm.

To achieve a high vascular contrast, the data acquisition has to be exactly timed to encompass the first passage of contrast medium through the circle of Willis with a start delay of 20 seconds, if possible before contrast medium has reached the venous sinus. If bolus tracking (BT) is not available, a test bolus should be injected to determine the individual circulation time. The following examination protocols can serve as guides for the visualization of the circle of Willis:

Type of spiral CT	Scan Mode	Voltage [kV] A	Voltage [kV] B	[mAs] A	[mAs] B	Coll. [mm]	Rot. Time [s]	Pitch	Recon Direction	ST [mm]	RI [mm]	Kernel	Window W/C [HU]
16-rows scanner	Spiral	80		93		16 x 0.7	0.8	1.50	axial/coro/sag	3.0	3.0	Hv36	700/80
32-rows scanner	Spiral	80		93		32 x 0.7	0.8	1.50	axial/coro/sag	3.0	3.0	Hv36	700/80
64-rows scanner	Spiral	90		82		64 x 0.6	0.33	1.50	axial/coro/sag	3.0	3.0	Hv36	700/80
128-rows scanner	Spiral	90		95		128 x 0.6	0.3	1.50	axial/coro/sag	3.0	3.0	Hv36	700/80
Dual Source 128	Spiral	100		123		128 x 0.6	0.28	0.60	axial/coro	4.0	4.0	Hv38	700/80
Dual Source 128	Dual Energy-Spiral	80	140Sn	178	98	64 x 0.6	0.5	0.70	axial/coro	4.0	4.0	Qr40	700/80
Dual Source 192	Spiral	90		133		128 x 0.6	0.25	0.60	axial/coro	4.0	4.0	Hv36	700/80
Dual Source 192	Dual Energy-Spiral	80	150Sn	100	67	64 x 0.6	0.25	0.70	axial/coro	4.0	4.0	Qr40	700/80

Table 178.1 Protocols for Intracranial Arteries

All scan protocols should be performed with automatic dose- and kV-modulation and with iterative recon with a mean strenght, if possible.

The subsequently reconstructed individual sections can display the vessels as seen from below with transverse MIP (Fig. 178.1b), from the front with coronal MIP (Fig. 178.1c) or from the side with sagittal MIP (Fig. 179.1b). The first two planes clearly show the major branches of the anterior (**91a**) and middle (**91b**) cerebral arteries.

Figure 178.1d shows a 3D VRT of another patient with an aneurysm (✎) arising from the anterior communicating artery. The junction of both vertebral arteries (**88**) to form the basal artery (**90**) and posterior cerebral arteries (**91c**) is clearly identified. Furthermore, the branches of the anterior circulation are identifiable: branches of the medial cerebral artery (**91b**) and the pericallosal arteries (**93**).

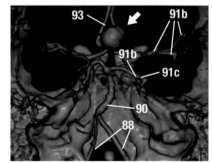

Fig. 178.1d

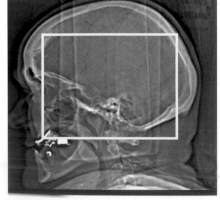

Fig. 178.1a

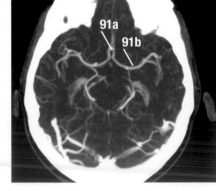

Fig. 178.1b

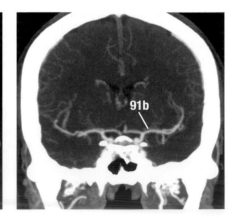

Fig. 178.1c

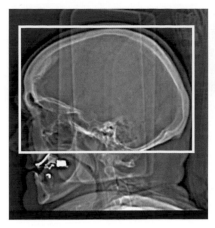

Fig. 179.1a

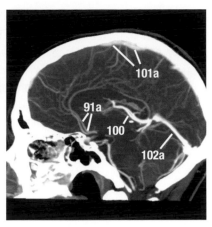

Fig. 179.1b

Venous Sinus

To visualize the venous channels, the FOV has to be extended to the sagittal cranial vault (Fig. 179.1a) and the start delay increased to about 100 seconds. Craniocaudal sections are recommended for both types of CTA (arterial and venous cerebral vessels). The sagittal plane (Fig. 179.1b) preferably shows contrast in the vein of Galen (**100**) and venous channels (**101a, 102a**).

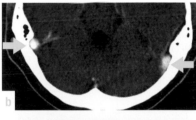

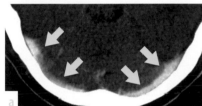

Fig. 179.2

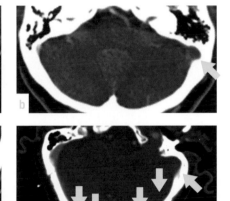

Fig. 179.3

Venous Sinus Thrombosis

In cases of normal venous flow in the cerebral sinuses, you will find hyperdens lumina of both transverse sinuses (in Fig. 179.2a) as well as both sigmoid sinuses (in Fig. 179.2b) without any filling defects in contrast-enhanced images.

In contrast to this, Fig. 179.3 shows unilateral thombosis of the left sigmoid sinus ( ) and bilateral thrombosis of both transverse sinuses ( ).

3D-reconstructions and MIPs might be time-consuming to create, because of the adjacent hyperdense skull, which has to be eliminated first by the investigator at the workstation, before the reconstructions can be done – and they often do not provide useful additional information.

„Triple-Rule Out" protocol

On pages 182-186, you will find special protocols to look for aortic aneurysm, coronary artery stenosis or calcifications and for pulmonary emboli. This protocol might be used to clarify all three issues with only one spiral scanning.

Type of spiral CT	Scan Mode	Voltage [kV] A	Voltage [kV] B	[mAs] A	[mAs] B	Coll. [mm]	Rot. Time [s]	Pitch	Recon Direction	ST [mm]	RI [mm]	Kernel	Window W/C [HU]
64-rows scanner	Spiral	100		47		64 × 0.6	0.33	0.31	axial/coro/sag	3.0	3.0	Bv36	600/200
128-rows scanner	Spiral	100		55		128 × 0.6	0.3	0.31	axial/coro/sag	3.0	3.0	Bv36	600/200
Dual Source 128	Dual Source-Spiral	120		320		128 × 0.6	0.28	3.20	axial/oblique	3.0	3.0	Bv38	600/200
Dual Source 192	Dual Source-Spiral	100		288		192 × 0.6	0.25	3.20	axial/oblique	3.0	3.0	Bv36	600/200

Table 179.4 Tripel Rule Out: Aorta - Pulmonary Embolism - Coronary Arteries (feed/rotation and pitch depending on heart rate)

Carotid Arteries

Important criteria for stenotic processes of the carotid arteries are the exact determination of the severity of the stenosis. It is for this reason that the examination is carried out with thin sections, for instance, 4 x 1 mm or 16 x 0.75 mm, allowing direct planimetric quantification of the stenosis with adequate accuracy on individual axial sections. Furthermore, the sagittal and coronal MIP (0.7 – 1.0 mm RI with 50% sectional overlapping) shows no major step deformity (see page 8).

The best reconstruction with maximal contrast of the carotid artery is achieved with minimal contrast in the jugular vein. Therefore, the use of a bolus tracking program is strongly advised. If a preceding Doppler examination suggests a vascular process at the bifurcation, transverse images in caudocranial direction are recommended. For processes near the cranial base, a craniocaudal direction can be superior. VRT often proves helpful to get oriented (Figs. 180.1d, 180.2b).

Type of spiral CT	Scan Mode	Voltage [kV] A	Voltage [kV] B	[mAs] A	[mAs] B	Coll. [mm]	Rot. Time [s]	Pitch	Recon Direction	ST [mm]	RI [mm]	Kernel	Window W/C [HU]
16-rows scanner	Spiral	110		110		16 x 0.7	0.8	1.20	sag/coro/axial	3.0	3.0	Bv36	700/80
32-rows scanner	Spiral	110		110		32 x 0.7	0.8	1.20	sag/coro/axial	3.0	3.0	Bv36	700/80
64-rows scanner	Spiral	100		113		64 x 0.6	0.33	1.20	sag/coro/axial	3.0	3.0	Bv36	700/80
128-rows scanner	Spiral	100		130		64 x 0.6	0.3	1.20	sag/coro/axial	3.0	3.0	Bv36	700/80
Dual Source 128	Spiral	120		84		128 x 0.6	0.28	1.20	axial/coro	3.0	3.0	Bv38	700/80
Dual Source 128	Dual Energy-Spiral	100	140Sn	83	83	128 x 0.6	0.28	0.70	axia /coro	3.0	3.0	Qr40	700/80
Dual Source 192	Spiral	120		84		128 x 0.6	0.25	1.20	axial/coro	3.0	3.0	Bv36	700/80
Dual Source 192	Dual Energy-Spiral	90	150Sn	90	69	192 x 0.6	0.25	0.70	axial/coro	3.0	3.0	Qr40	700/80

Table 180.1 Protocols for Carotid Arteries

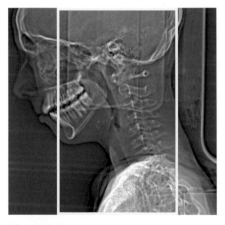
Fig. 180.1a

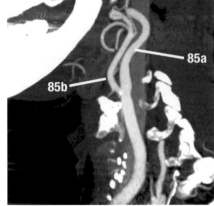
Fig. 180.1b

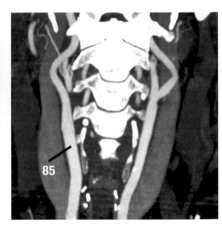
Fig. 180.1c

Figure 180.1 shows the lateral topogram (**a**) for positioning of the FOV as well as lateral (**b**) and anterior (**c**) images of an MIP and an image in VRT (**d**), showing normal findings. In contrast, Figure 180.2 shows images of sagittal MIP and VTR that reveal two indentations of the vascular contrast column at

the typical site for a carotid stenosis: The left ACI (**85a**) shows a short segment of a severe luminal narrowing just distal to the bifurcation ( ) after a preceding bulbar stenosis ( ) of the ACC (**85**) at the origin of the ACE (**85b**).

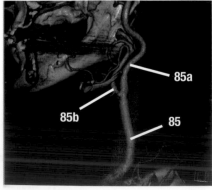
Fig. 180.1d

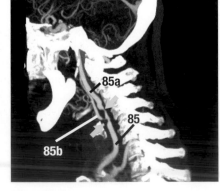
Fig. 180.2a

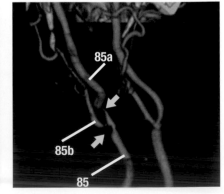
Fig. 180.2 b

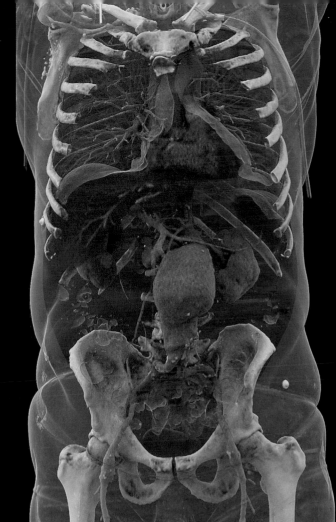
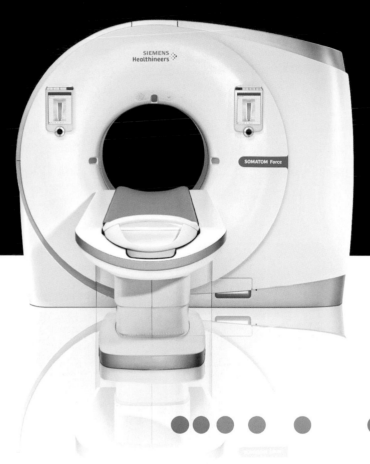
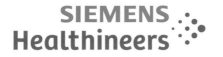

Aorta

The CT angiography of the aorta must above all exclude aneurysms, isthmus stenoses and possible dissection, and if present, visualize their extent. Automatic bolus tracking (BT: ROI placed over the aorta) is advisable, especially in patients with cardiac diseases who have variable pulmonary circulation times of contrast medium. Imaging in caudocranial direction can minimize the respiration-induced motion artifacts that primarily affect the regions close to the diaphragm since involuntary respiratory excursions are more likely at the end of the examination. Furthermore, caudocranial imaging avoids the initial venous inflow of contrast medium through the subclavian and brachiocephalic veins and any superimposition on the supra-aortic arteries.

Type of spiral CT	Scan Mode	Voltage [kV] A	Voltage [kV] B	[mAs] A	[mAs] B	Coll. [mm]	Rot. Time [s]	Pitch	Recon Direction	ST [mm]	RI [mm]	Kernel	Window W/C [HU]
16-rows scanner	Spiral	110		57		16 x 0.7	0.8	1.50	sag/coro/axial	5.0	5.0	Bv36	700/80
32-rows scanner	Spiral	110		57		32 x 0.7	0.8	1.50	sag/coro/axial	5.0	5.0	Bv36	700/80
64-rows scanner	Spiral	100		62		64 x 0.6	0.33	1.50	sag/coro/axial	5.0	5.0	Bv36	700/80
128-rows scanner	Spiral	100		72		64 x 0.6	0.3	1.50	sag/coro/axial	5.0	5.0	Bv36	700/80
Dual Source 128	Spiral	100		112		128 x 0.6	0.28	2.20	axial oblique	3.0	3.0	Bv38	700/80
Dual Source 128	Dual Energy-Spiral	100	140Sn	95	74	128 x 0.6	0.33	0.70	axia /oblique	3.0	3.0	Qr40	700/80
Dual Source 192	Spiral	80		174		192 x 0.6	0.25	1.90	axial/oblique	3.0	3.0	Bv36	700/80
Dual Source 192	Dual Energy-Spiral	90	150Sn	95	59	192 x 0.6	0.25	0.70	axial/oblique	3.0	3.0	Qr40	700/80

Table 182.1 Protocols for Aorta

As reconstruction images, MIP and MPR (Figs. 182.3, 182.4) often allow an exact quantification of the vascular pathology as survey images in VRT (Fig. 182.5), as seen here as an example of an infrarenal aneurysm of the abdominal aorta: The aneurysmal dilatation (**171**) begins immediately distal to the renal arteries (**110**) and spares both the superior mesenteric artery (**106**) and iliac arteries (**113**).

For planning any vascular surgery, it is crucial to know any involvement of visceral and peripheral arteries and any possible associated dissection. Furthermore, the level of the aortic origin of the artery of Adamkiewicz, which supplies the thoracospinal transition of the spinal cord, must be considered for aneurysms of the descending thoracic aorta.

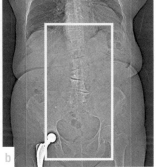

Fig. 182.2

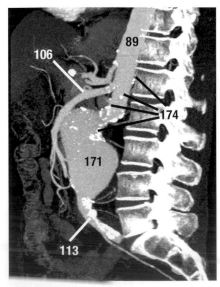

Fig. 182.3

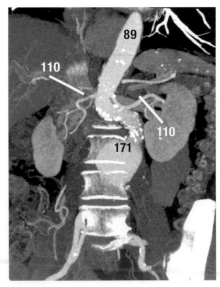

Fig. 182.4

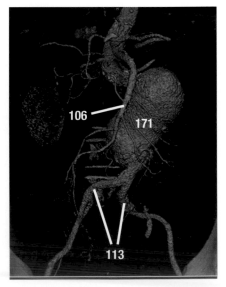

Fig. 182.5

Frequently, a cine mode review of the coronal or sagittal MPR images on a second monitor can be helpful for a quick and convincing determination of the extent of a pathologic finding, as shown here in a case of thrombosis within an abdominal aortic aneurysm. The cine mode of the coronal MPR images reveals not only an infrarenal thrombus (**173**) along the left lateral wall (Fig. 183.1) but also a second thrombus further cranial along the right lateral wall at the level of the origin of the right renal artery (**110**) (Fig. 183.1), which is still perfused (Fig. 183.3). The individual axial sections (Figs. 183.4, 5) allow a planimetric quantification of the stenosis, and the sagittal MPR (Fig. 183.6) a clear separation from the origin of the anterior mesenteric artery (**106**).

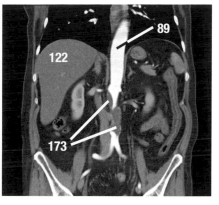

Fig. 183.1

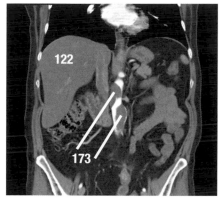

Fig. 183.2

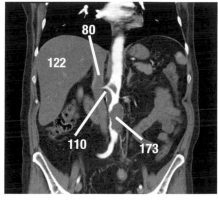

Fig. 183.3

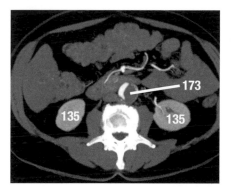

Fig. 183.4

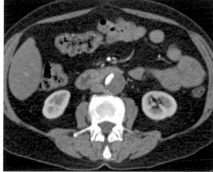

Fig. 183.5

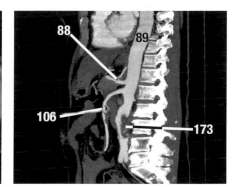

Fig. 183.6

Of course, the benefit of the three-dimensional visualization by means of VRT also depends on the viewing angle. While viewing from an angle (Fig. 183.7) can underestimate the extent of the thrombus and easily mistake it for a soft plaque, the extent is much better appreciated if seen from different viewing angles (Figs. 183.8 and 183.9). The final images illustrate the effect of a careful elimination of interfering superimposed osseous structures. Because of its high density, the lumbar spine dominates the initial image (Fig. 183.8), and the vascular findings are only fully appreciated after subtraction of the lumbar spine (Fig. 183.9).

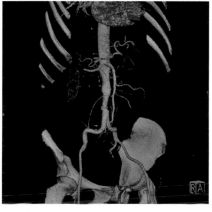

Fig. 183.7

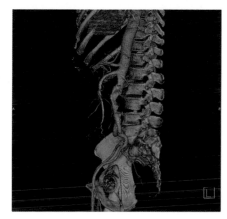

Fig. 183.8

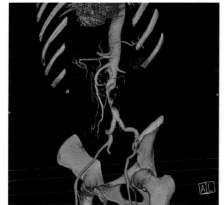

Fig. 183.9

Pulmonary Vasculature (Pulmonary Emboli)

FOV and volume to be scanned are marked on the topogram (Fig. 186.2), beginning from just above the aortic arch, to visualize primarily the central hilar vessels and the heart with the right atrium (a possible source of emboli). Lateral and apical regions of the lung are dispensable. The total acquisition time should not exceed 15 seconds in order to complete the examination during a single breath hold without artifacts. The images are best obtained from caudal to cranial, to have the motion-sensitive areas close to the diaphragm already completed during the end phase and to minimize the artifacts caused by the venous inflow of contrast medium through brachiocephalic veins and superior vena cava. Exact timing with bolus tracking (BT, ROI over the pulmonary outflow tract) is strongly advised. The reconstructed sections should not be less than 3 mm in width. The sections for the MIP should be close to 1.0 mm to avoid overlooking small subtle pulmonary emboli.

Type of spiral CT	Scan Mode	Voltage [kV] A	Voltage [kV] B	[mAs] A	[mAs] B	Coll. [mm]	Rot. Time [s]	Pitch	Recon Direction	ST [mm]	RI [mm]	Kernel	Window W/C [HU]
16-rows scanner	Spiral	110		57		16 x 0.7	0.80	1.50	sag/coro/axial	3.0	3.0	Bv36	700/80
32-rows scanner	Spiral	110		57		32 x 0.7	0.80	1.50	sag/coro/axial	3.0	3.0	Bv36	700/80
64-rows scanner	Spiral	100		62		64 x 0.6	0.33	1.50	sag/coro/axial	3.0	3.0	Bv36	700/80
128-rows scanner	Spiral	100		72		64 x 0.6	0.3	1.50	sag/coro/axial	3.0	3.0	Bv36	700/80
Dual Source 128	Dual Source-Spiral	100		120		128 x 0.6	0.28	2.20	axial/oblique	3.0	3.0	Bv38	700/80
Dual Source 192	Dual Source-Spiral	100		120		192 x 0.6	0.25	1.90	axial/oblique	3.0	3.0	Bv36	700/80

Table 186.1   Protocols for Pulmonary Embolism

The vascular lumina contrast well with the pulmonary tissue (Figs. 186.3 - 186.6) and extend all the way to the periphery. Acute pulmonary emboli (Figs. 186.7 and 186.8) cause intravascular defects representing thrombi (**173**), located in this case in the right pulmonary artery (**90a**).

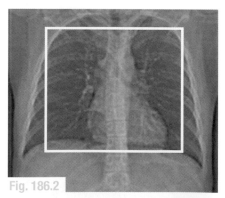

Fig. 186.2

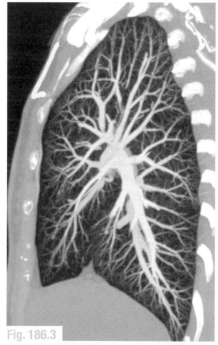

Fig. 186.3

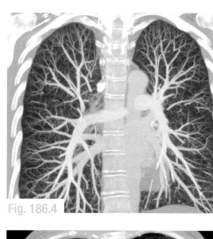

Fig. 186.4

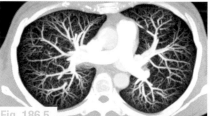

Fig. 186.5

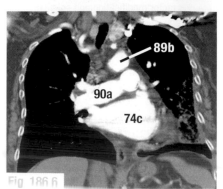

Fig. 186.6

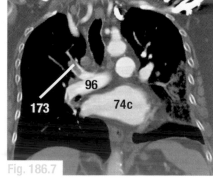

Fig. 186.7

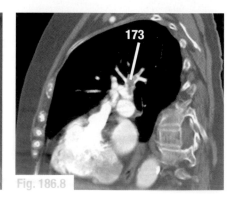

Fig. 186.8

Abdominal Vessels

Most pathologic vascular processes are located close to the center at the origin of major vascular branches, allowing the FOV to be confined to the central two thirds of the abdominal space on the topogram (Fig. 187.2). The origins of the vessels arising from the abdominal aorta are visualized on axial sections and on MIP and MPR images. If a larger volume needs to be acquired on the z-axis, a four-slice CT needs a collimation of 4 x 2.5 mm to achieve an acceptable acquisition time during one breath hold. In contrast, a suspected renal artery stenosis requires a reduction of the acquisition volume to the

renal region. To achieve an adequate visualization of possible stenoses in thin renal arteries, the examination should be performed with thin sections of, for instance, 6 x 1 mm and with an RI of only 0.6 mm.

Since the individual circulation times often vary, a fixed delay of the injection of contrast medium is not recommended, and the use of a test bolus or bolus tracking is suggested instead. The ROI to register the increase in density (arrival of the contrast medium = commencement of the measurement) is best placed over the lumen of the descending aorta (see page 176).

Type of spiral CT	Scan Mode	Voltage [kV] A	Voltage [kV] B	[mAs] A	[mAs] B	Coll. [mm]	Rot. Time [s]	Pitch	Recon Direction	ST [mm]	RI [mm]	Kernel	Window W/C [HU]
16-rows scanner	Spiral	110		94		16 x 0.7	0.8	1.50	sag/coro/axial	5.0	5.0	Bv36	700/80
32-rows scanner	Spiral	110		94		32 x 0.7	0.8	1.50	sag/coro/axial	5.0	5.0	Bv36	700/80
64-rows scanner	Spiral	100		103		64 x 0.6	0.33	1.50	sag/coro/axial	5.0	5.0	Bv36	700/80
128-rows scanner	Spiral	100		118		64 x 0.6	0.3	1.50	sag/coro/axial	5.0	5.0	Bv36	700/80
Dual Source 128	Spiral	120		84		128 x 0.6	0.5	1.20	axial/coro	5.0	5.0	Bv38	700/80
Dual Source 128	Dual Energy-Spiral	100	140Sn	95	74	128 x 0.6	0.33	0.70	axial/coro	5.0	5.0	Qr40	700/80
Dual Source 192	Spiral	110		90		192 x 0.6	0.5	1.20	axial/coro	5.0	5.0	Bv40	700/80
Dual Source 192	Dual Energy-Spiral	90	150Sn	95	59	192 x 0.6	0.25	0.70	axial/coro	5.0	5.0	Qr40	700/80

Table 187.1 Protocols for Abdominal Vessels

The FOV is placed over the central abdominal space (Fig. 187.2). Normally, the visceral branches of the abdominal aorta show a good luminal contrast without filling defects, including the branches of the mesenterial vessels as shown in Figures

187.3 and 187.4. In case of an occlusion of the superior mesenteric artery (**106**), the interrupted vascular lumen (←) and the collateral vessels (⬈) are easily recognized on VRT and MIP images (Figs. 187.5-7).

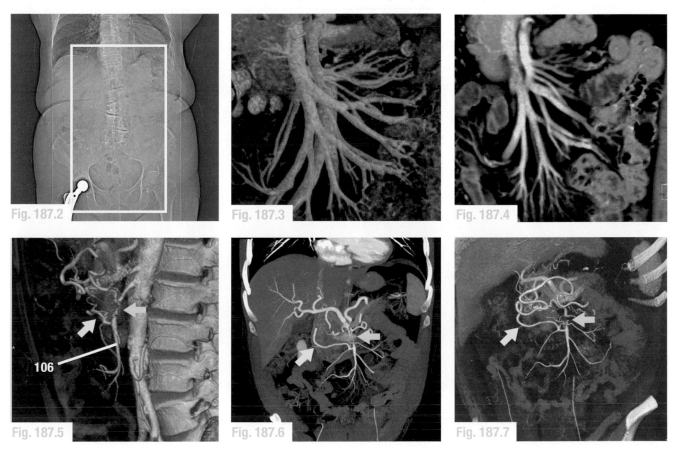

Fig. 187.2

Fig. 187.3

Fig. 187.4

Fig. 187.5

106

Fig. 187.6

Fig. 187.7

Iliofemoral Vessels

For CT angiography of the iliofemoral vessels, the patient is placed feet first on the table. The length of the relevant body region along the z-axis is critical (Fig. 188.3), and therefore it is generally preferred to use a wide collimation of 4 x 2.5 mm or 16 x 1.5 mm (instead of 4 x 1 mm or 16 x 0.75 mm), which allows a faster table feed. Narrow overlapping reconstructions should guarantee the quality of the final images.

Problems can arise with the timing of the injection of CM, especially with unilateral high-degree stenoses because of the slow flow (see below) in the peripheral vessels of the affected side. If bolus tracking (BT) is used, the ROI is placed over the descending thoracic aorta or abdominal aorta to register the increase in the contrast medium-induced density (see page 176). Already VRT images allow a good overview from the aortic bifurcation to the ankle in most cases (Fig. 188.2).

Type of spiral CT	Scan Mode	Voltage [kV] A	Voltage [kV] B	[mAs] A	[mAs] B	Coll. [mm]	Rot. Time [s]	Pitch	Recon Direction	ST [mm]	RI [mm]	Ker-nel	Window W/C [HU]
16-rows scanner	Spiral	110		110		16 x 0.7	0.8	1.50	sag/coro/axial	5.0	5.0	Bv36	700/80
32-rows scanner	Spiral	110		125		32 x 0.7	0.8	1.00	sag/coro/axial	5.0	5.0	Bv36	700/80
64-rows scanner	Spiral	100		136		64 x 0.6	0.33	0.35	sag/coro/axial	5.0	5.0	Bv36	700/80
128-rows scanner	Spiral	100		157		128 x 0.6	0.5	0.35	sag/coro/axial	5.0	5.0	Bv36	700/80
Dual Source 128	Spiral	120		84		128 x 0.6	0.50	0.60	axial/coro	5.0	5.0	Bv38	700/80
Dual Source 128	Dual Energy-Spiral	80	140Sn	184	78	64 x 0.6	0.33	0.70	axial/coro	5.0	5.0	Qr40	700/80
Dual Source 192	Spiral	110		90		128 x 0.6	0.50	0.60	axial/coro	5.0	5.0	Bv40	700/80
Dual Source 192	Dual Energy-Spiral	80	150Sn	120	67	128 x 0.6	0.25	0.70	axial/coro	5.0	5.0	Qr40	700/80

Table 188.1 Protocols for Iliofemoral Vessels

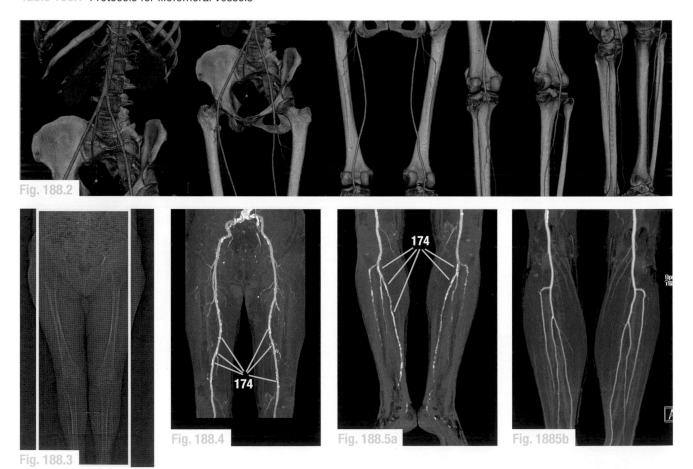

Fig. 188.2

Fig. 188.3

Fig. 188.4

Fig. 188.5a

Fig. 1885b

In cases of peripheral arterial occlusive disease, both arterio-sclerotic plaques (**174**) and luminal narrowing with impaired flow distally (Fig. 188.5a) are clearly recognized in comparison with a normal post-stenotic flow in the tibioperoneal vessels

(Fig. 188.5b). In high-degree peripheral arterial occlusive disease examined with a table feed of > 3 cm/sec, the flow can be so much delayed that the craniocaudal acquisition leaves the bolus behind.

Vascular Prothesis

CT angiography is also suitable to follow implanted stents or vascular prostheses (**182**) that interfere with the assessment of mural calcifications because of acoustic shadowing (Fig. 189.1-3) in color duplex sonography images.

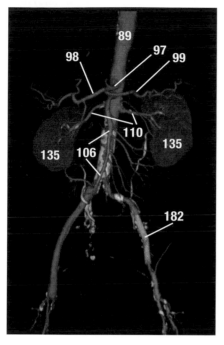

Fig. 189.1

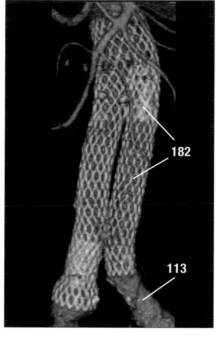

Fig. 189.2

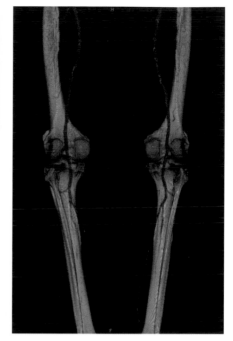

Fig. 189.3

Outlook

CT angiography undergoes rapid technical changes and its advancement can be expected to escalate due to more chip capacity and increasing computer power. It is foreseeable that separate work stations with user-friendly software and partially automated programs will shorten reconstructions using VRT further. Generating images of the descending aorta (Fig. 189.4) or major thoracic vessels (Fig. 189.5) with VRT and MIP as illustrated here will become ever more effortless. This represents a challenge for the user to stay abreast with the technical developments and to keep the departmental protocols of the various CTA applications up to date.

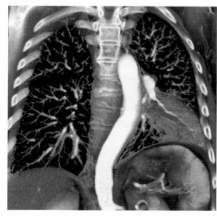

Fig. 189.4

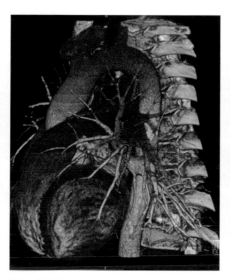

Fig. 189.5a

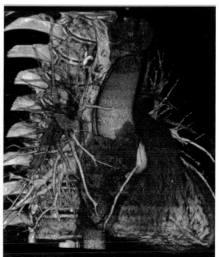

Fig. 189.5b

When unpacking and connecting the lines between the infusion pump and the patient, be sure to practice sterile technique and either wear gloves or use a hand sanitizer (Fig. 192.1). If your hands are wet with alcohol, do <u>not</u> touch the adapters or connectors because contact with alcohol will make them brittle and may cause them to crack (Fig. 192.2). This cannot happen if you let your hands dry briefly after sanitizing them. Next remove the two injection syringes from their package and insert them (⇧) with the plunger head down (☆, weakest part of the system) into their holders ↘ in Fig. 192.3.

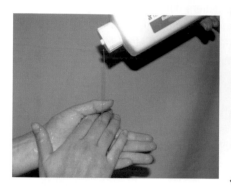

Fig. 192.1 Use a hand sanitizer

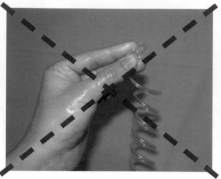

Fig. 192.2 Do not grasp with wet hands

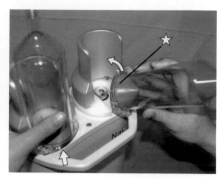

Fig. 192.3 Install the syringes

Place the injector in a vertical position (Fig. 192.4). Then enter the syringe type that is being used (↘ , Fig. 192.5). Generally the filling speed for the contrast syringe should not exceed 3 mL/s (⇦ ,Fig. 192.6). If drawn at a faster speed, the viscous CM could create foam, making it harder to remove the air from the system later on.

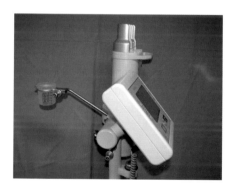

Fig. 192.4 Position the injector upright

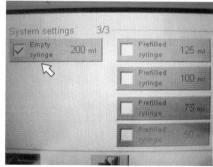

Fig. 192.5 Enter the syringe type

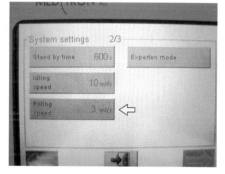

Fig. 192.6 Fill speed ≤ 3 mL/s

Push the button that raises the plunger (shown here in blue) to the "ready to fill" position (Fig. 192.7) and confirm that the patient is not yet connected (precaution against air embolism, Fig. 192.8). Use this time to remove the tubing from the set and connect it.

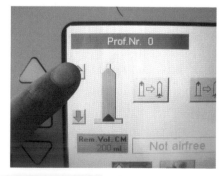

Fig. 192.7 Raise plunger to "ready to fill" position

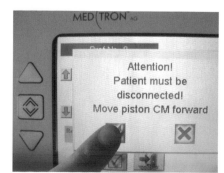

Fig. 192.8 Confirm that the patient is not yet connected

While the plungers are being raised, connect the two lines to the built-in valves (shown here in green, Fig. 193.1) by twisting them 180° clockwise (↻). Do not overtighten the connectors; otherwise they may be very difficult to disconnect later since the CM is somewhat viscous and may acquire a sticky consistency when exposed to air. Connect the tubing for the CM (in this case green-coded) on the left side and the white-coded pressure tubing for the saline on the right side. Figure 193.2 illustrates how the setup should look. The built-in valves permit flow in one direction only: either from the solution bottle toward the syringes (⚠) or from the syringes toward the patient (⇧⇧ in Fig. 193.3). If the plungers are still moving when the hookups are being made, air flow through the valves may produce a whistling sound; this is a normal occurrence and is no cause for concern.

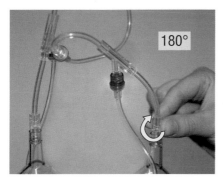

Fig. 193.1 Connect the tubing

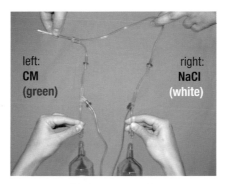

Fig. 193.2 Tubing connections

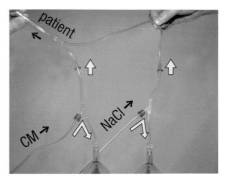

Fig. 193.3 Possible flow directions

Now connect the green-coded line to the CM bottle by first removing the protective cap (✎), inserting the spike (⇧ in Fig. 193.4), opening the vent valve (↶ in Fig. 193.5), and squeezing the drip chamber two or three times (⇨◁⇦) to fill it one-third to one-half full (Fig. 193.6). Do the same on the other side with the saline bottle. Then press the button to draw CM into the syringe (Fig. 193.7). Enter the desired fill volume, activate the plunger-down sequence (Fig. 193.8), and repeat these steps on the right side for drawing saline into the second syringe (Fig. 193.9).

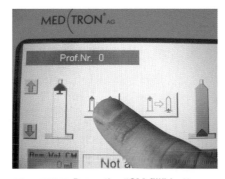

Fig. 193.4 Remove cap and insert spike

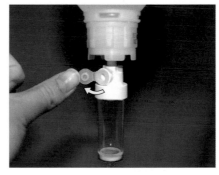

Fig. 193.5 Open the vent valve

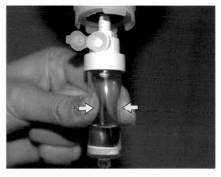

Fig. 193.6 Prime the drip chamber to half-full

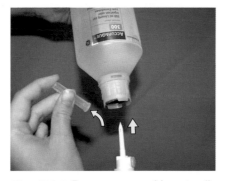

Fig. 193.7 Press the "CM fill" button

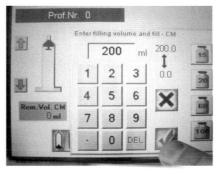

Fig. 193.8 Enter the desired volume

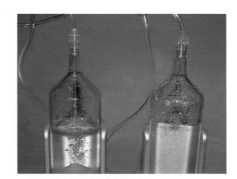

Fig. 193.9 Draw CM or saline into the syringe

Next connect the (straight or coiled) patient line (Fig. 194.1) so that all air can be removed from the system. With the injector in a vertical position, press the yellow button to remove the air from the CM limb before the patient is connected. This triangular button (▷) activates a very slow forward flow that can be stepped up if necessary by pressing the square yellow button (◁) one or more times (Fig. 194.2). Meanwhile hold the end of the line over a collection vessel until all the air has been expelled (Fig. 194.3). Do the same on the right side for the saline limb of the system (Figs. 194.4, 194.5), then hang the sterile end of the tubing on the special holder (Fig. 194.6) without touching it.

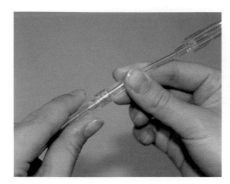

Fig. 194.1 Connect the patient line

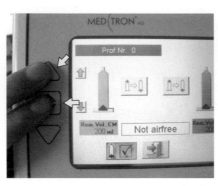

Fig. 194.2 Remove air on the CM side

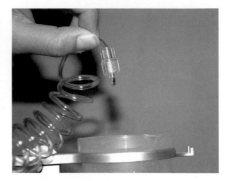

Fig. 194.3 Collection vessel

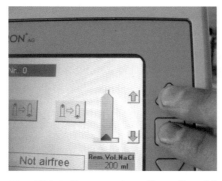

Fig. 194.4 Remove air on the saline side

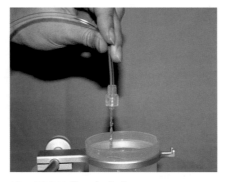

Fig. 194.5 Expel all air …

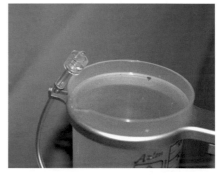

Fig. 194.6 … and hang the sterile (!) tip on its holder

Given the importance of avoiding IV air injection (risk of air embolism!), confirm twice on the unit that all air has been expelled from the system (Figs. 194.7, 194.8). Then invert the injector (↻), tilting it down from the vertical fill position to the injection position (Fig. 194.9). Make sure that the tip of the injector is level with the arm of the supine patient (it should not be higher or lower, if possible).

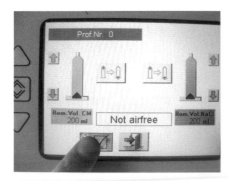

Fig. 194.7 Confirm air removal on the unit

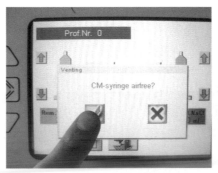

Fig. 194.8 Reconfirm

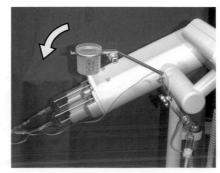

Fig. 194.9 Invert the injector

Before you connect the high-pressure tubing to the IV catheter in the patient's arm, make sure that the catheter is within the vessel and can tolerate the proposed flow rate. Many radiology departments do this by preparing kidney basins that are stocked with airless high-pressure tubing in addition to a 5- or 10-mL manual syringe filled with sterile isotonic saline (Fig. 196.1). Inject this test bolus briskly (⇧) into the IV catheter (Fig. 196.2) and watch closely to see if the saline passes freely through the catheter and into the vein, or if it extravasates and forms a subcutaneous wheal (✐ , Fig. 196.3). In the latter case the catheter should be removed (⇨) and a new IV access should be established.

Using the test-bolus function of some injection systems may be problematic if the test is done from an adjacent room without having a colleague directly observing the venipuncture site to see if extravasation occurs.

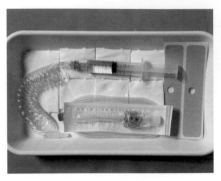

Fig. 196.1   Saline test bolus

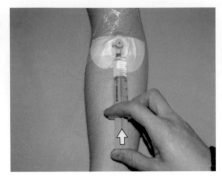

Fig. 196.2   Test injection OK?

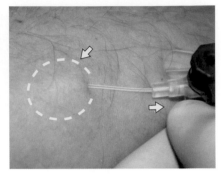

Fig. 196.3   Extravasation?
Replace IV catheter!

The line connected to the IV catheter may be straight (Fig. 196.4, right side), or coiled high-pressure tubing may be used as an alternative (Fig. 196.4, left side). The advantage of coiled tubing is that it is more compliant and less likely to become trapped, for example, between the moving CT gantry and the patient table.

Never use "ordinary" extension tubing because it may lack the necessary pressure stability (thinner, softer wall) and may even burst during the injection (Fig. 196.5). If you have ever had to clean up sticky contrast material that has been sprayed all over the scan room by pressure from the infusion pump, you will appreciate the importance of heavy-duty tubing.

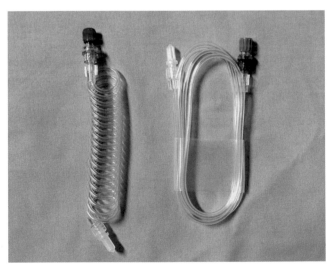

Fig. 196.4   Types of pressure tubing

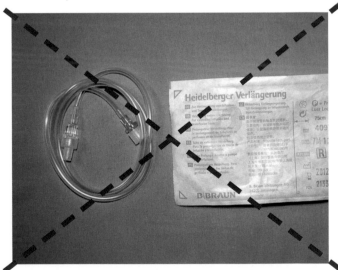

Fig. 196.5   Do not use "ordinary" extension tubing!

Start and User Options

A major advantage of the power injector is the ability to store different contrast injection profiles and quickly access the profile that is best for a specific investigation or body region; particularly in multiphase contrast prot cols, such as a brief injection phase at a relatively high flow rate followed by a sec-

ond phase at a lower flow rate and a saline chaser (Fig. 197.1). This memory option will spare the user from having to reenter all essential settings (volume, concentration, flow rate, delay options, etc.). The monitor image on the operating console has a similar display (Fig. 197.2).

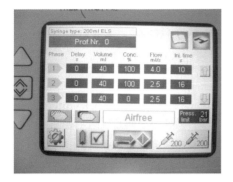

Fig. 197.1 Example of a multiphase protocol

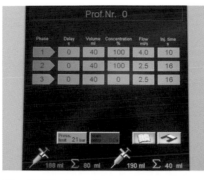

Fig. 197.2 Operating console

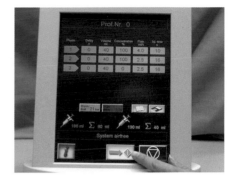

Fig. 197.3 Start screen

After you have selected the desired profile for the current patient and made any necessary modifications, go to the start screen (Fig. 197.3) and initiate the automatic contrast injection (Fig. 197.4). If you are not using bolus tracking for automatic start and data acquisition, do not forget to initiate

the scan after a suitable delay time. Of course, you can track the progress of the individual injections on the monitor (Fig. 197.5) or stop the injection at any time if problems arise (disconnected IV line, patient distress, etc.) (Fig. 197.6).

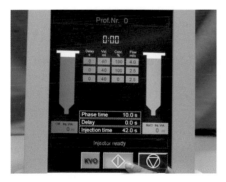

Fig. 197.4 Start contrast injection

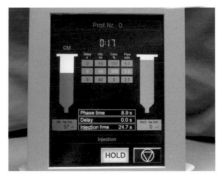

Fig. 197.5 Check progression of phases

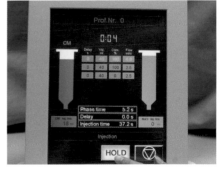

Fig. 197.6 Stop, end procedure

The KVO (keep vein open) function is of interest in longer procedures such as CT-guided biopsies (see p. 168). This function automatically flushes the IV catheter with 0.5 mL saline every 2 minutes to maintain access for later contrast injections or for some other, subsequent use of the IV line.

For special investigations, the concentration of the CM drawn into the syringe can be diluted during any injection phase by automatically adding isotonic saline to the medium while it is still in the syringe. This option eliminates the need to completely replace the syringe contents during the study.

z-Flying Focal Spot

Several techniques have been established that can provide submillimeter resolution with short breath holds, even in routine protocols. The entire x-ray tube rotates in an oil bath, so that the anode is in direct contact with the cooling oil. The central cathode rotates as well. In recent years, further improvements in spatial and temporal resolution have been achieved by adding periodic motion of the focal spot in the longitudinal direction (z-axis).

Permanent electromagnetic deflection of the electron beam is used to control the shape and position of the focal spot. In this way the focal spot is made to "fly" back and forth between two different positions on the anode (indicated by the two asterisks in Fig. 198.1). Since the anode plate is typically angled by approximately 7-9°, this deflection translates into motion of the x-rays in both the z-axis direction and the radial direction.

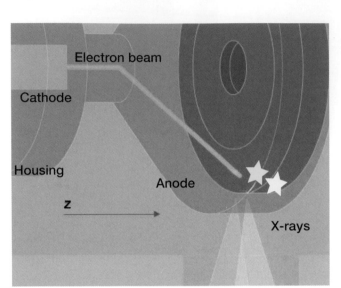

Fig. 198.1

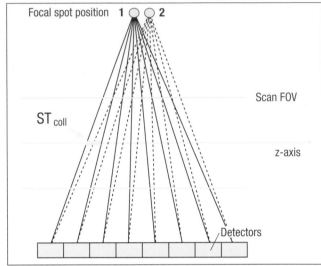

Fig. 198.2

Applied to a 64-slice CT scanner, this technology can double the number of simultaneously acquired slices, say, to 64 overlapping 0.6-mm slices per rotation, similar to the sampling scheme of a 64 x 0.3-mm detector (Fig. 198.2). The periodic motion of the focal spot on the z-axis can achieve a resolution equal to just half the collimated slice thickness at the isocenter ($ST_{coll}/2$). This double-z sampling is no longer optimal at greater distances from the isocenter, however, and

so ultimately the highest z-axis resolution that can be achieved is approximately 0.33–0.36 mm (14–15 lp/cm [47, 48].

The focal spot can also be deflected within the axial scan plane (for clarity, not shown here) to improve in-plane resolution. When this deflection is added to the scan, the focal spot flies within a roughly rectangular area that is constantly controlled by the electromagnetic deflection of the electron beam.

Data Acquisition System

The dual source CT technique was introduced onto the market by Siemens Healthineers. These systems, called Somatom Definition, Flash, Drive and Force, incorporate two detector systems: one with a 50-cm FOV and almost 88,000 detector elements, and a smaller array. It also has two separate x-ray tubes, which can be operated in different modes. Most routine examinations can be performed with only one tube/detector pair. But cardiac patients, trauma patients, and very obese patients can be scanned at a tube output of 2 x 80 kW. This dual power mode combines the output of two x-ray tubes to obtain high performance and/or high scan speeds when specifically needed, as in CT angiography of the iliofemoral, pulmonary, and abdominal vessels (see pp. 186–188) or the coronary arteries (see pp. 184–185).

Another advantage of these new scanner systems is their speed: The shorter gantry rotation time up to 0.25 seconds can provide temporal resolutions as high as 62 ms with ECG-gated reconstruction. This feature is particularly useful in cardiac examinations at a high pulse rate, as it can reduce the number of patients who would otherwise require pharmacologic reduction of their heart rate. This new generation of scanners can completely cover the chest (approximately 35 cm) with submillimeter resolution in approximately 1 second. As a result, this innovative technology can significantly shorten the usual breath-hold times while reducing respiratory artifacts.

Detector Design

The principle of adaptive detector design was previously described on pages 10 and 11. At the time of this writing, Dual Source systems manufactured by Siemens employ a 96-row detector, which can also be used as 192-row detector (with application of z-flying focal spot, cf. p. 198). It has a collimated z-axis slice width of 0.6 mm each, resulting in a total z-axis coverage of approximately 58 mm (Fig. 199.1).

As described on the previous page, the amplitude of the periodic z-axis motion of the focal spot is adjusted in such a way that two subsequent data acquisitions are shifted by one-half the collimated slice thickness along the z-axis.

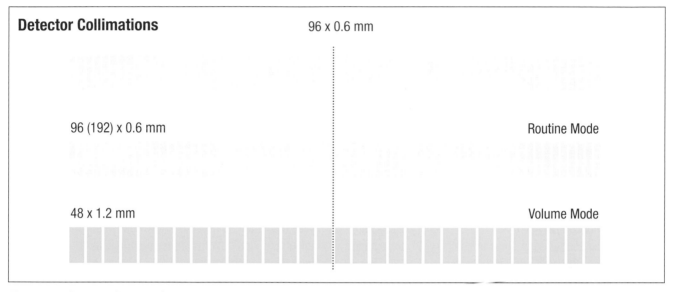

Detector Collimations

96 x 0.6 mm

96 (192) x 0.6 mm

48 x 1.2 mm

Routine Mode

Volume Mode

Fig. 199.1　Detector Design of Dual Source Scanner (duplication of rows by the use of z-flying focal spot, cf. p. 198)

Dual Energy Mode

When both tube/detector pairs are operated simultaneously at different energy levels (e.g. one at 90 kV and one at 150 kV with Sn filter), the two resulting data sets can be combined to yield a variety of information that goes beyond the usual attenuation values (in HU). Imaged tissues can be characterized, differentiated, and isolated based on differences in their chemical composition. Clinical applications range from accurate bone subtraction in CT angiography to the selective removal of contrast medium from images. This can provide virtual unenhanced scans of kidney stones, for example. Initial studies suggest that other promising new applications will be developed in the future.

Reduction of Spiral Artifacts

In the past, other techniques have required protocols with low pitch values in order to reduce spiral artifacts. The z-flying focal spot technique (see p. 198) makes it possible to control typical "windmill" arti-facts (⬆ in Fig. 199.3) despite higher pitch values while obtaining greater volume coverage, even under difficult conditions (Fig. 199.4).

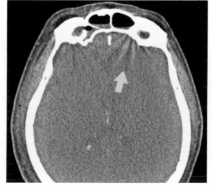

Fig. 199.3

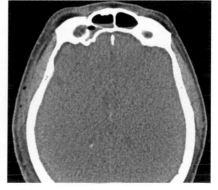

Fig. 199.4

The technique, which we have described on the preceding pages, allows the visualization of large tissue volumes with improved spatial resolution: Thus, especially in CT angiography, the extension of dissected aortic aneurysm in z-axis can be demonstrated much more accurately (Fig. 200.1a). In addition, it is easier to determine, which of the two renal arteries originates from the true and the false aortic lumen (Fig. 200.1b). Even the evaluation of smaller aortic branches, like lumbar arteries (Fig. 200.1c), or the Adamkiewicz artery for the spinal perfusion comes within our reach. *(Images 200.1 a-c are courtesy of Centre Cardio-Thoracique de Monaco.)*

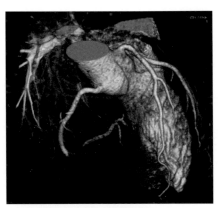

Fig. 200.1a Aortic dissection

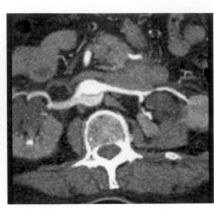

Fig. 200.1b Renal orifices

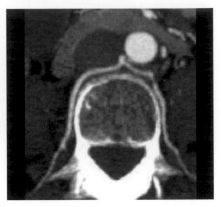

Fig. 200.1c Lumbar arteries

The detection of coronary stenoses and of coronary calcifications is improved by shorter scan times in coronary CT angiography: overviews (Fig. 200.2b), 3D reconstructions (Fig. 200.2a) or more detailed views (Fig. 200.2c/d) are achievable with higher spatial resolution, compared to previous years. Therefore, CT angiography will become more important as a non-invasive alternative to catheter-based DSA techniques.
(Fig. 200.2 courtesy of German Herzzentrum Munich.)

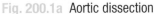

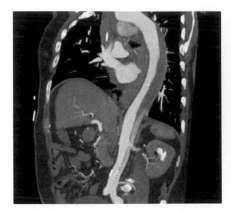

Fig. 200.2a 3D - overview

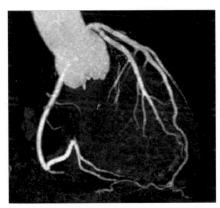

Fig. 200.2b Multiplanar reconstruction

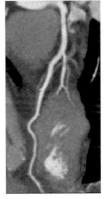

Fig. 200.2c/d Detailed views

Functional imaging to evaluate coronary perfusion defects (⇧), here at the posterior cardiac wall, can be performed within shorter scan times und can be easily visualized from several views (Fig. 200.3). *(Courtesy of Univ. of South Carolina, Charleston, USA.)*

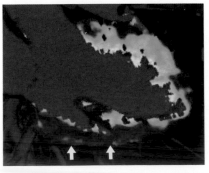

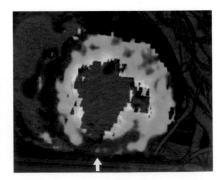

Fig. 200.3a Coronary perfusion defects   Fig. 200.3b Short axis view

The pulmonar vessel tree can be examined far out into its periphery (Fig. 201.1a) and the quantification of pulmonary perfusion defects (Fig. 201.1b) in cases of pulmonary embolism or in cases of tumor-induced bronchial occlu-sion (⇨ in Fig. 201.1c) can be improved significantly: *(Images 201.1a-c Courtesy of Inst. for Medical Physics, Univ. Erlangen-Nürnberg / Univ.-Hosp. Frankfurt, Germany)*

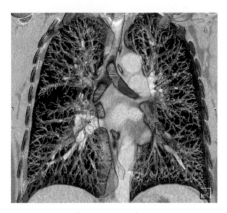

Fig. 201.1a Lung vessels

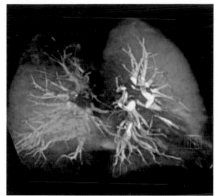

Fig. 201.1b Perfusion defect RUL

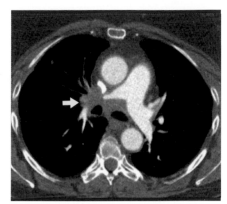

Fig. 201.1c Bronchial occlusion

Nowadays, with the new generation of dual-source-scanners, the examination of cerebral (brain) perfusion is achievable much less time-consuming, comparable to functional MRI-examinations: Fig. 201.2b / c shows cerebral perfusion defects with a data acquisition time of as low as 36 seconds in this case (collimation of e.g. 32 x 1,2 mm), which would not have been detectable in conventional CT imaging (Fig. 201.2a): *(Images. 201.2-3 Courtesy of Univ.-Clinic, Großhadern, Munic, Germany)*

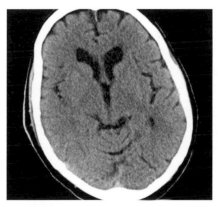

Fig. 201.2a Conventional

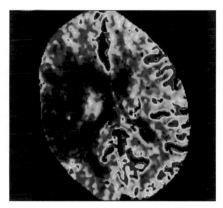

Fig. 201.2b Perfusion defect

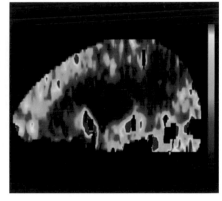

Fig. 201.2c Perfusion defect

The new dual-energy-technique opens up promising approaches to differentiate different kinds of tissue according to their different chemical attributes: For example, different kinds of kidney stones can be visualized in different colors, e.g. uric acid stones (⇩) in red (Fig. 201.3a) and calcium oxalate stones (⬈) in blue (Fig. 201.3b). This ability will be used in the future to differentiate tumorous or metastatic infiltrations of the liver (Fig. 201.4) and other organs. (*Fig. 201.4 Courtesy of Nara Medical University, Japan*)

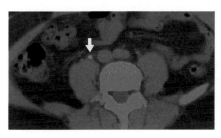

Fig. 201.3a Uric acid stone

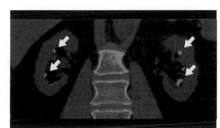

Fig. 201.3b Calcium oxalate stones

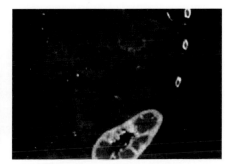

Fig. 201.4 Liver metastases

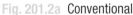

A PET/CT diagnostic study combines functional biochemical imaging (PET = Positron Emission Tomography) with morphologic imaging (CT) in a single examination. The examination makes it possible to simultaneously document metabolic information and the anatomy of healthy and pathologic tissue. Various radionuclides (known as tracers) are used depending on the specific clinical line of inquiry and the target organ.

Uptake Mechanism of Radioactive Tracers
The most commonly used tracer is fluorine-18-FDG (fluorodeoxyglucose), in which one of the oxygen atoms in the glucose molecule has been replaced with a fluorine-18 isotope (Fig. 202.1). During its half-life of about 110 minutes, the fluorine isotope emits measurable radiation that accumulates and can be measured at those locations at which the altered glucose molecule concentrates. This occurs not only in the brain, the working skeletal and cardiac musculature, the larynx and pharynx (after speech), the liver, the bowel, the kidney, and the urinary tract (✱ in Fig. 202.2); it also occurs in acutely inflamed tissues (such as in arthritis or gingivitis) with increased metabolism – or in metastases such as the right axillary one shown here (✱✱).

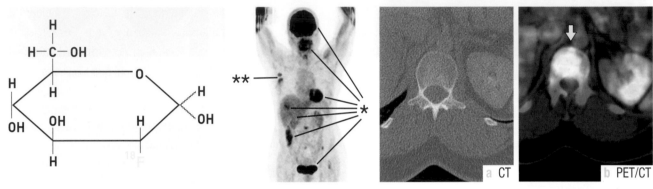

Fig. 202.1 FDG molecule with fluorine-18 isotope

Fig. 202.2 FDG uptake

Fig. 202.3 Metastasis visible only on PET scan

a CT   b PET/CT

The glucose molecule is phosphorylated during glycolysis by the enzyme hexokinase in the mitochondria, particularly in the rapidly growing cells of malignant tumors or their metastases. The fluorine-18 isotope then impedes the further breakdown of glucose for some time, causing FDG molecules to accumulate more in malignant cells than in healthy tissues. This means that relatively increased FDG uptake can also indicate tumor metastases (⇩ in Fig. 202.3b) that would escape detection on conventional CT images (Fig. 202.3a).

Patient Preparation
After the indication has been verified and the physician has obtained the patient's informed consent to the planned examination, the specific examination protocol for PET and CT is determined (i.e., IV, oral, rectal administration of contrast; arterial and portal venous phase). The patient is informed of possible risks and side effects that can occur within the scope of the examination (for example, contrast agent allergy). Then the blood glucose level is measured, which should be lower than 150 mg/dL so that the body's cells take up a sufficient quantity of the injected FDG (for this reason patients should fast for about 4 to 6 hours before the examination begins).
The quantity of intravenous FDG is calculated from the respective body surface area and the patient's body weight. The examination is performed following a waiting period of 60 minutes on average during which the FDG can circulate in the bloodstream, be taken up, and become phosphorylated. During the waiting period patients should rest (not walk around) and speak as little as possible (not talk on the phone or chew gum). This is to avoid increased FDG uptake in the neck and facial musculature that later might be difficult to distinguish from cervical metastases (Fig. 202.2). Where orbital metastases of a neoplasm such as malignant melanoma on the head are to be excluded, patients should also not be allowed to read during the waiting period as otherwise the posterior ocular muscles could show increased uptake. The best solution is to have patients wear a blindfold and listen to music. It is important to ensure a sufficiently warm ambient temperature in the waiting room for all patients, but particularly for slender ones, and to provide warm blankets on the couches so that patients do not shiver. Shivering of the skeletal musculature can easily be overlooked but leads to increased uptake in the musculature and in brown fat. This increased uptake would later make it unnecessarily difficult to distinguish tumors in the local and regional lymph nodes or muscles. The quantity measured is the so-called SUV_{max} (maximum standardized uptake value), which is the correlate of the radionuclide taken up in the target tissue. While the measurements are being taken, it is important for the patient to lie as still as possible in order to facilitate subsequent fusion of the CT and PET images.

Exposure to Ionizing Radiation

For a full body scan about 200 to 400 mBq is applied intravenously depending on the patient's body surface area and body weight. At about 0.02 mSv/mBq of radiation exposure, this corresponds to a total of about 7 to 10 mSv including the radiation dose of the CT scan. Note that the dose of radiation varies among the different organs. Accumulation of the tracer in urine means that at about 0.17 mSv/mBq the bladder receives a significantly higher dose than the other organs (see pp. 174–177).

Indications and Selection of Tracer

Aside from primary staging (extent of the primary tumor, detection of lymph node metastases and remote metastases), PET/CT can also be performed in the setting of restaging where there is cause to suspect recurrence and within the scope of follow-up (response evaluation). In these cases it is helpful in differentiating scar tissue from viable residual tumor tissue. In addition to tumor diagnostics, PET/CT is also used in specific neurologic and cardiologic settings. Most recently, PET/CT is increasingly being used in the diagnostic workup of specific cases of inflammatory disorders (vasculitis). FDG (see p. 202) is not particularly well suited as a tracer with slowly progressive types of tumors, well-differentiated tumors, or mucinous tumor components (such as prostate tumors, low-grade brain tumors, well-differentiated hepatocellular carcinoma, mucinous gastric or ovarian carcinoma). In these cases, other radionuclides are preferred (see the following pages).

Brain Tumors

Brain tissue invariably exhibits a high level of glucose metabolism. As a result, it is often not possible to draw a clear distinction between moderately malignant grade I astrocytomas and healthy brain tissue (see high cerebral FDG uptake in Fig. 203.2), leading to false negative findings. For this reason radioactively labeled amino acids (carbon-11-methionine or fluorine-18-ethylene thyrosine (FET) are preferred when the line of inquiry does not involve highly malignant undifferentiated gliomas that can visualized with FDG.

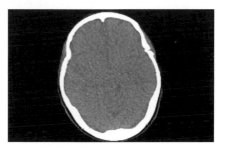 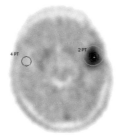 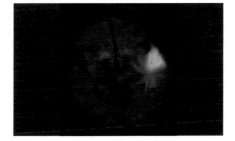

Fig. 203.1a Normal low-dose CT   Fig. 203.1b Left temporal lesion on PET   Fig. 203.1c Fused PET/CT image

Fig. 203.1 shows the comparison with an unremarkable low-dose CT of a patient with a suspected brain tumor: Because MRI (not shown here) had detected a left temporal edema, a PET/CT study was ordered which demonstrated focal 18F-FET uptake at that location and confirmed the suspected tumor.

Differential Diagnosis of Lymph Nodes

The CT morphologic criteria of enlarged lymph nodes do not always match up as they do in Fig. 203.2: In the right axillary region (⟰) there is a benign lymph node with a hilum fat sign but without FDG uptake. However, in the left axillary region (⟰) there are two lymph node metastases with pathologic FDG uptake. Fig. 203.3 shows exactly the opposite: In this patient only a small 5-mm lymph node with a hilum fat sign (Fig. 203.3a) shows increased uptake. Surprisingly, it is this node which represents a metastasis (⟰), whereas the larger 12-mm lymph node (with suspicious CT morphology) in another patient does not show increased uptake (⟰) and on PET/CT must be classified as benign (Fig.203.3b).

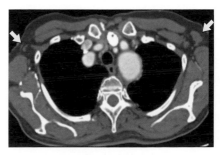 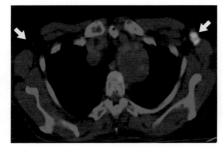 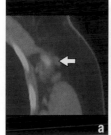 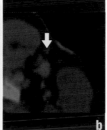

Fig. 203.2a Axillary lymph nodes on CT   Fig. 203.2b Different uptake on each side on PET/CT   Fig. 203.3 Nodal metastasis vs. benign node

Tumors of the Gastrointestinal Tract

After a minimum interval of 3–4 months after surgery, chemotherapy, or irradiation of a tumor, PET/CT can very precisely distinguish a local recurrence (↗) from a postoperative scar; for example, in cases where laboratory tumor markers are increase or imaging findings suggest recurrence. Figs. 204.1b,c show a recurrent rectal carcinoma in a presacral scar plate, whereas conventional CT images (Fig. 204.2a) do not always allow this differentiation.

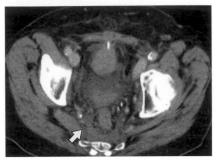

Fig. 204.1a   CT 6 months after treatment

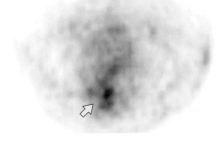

Fig. 204.1b   PET showing focal uptake

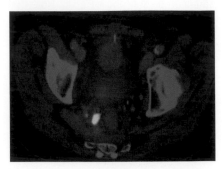

Fig. 204.1c   Fused PET/CT image

The following figures (Figs. 204.2a–c) show preoperative images of an esophageal carcinoma (↗) with increased FDG uptake but without evidence of a liver metastasis (upper row). In comparison, these images after combined radiation and chemotherapy (Figs. 204.2d-f) show complete remission without residual uptake (lower row).

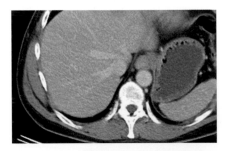

Fig. 204.2a   Esophageal carcinoma on CT

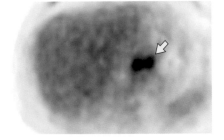

Fig. 204.2b   Focal FDG uptake

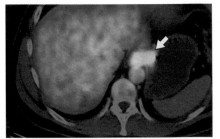

Fig. 204.2c   Fused PET/CT image

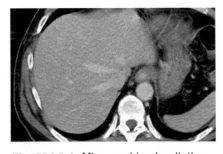

Fig. 204.2d   After combined radiation and chemotherapy

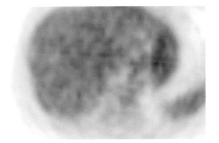

Fig. 204.2e   FDG uptake has disappeared

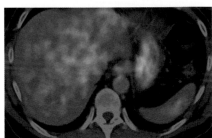

Fig. 204.2f   Fused PET/CT image

In the case of intrahepatic tumors or metastases, for example after TACE (transarterial chemoembolization), PET/CT can play an important role by helping to ascertain whether viable tumor components (⇓) are still present and thus determine the appropriate therapy in applicable cases (Fig. 204.3).

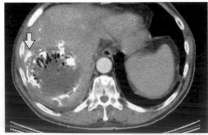

Fig. 204.3a   CT follow-up examination after

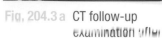

Fig. 204.3b   ... chemoembolization

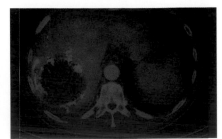

Fig. 204.3c   FDG uptake on PET/CT

Pulmonary Tumors

FDG-PET/-CT is highly accurate in detecting malignant pulmonary tumors (⇩) and their metastases in lymph nodes, adrenal glands, liver, and bone: Depending on the vertical extent of a bed position (scanning field), the duration of the measurement can lead to an increased cardiac signal (↖)

(Fig. 205.1). Some suspicious solid round focal pulmonary lesions (↗) are identified as benign lesions by the absence of pathologic FDG uptake (Fig. 205.2) and therefore do not require surgery or invasive treatment.

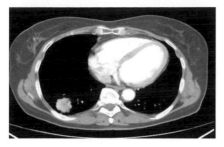

Fig. 205.1a Peripheral bronchial carcinoma

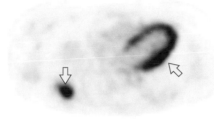

Fig. 205.1b Increased FDG uptake

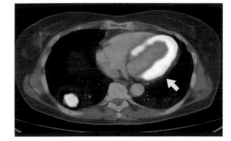

Fig. 205.1c Left ventricular activity

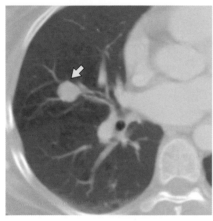

Fig. 205.2a Suspicious round focal pulmonary lesion on CT

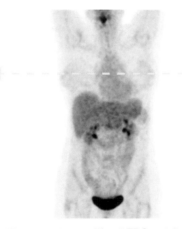

Fig. 205.2b ... without FDG uptake

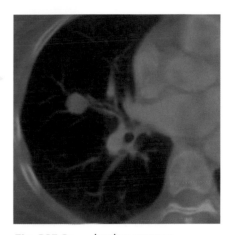

Fig. 205.2c ... benign process

Staging and TNN classification and consequently the choice of therapy for lymph nodes of borderline size in the hilum (↘) or in the mediastinum along the esophagus (↗ in Fig. 205.3) are rendered considerably easier by pathologic SUV$_{max}$ values

on PET/CT (Figs. 205.3b,c). However, a differential diagnosis must consider that reactive inflammatory lymph nodes in bronchitis or nodes in the setting of sarcoidosis can also lead to increased FDG uptake.

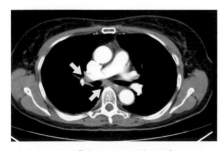

Fig. 205.3a Primary staging of a bronchial carcinoma

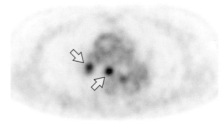

Fig. 205.3b FDG uptake in lymph node

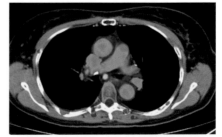

Fig. 205.3c Classification by location on fused PET/CT image

Other common sites of metastases of a bronchial carcinoma include the skeleton and adrenal glands. PET/CT can also demonstrate bone metastases (⇨) (Figs. 206.1b,c) that would go undetected on conventional CT (Fig. 206.1a). MRI

or PET/CT can also clarify whether enlargement of an adrenal gland is due merely to an adrenal adenoma (⇧ in Fig. 206.2a) or an adrenal metastasis (↖ in Fig. 206.2b).

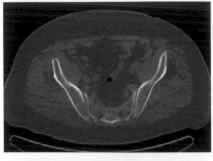

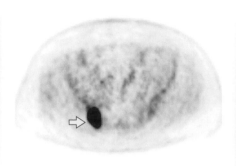

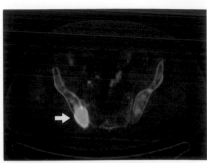

Fig. 206.1a Unremarkable pelvic bones   Fig. 206.1b Focally increased FDG uptake   Fig. 206.1c Pelvic metastasis

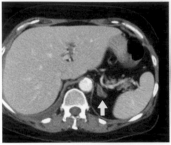

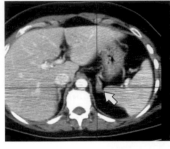

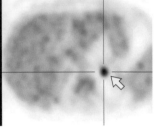

Fig. 206.2a Adrenal adenoma without uptake   Fig. 206.2b Adrenal metastasis with FDG uptake

This additional information from PET/CT is particularly helpful in cases where neither CT densitometery (see p. 131) nor MRI can unequivocally determine whether or not adrenal thickening is malignant. No other modality can predict with the same precision whether or not a pulmonary carcinoma is operable. Fig. 206.3 shows a central paramediastinal tumor whose "true" extent includes only the medial portion (⬦), whereas what appears to be its lateral portion here actually represents poststenotic atelectasis (⬦). With operable tumors, such

findings can of course influence the surgical strategy; with inoperable tumors, they can determine the size of the irradiated field. Physiologic renal uptake in both kidneys and the bladder (⬅) must not be confused with pathologic metastases (⬆). A more recently developed modality, virtual PET/CT bronchoscopy, can localize tumor tissue (⬦) so precisely in its proximity to the bronchial wall that a bronchoscopic transbronchial biopsy can be performed considerably more easily (Fig. 206.4).

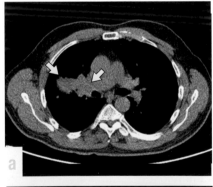

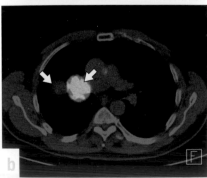

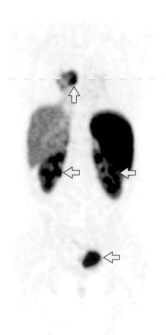

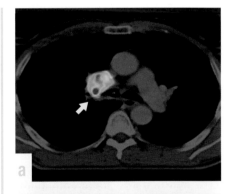

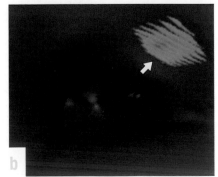

Fig. 206.3 Bronchogenic carcinoma with atelectasis

Fig. 206.4 Virtual bronchoscopy

Tumors of the Prostate Gland

As prostate carcinomas frequently grow slowly, carbon-11-choline (an important building block of cell membranes), and recently gallium-68-labeled PSMA (see below) as well, are often preferred over FDG with this type of tumor. These radionuclides are used both for primary staging and in follow-up studies after surgery; after combined hormone therapy, radiation, and chemotherapy where a recurrence of the tumor is suspected; and where there is an unexplained increase in PSMA. Fig. 207.1 shows a prostate tumor that cannot be identified on CT (Fig. 207.1b). The focal decreased signal (⬚) on MRI (Fig. 207.1e) provides a significantly better correlate to the increased choline uptake (◥) on the PET image (Figs. 207.1a,d), which on PET/MRI can clearly be attributed to the suspicious lesion (Fig. 207.1f).

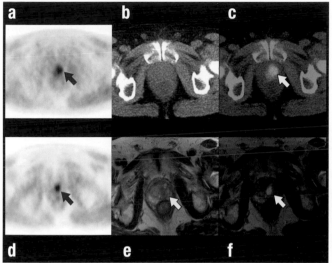

Fig. 207.1 Prostate carcinoma: PET/CT compared with PET/MRI

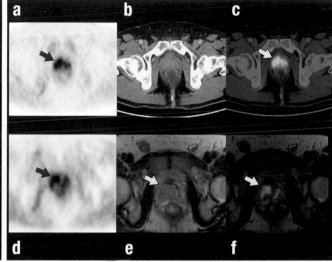

Fig. 207.2 The same for benign prostate hyperplasia

An important fact to consider in a differential diagnosis is that benign prostate hyperplasia (Fig. 207.2) also shows significant choline uptake (◥) and can be mistaken for a carcinoma where corresponding signal changes are present on MRI (◺). For this reason a new tracer to prostate-specific membrane antigen (PSMA), which is only expressed by cancer cells, is currently being tested.

Depending on the stage of the tumor or size of the metastases, bone metastases may not yet be detectable on CT (Fig. 207.3b), whereas they can already be identified on MRI (Fig. 207.3e). The fused image of the PET signals (Figs. 207.3a,d) with the CT or MRI scans (Figs. 207.3b,e) allows more precise anatomic correlation (⬚) of the suspicious areas of focal uptake (◢) in uncertain cases. As with FDG, tracer uptake regularly occurs in the liver, spleen, and bowel lumen and should be regarded as physiologic (Fig. 207.4a). However, it is often difficult to classify smaller para-iliac lymph nodes (⇨ in Figs. 207.4b,e) as benign or malignant on CT or MRI. Only when the image is fused with the PET signals (◥) can one tentatively diagnose a right para-iliac lymph node metastasis (⇦ in Figs. 207.4c,f).

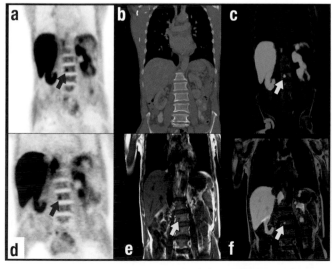

Fig. 207.3 Bone metastasis: PET/CT ⟷ PET/MRT

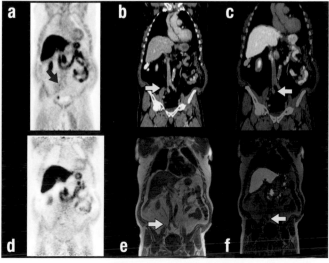

Fig. 207.4 Evaluation of suspicious lymph node on PET/CT/ and PET/MRI

Neuroendocrine Tumors

Gallium-68-labeled DOTANOC or DOTATOC (Edotreotid) is a tracer for neuroendocrine tumors arising from nerve ganglia, the pancreas, or the ileum, and expressing large quantities of somatostatin-2 receptors. This tracer consists of two components: The chelating agent DOTA is combined with the octapeptide TOC. Replacement of one amino acid prevents premature breakdown so that DOTATOC has a significantly longer half-life (1.5 to 2 hours) than somatostatin, whose half-life is a few minutes. The longer half-life can be used to measure the beta radiation emitted by the gallium isotope. Fig. 208.1 shows a residual metastasis of a neuroendocrine tumor (⬇) along with the residues of chemoembolization (⬈). This residual tumor was not clearly delineated on CT (Fig. 208.1a) and could only be definitively identified on the PET/CT fused image (Fig. 208.1c).

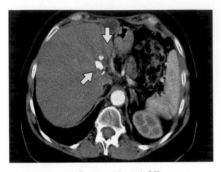

Fig. 208.1a Conventional CT

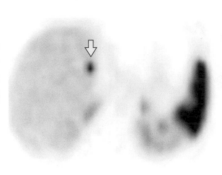

Fig. 208.1b Focal DOTATOC uptake

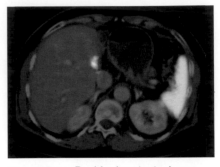

Fig. 208.1c Residual metastasis on PET/CT

A differential diagnosis must consider that even normal pancreatic tissue has many SST2 receptors and can therefore show increased uptake of DOTATOC (⬉) even without having been invaded by the tumor, in this case a neuroendocrine carcinoma of the small bowel (Fig. 208.2).

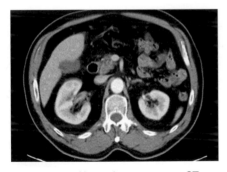

Fig. 208.2a Normal pancreas on CT

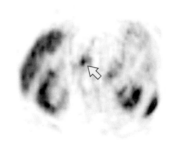

Fig. 208.2b Focal DOTATOC uptake ...

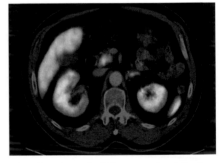

Fig. 208.2c ... in this case physiologic

Even in complex uncertain cases (Fig. 208.3a), this highly selective tracer can be used to differentiate suspiciously enlarged lymph nodes in the mediastinum (⇨) and the perihilar region (⬉) from actual metastases of neuroendocrine tumors (⇦ in Fig. 208.3b). In this case only one of the lymph nodes showed metastatic infiltration.

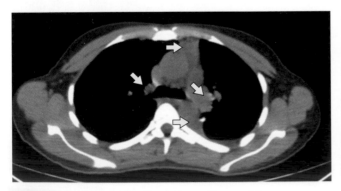

Fig. 208.3a Neuroendocrine tumor with suspicious lymph nodes on CT

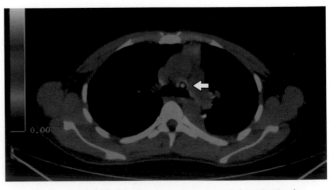

Fig. 208.3b Yet PET/CT shows only one nodal metastasis

The images on the next four pages illustrate the sectional anatomy of the abdomen as it appears in coronal reconstructions. These multiplanar reconstructions (MPRs) can be generated from the original three-dimensional data set in any desired slice thickness and with any interval or degree of overlap between adjacent slices. Only the initial collimation sets the limits of the spatial resolution along the Z-axis that can be achieved in the reconstructions (see p. 9).

The numerical labels are keyed to the "Thoracic and Pelvic Diagrams" fold-out key on the back cover flap of this book. Sections through the anterior abdominal skin and subcutaneous tissue are omitted here so that portions of the air- (**4**) filled stomach (**129**) and colon (**143**) and a partial anterior section of the liver (**122**) are directly displayed in Fig. 210.1. Sections of the mesenteric vessels (**108**) are found between the loops of small bowel (**140**) and the ascending, transverse, and descending limbs of the colon.

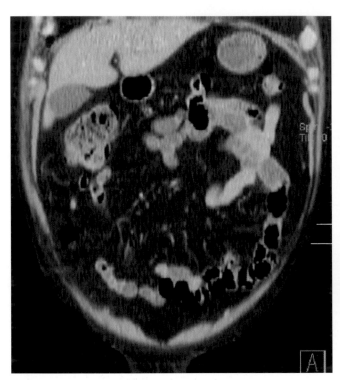

Fig. 210.1a

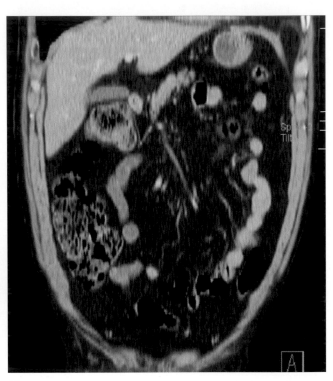

Fig. 210.2a

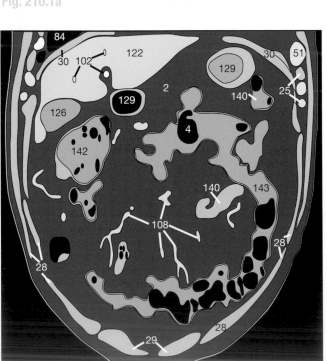

Fig. 210.1b

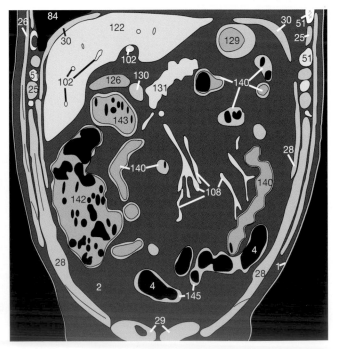

Fig. 210.2b

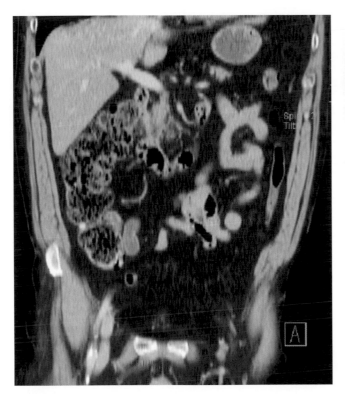

Fig. 211.1a

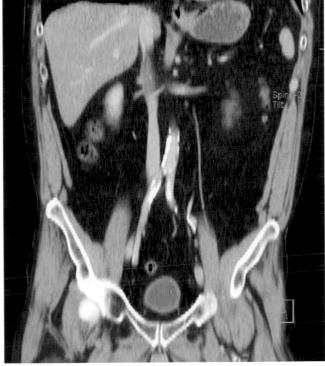

Fig. 211.2a

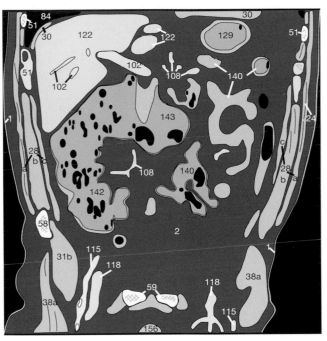

Fig. 211.1b

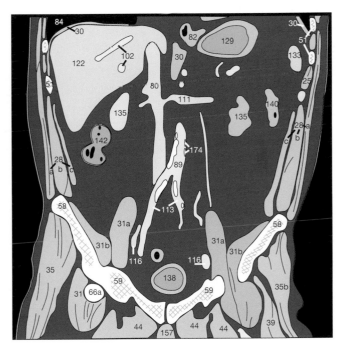

Fig. 211.2b

Please note significant calcifications (**174**) of the arterial walls of the infrarenal part of the aorta (**89**) and both common iliac arteries (**113**) on both sides (Fig. 211.2), which can be found frequently in elder patients.

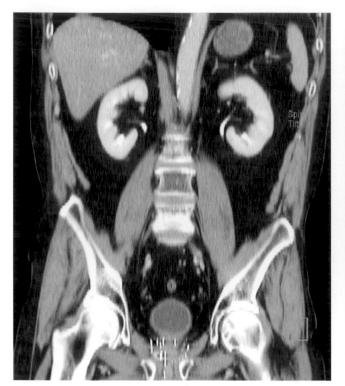

Fig. 212.1a

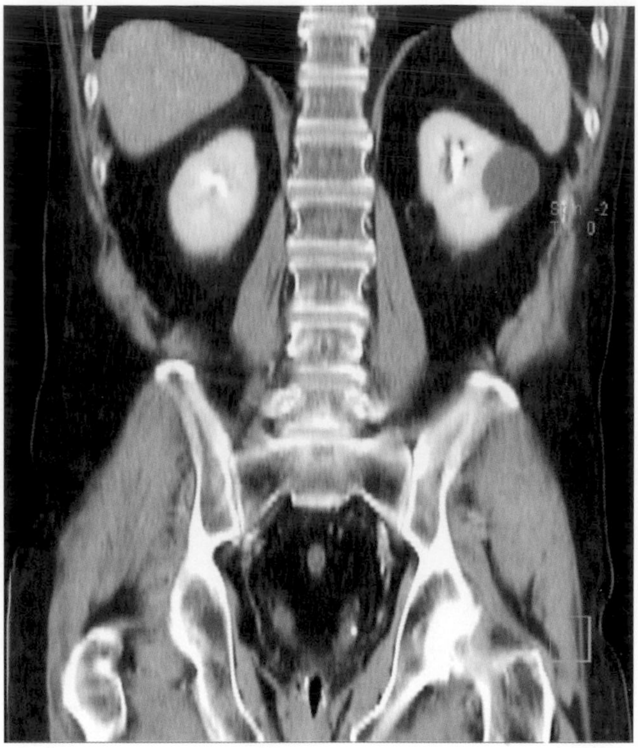

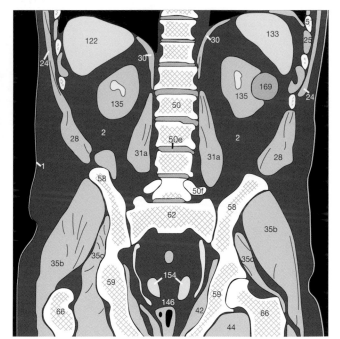

Fig. 212.2a

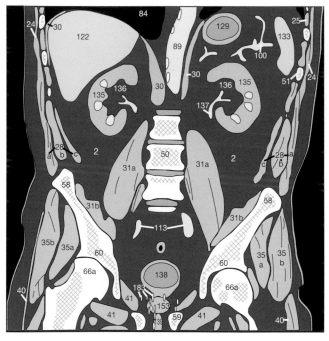

Fig. 212.1b

Fig. 212.2b

In coronal views, the width of renal parenchyma (**135**) can be evaluated – and eventual side differences (not presented here) could be detected more easily. Fig. 212.2 shows a common finding of a benign renal cyst (**169**) at the lateral border of the left kidney (**135**) with a sharp outline towards the perirenal fatty tissue (**2**).

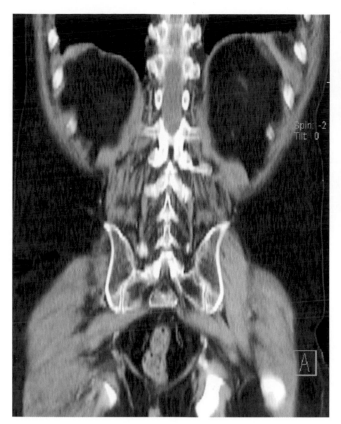

Fig. 213.1a

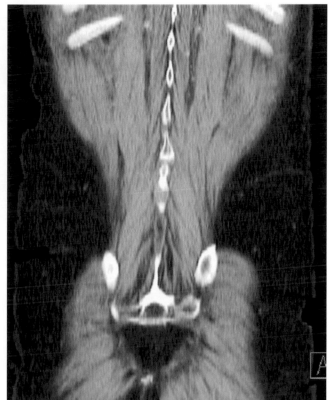

Fig. 213.2a

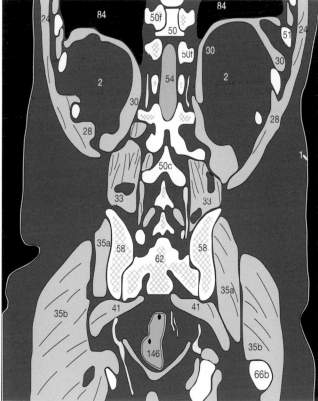

Fig. 213.1b

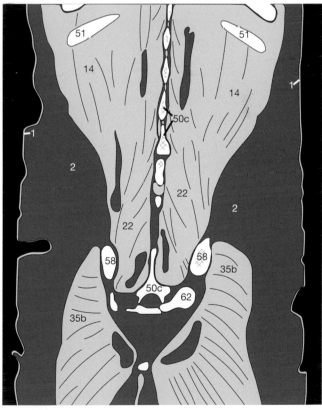

Fig. 213.2b

The images on the next seven pages illustrate the sectional anatomy of the chest and abdomen as it appears in a right-to-left series of sagittal reconstructions.

The first sagittal plane (Fig. 214.1) through the far right side of the body shows the oblique muscles of the abdominal wall (**28**), sections of the ribs (**51**) with the intercostal muscles (**25**), and a section of the scapula (**53**) with the subcostal muscle (**18**) and infraspinatus muscle (**20**). The next image in a slightly more medial plane (Fig. 214.2) displays the right lobe of the liver (**122**) and a section of the ascending colon (**142**). The numerical labels are keyed to the "Thoracic and Pelvic Diagrams" fold-out key on the back cover flap of this book.

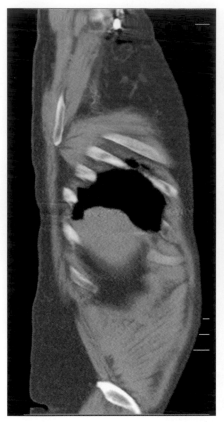

Fig. 214.1a

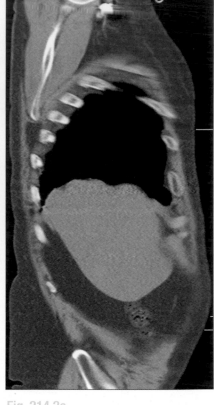

Fig. 214.2a

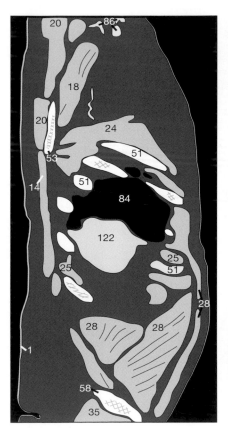

Fig. 214.1b

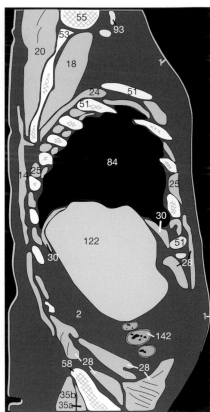

Fig. 214.2b

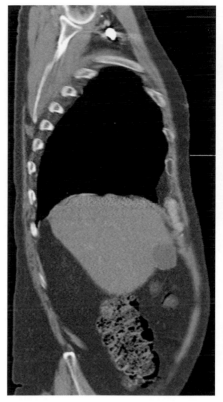

Fig. 215.1a

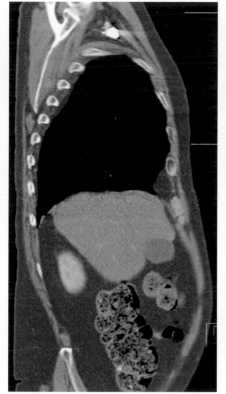

Fig. 215.2a

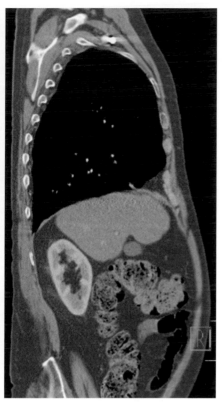

Fig. 215.3a

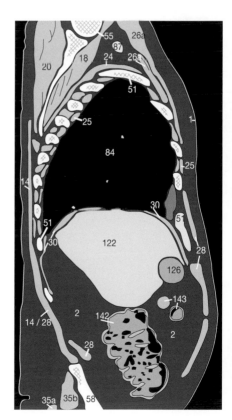

Fig. 215.1b

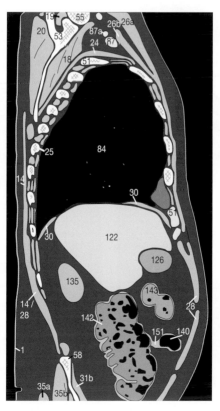

Fig. 215.2b

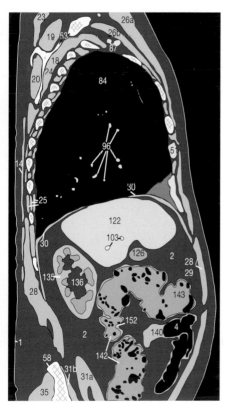

Fig. 215.3b

These images (Figs. 215.1–3) display the gallbladder (**126**), the parenchyma of the right kidney (**135**) with the renal pelvis (**136**), and the transverse colon (**143**). Please note the appearance of thin colon walls, sharply outlined towards surrounding mesenteric fat (**2**). A blurred appearance of colon walls would suggest either an inflammatory process or an infiltration by a malignant tumor.

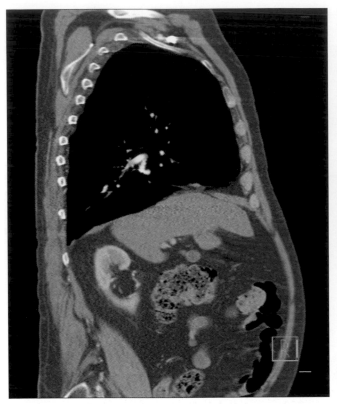

Fig. 216.1a

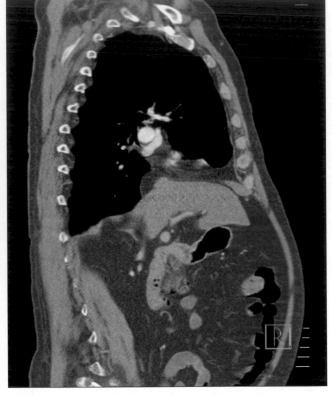

Fig. 216.2a

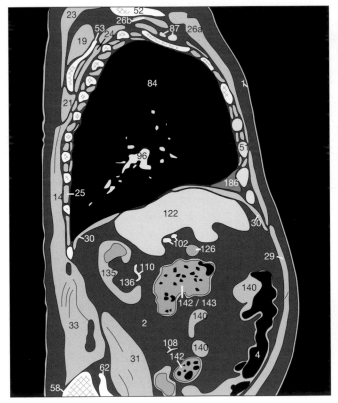

Fig. 216.1b

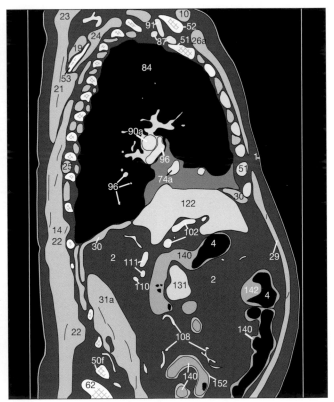

Fig. 216.2b

Like in transverse sections, you might also come across a subtle partial volume effect of the renal pelvis (**136**), filled with branches of renal vessels (**110, 111**) and dark fat (**2**), which should not be confounded with renal tumors. The more we move from right to left, the smaller the size of subdiaphragmatic hepatic segments (**122**) will appear (Figs. 216.1 and 2).

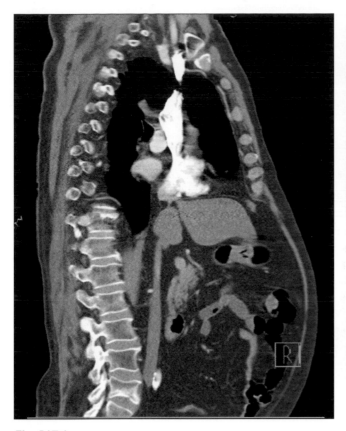

Fig. 217.1a

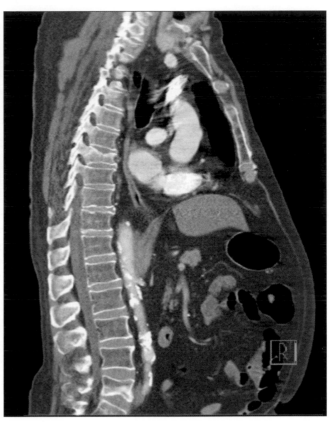

Fig. 217.2a

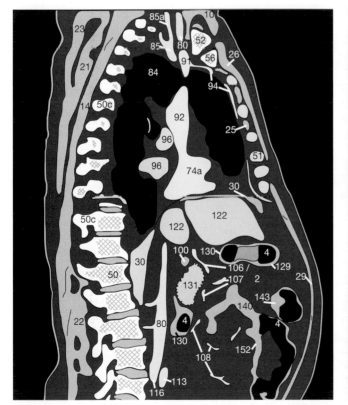

Fig. 217.1b

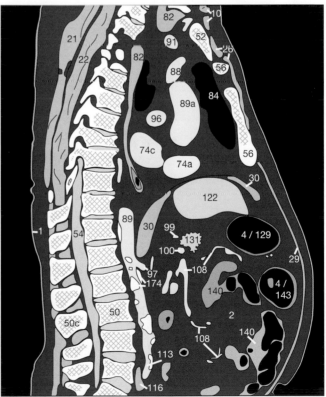

Fig. 217.2b

On this page, we approach the paramedian sagittal image level with the inferior vena cava (**80**) and the abdominal aorta (**89**). Again, you can see here moderate to severe arteriosclerotic plaques (**174**) attached to the aortic wall (Fig. 217.2), which narrow or might even occlude the vascular lumen (see Fig. 211.2, same patient).

Above the diaphragm (**30**), you can identify the ascending aorta (**89a**), pulmonary blood vessels (**96**) and heart chambers (**74a-c**).

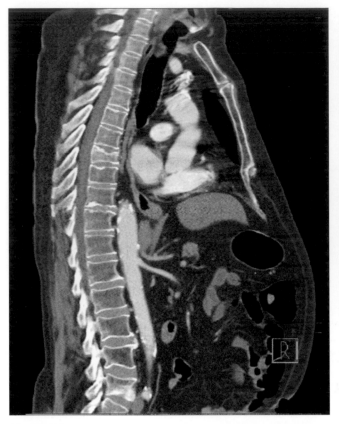

Fig. 218.1a

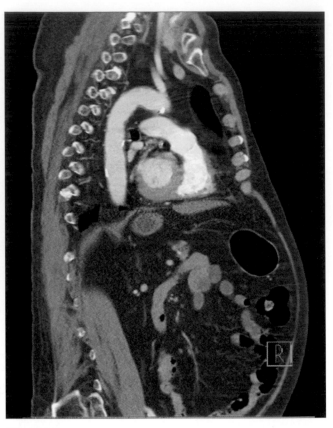

Fig. 218.2a

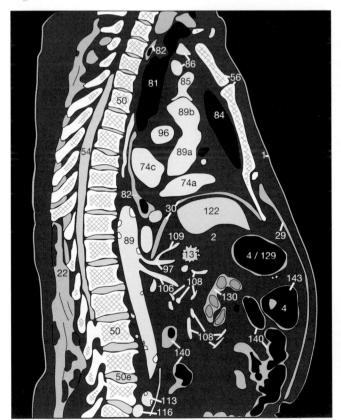

Fig. 218.1b

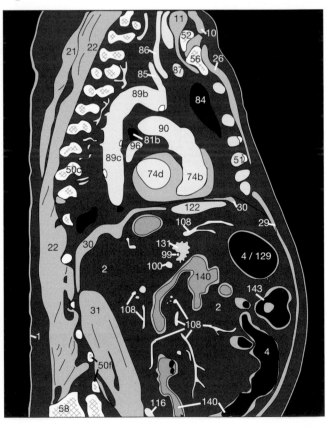

Fig. 218.2b

While we move further towards the left paramedian side, the ascending aorta (**89a**), aortic arch (**89b**) and descending aorta (**89c**) come into our field of view, as well as the left ventricle (**74d**). In Fig. 218.1, we can identify the celiac trunk (**97**) with left gastric artery (**109**) and superior mesenteric artery (**106**),

originating from the suprarenal part of the abdominal aorta (**89**). In the center of the mesenteric root, we see branches of small mesenteric blood vessels (**108**) running towards small bowel loops (**140**) and colon (**143**), which is partially filled with gas (**4** in Fig. 218.2).

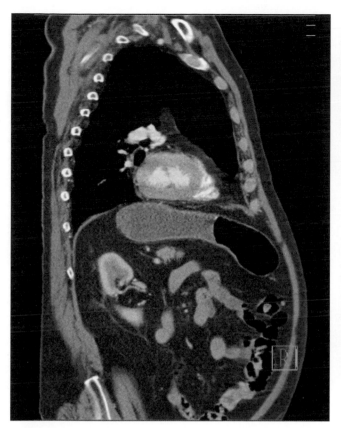

Fig. 219.1a

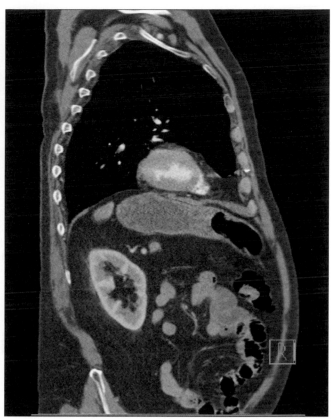

Fig. 219.2a

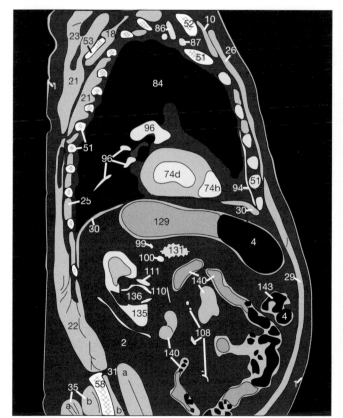

Fig. 219.1b

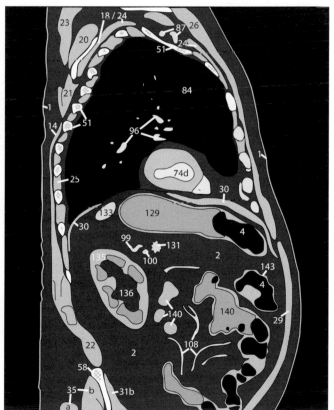

Fig. 219.2b

Further to the left, the stomach (**129**) with usually thin gastric walls and the left renal pelvis (**136**) are visualized. Please note that the myocardial wall of the left ventricle (**74d** in Figs. 219.1–2) is significantly thicker compared to right ventricular walls (**74b** in Fig. 218.2). In normal findings, both bowel walls (**140, 143**) and renal borderlines are sharply defined by adjacent mesenteric fatty tissue (**2**).

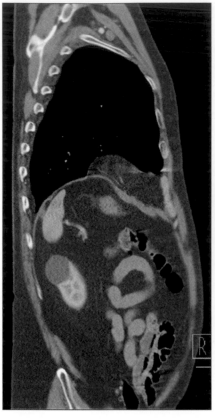

Fig. 220.1a

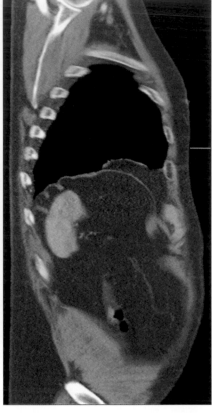

Fig. 220.2a

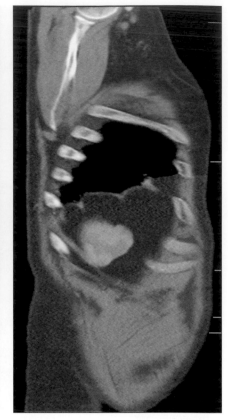

Fig. 220.3a

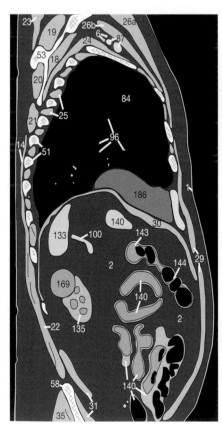

Fig. 220.1b

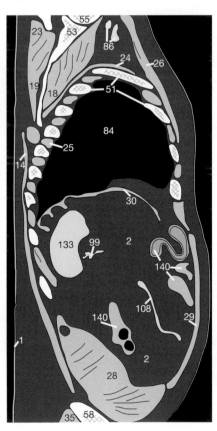

Fig. 220.2b

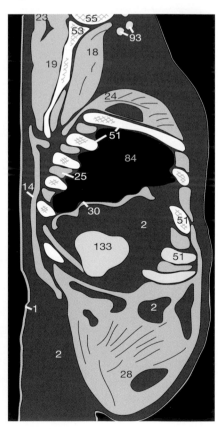

Fig. 220.3b

In elder patients, not only obesity, but also benign renal cysts (**169**) can often be observed (Fig. 220.1) and fat and post-inflammatory scar tissue (**186**) in the lower parts of the pleural cavity, close to the diaphragm (**30**). Posteriorly, just under the diaphragm, we find the spleen (**133**), which might appear inhomogeneous in early arterial phases of CM-enhanced images (Figs. 220.1–3), but should be homogenous in late venous perfusion phases (see p. 127).

The exercises and solutions have been numbered consecutively. Some of the exercises have several different correct solutions. If the exercises can be solved simply by referring to the chapters in the book, I have indicated where you will find the necessary information.

After you have completed the exercises, compare your score and results with those of your colleagues. The score on the right gives you an impression of the degree of difficulty. Enjoy the challenge!

Solution to exercise 1 (p. 32): 9 Points

You will find the sequence for interpreting CCTs on page 26. Each step gives you $1/2$ point with 3 extra points for the correct sequence, which adds up to 9.

Solution to exercise 2 (p. 45): 9 Points

	Level	Width	Gray scale	
Lung/pleural window	- 200 HU	2000 HU	-1200 HU to + 800 HU	3
Bone window	+300 HU	1500 HU	- 450 HU to +1050 HU	3
Soft-tissue window	+ 50 HU	350 HU	- 125 HU to + 225 HU	3

Solution to exercise 3 (p. 45): 10 Points

a)	Barium sulfate	Routine for abdominal/pelvic CT if there are no contraindications	30 min before CT of upper abdomen 60 min before full abdominal CT	4
b)	Gastrografin	Water soluble, but expensive; if perforation ileus or fistulas are suspected; prior to surgery	20 min before CT of upper abdomen 45 min before full abdominal CT	4 / 1

No oral CM shortly after surgery for an ileal conduit! 1

Solution to exercise 4 (p. 45): 6 Points

a)	Renal failure (creatinine, possibly creatinine clearance, function following kidney transplant or nephrectomy)	2
b)	Hyperthyroidism (clinical signs? if yes, hormone status, possibly thyroid ultrasound and scintigraphy)	2
c)	Allergy to CM (has CM-containing iodine already been injected? Are there any known previous allergic reactions?)	2

Solution to exercise 5 (p. 45): 2 Points

Tubular and nodular structures can be differentiated by comparing a series of images.

Solution to exercise 6 (p. 45): 3 Points

Vessels in which beam-hardening artifacts occur because of CM inflow are the superior vena cava, inferior vena cava, and the subclavian vein.

Solution to exercise 7 (p. 48): 3 Points

Fractures, inflammatory processes, and tumors or metastases can cause swelling of mucous membranes and retention of fluids in the mastoid sinuses and middle ear; these are normally filled with air.

Solution to exercise 8 (p. 57): 18 Points

This image requires careful study. You will discover several types of intracranial hemorrhage and the complications resulting from them.

- Bruising of the left frontoparietal soft tissues (extracranial, indicative of trauma to the head) — 1
- Subdural hematoma over the right hemisphere extending to occipital levels (hyperdense) — 2
- Edema in the right frontoparietal areas, possibly accompanied by an epidural hematoma — 2
- Signs of subarachnoid bleeding in several sulci in parietal areas on the right, adjacent to the falx — 2
- The hematoma has penetrated into the right lateral ventricle, which is practically obliterated — 4
- Choroid plexus in the left lateral ventricle appears normal — 1
- There is a midline shift toward the left, and edema surrounds the periventricular white matter on the right — 2
- Raised intracranial pressure (obstructed ventricle) and herniation of the brain (edema) can be expected — 4

Solution to exercise 9 (p. 72): 9 Points

Gray and white matter appear well defined on narrow brain windows.

	Level	Width	Gray scale	
	+ 35 HU	80 HU	- 5 HU to + 75 HU	3

CCT sections are normally oriented parallel to the orbitomeatal line, | 2

so that initial and follow-up studies can be precisely compared. | 2

2-mm sections at 4-mm increments are acquired through the petrosal bone, | 2

then thickness and table movement are set at 8 mm. | 2

Solution to exercise 10 (p. 72): 16 Points

Intracerebral hemorrhage	in early phases hyperdense, often with hypodense peripheral edema	2
Subarachnoid hemorrhage	hyperdense blood instead of hypodense CSF in the sulci and cisterns	2
Subdural hemorrhage	hyperdense crescentic area close to the calvaria, concave toward the cortex, not limited by cranial sutures	4
Epidural hemorrhage	hyperdense, biconvex area close to the calvaria, smooth toward the cortex, always limited by cranial sutures	4
Complications	hemorrhage into a ventricle, CSF flow is obstructed, edema, danger of herniation	4

Solution to exercise 11 (p. 72): 2 Points

Subarachnoid hemorrhage in children may be visible only next to the falx or in the lateral (Sylvian) fissure.

Solution to exercise 12 (p. 72): 10 Points

Practice makes perfect!

Solution to exercise 13 (p. 72): 4 Points

Fracture of the right frontal bone and absent right frontal sinus (the latter is a congenital variation, not a hemorrhage, as indicated by the osseous trabeculae)

Solution to exercise 14 (p. 72): 8 Points

This was a difficult question. In the left internal jugular vein there is unusual sedimentation of the CM due to slow blood flow. The asymmetry of the jugular veins is not a sign of thrombosis. A left cervical abscess makes the neck muscles appear poorly defined.

Solution to exercise 15 (p. 73): 4 Points

In this patient the surface subarachnoid spaces are clearly too narrow and the ventricles distended. These signs indicate that CSF drainage is reduced or blocked and there is imminent danger of brain herniation. There is generalized brain edema. A neurosurgeon should be consulted about inserting an intraventricular shunt.

Solution to exercise 16 (p. 73): 3 Points

It is possible to mistake the subarachnoid hemorrhage around the left frontal lobe as an artifact. The left frontal cortex is outlined by blood. If you did not see any abnormality, return to the chapter about the head.

Solution to exercise 17 (p. 73): 6 Points

You have of course taken the hint about not giving up too soon; the right medial rectus muscle (**47c**) is thickened. It is the second muscle to become involved in endocrine ophthalmopathy.

If you cannot remember which muscle is affected first, return to page 61.

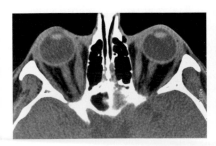
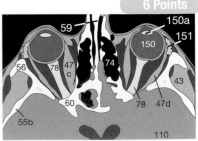

Fig. 222.1a   Fig. 222.1b

12 Points

Part of the question was misleading, but this was intentional, and I hope you take it in the right spirit. No fresh intracranial bleeding can be seen in this image (Fig. 73.4 is the same as Fig. 223.1). The abnormality in the left frontal lobe is an area of reduced attenuation representing an earlier hemorrhage (**180**) which has now reached the resorption phase (4 points). The extracranial swelling and bruising in the left frontoparietal area (1 point) is also 2 weeks old. In order to determine the nature of the hyperdense foci, particularly on the right side, you should of course ask to see adjacent images (4 points).

The next caudal section (Fig. 223.2) shows that these foci are formed by the orbital roofs (✳), the sphenoid bone (**60**), and the petrosal bone (✳✳) (1 point for each). These partial volume effects were discussed on page 53. If you misinterpreted them in the question, take it as a warning and you will be less likely to make this mistake again.

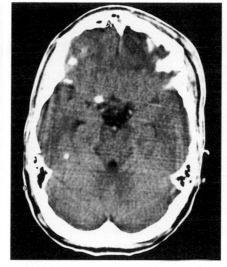

Fig. 223.1a

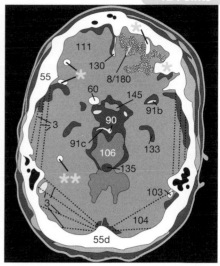

Fig. 223.1b

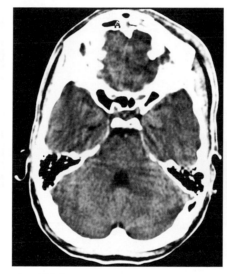

Fig. 223.2a

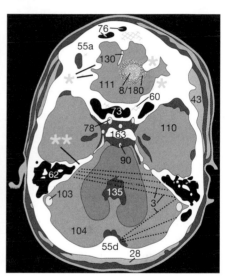

Fig. 223.2b

13 Points

Compare your checklist for CCT with the one on page 74.
As In exercise 1, each item is worth $1/2$ point and the correct sequence is worth 3 points.

4 Points

There is an area of low attenuation due to incomplete CM filling in the azygos vein, most likely because of a thrombosis (2 points). The esophagus is not well defined. There are hypodense lines crossing the pulmonary trunk and right pulmonary artery which are artifacts because they extend beyond the lumen of the vessels (2 points).

4 Points

Did you suggest doing bronchioscopy or biopsy in order to know more about the "lesion"? Then you must revisit the basic rules of CT interpretation. But if you remembered to look first of all at the other images in the series, as for example the one on the right, you will have seen that the "lesion" belongs to the sterno-clavicular joint (↖).
This is another example of a partial volume effect. There is degenerative change in this joint, but no pulmonary lesion or inflammation.

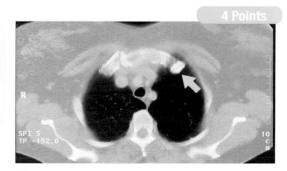

Fig. 223.3

Solution to exercise 22 (p. 100):

The cause of sudden back pain in this patient was the dissection (**172**) of the aortic aneurysm (1 point). At this level, both the ascending (**89 a**) and the descending (**89 c**) aorta (1 point each) show a dissection flap. It is a de Bakey type I dissection (1 point).

4 Points

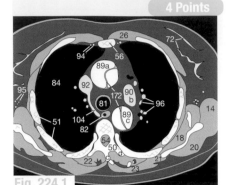

Fig. 224.1

Solution to exercise 23 (p. 100):

This is a case of bronchial carcinoma (the bronchial obstruction is not seen at this level). There is atelectasis of the entire left lung (**84**) (2 points) and an effusion (**8**) fills the pleural spaces (2 points). Did you detect the metastatic mediastinal LN (**6**)? (2 points).

6 Points

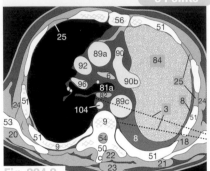

Fig. 224.2

Solution to exercise 24 (p. 101):

The most obvious abnormality is the bronchial carcinoma (**7**) in the left lung. The right lung shows emphysematous bullae (**176**). CT-guided biopsy of the tumor should be possible without causing a pneumothorax because it has a broad pleural base (2 points).

6 Points

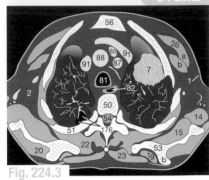

Fig. 224.3

Solution to exercise 25 (p. 101):

The small metal clip (**183**) is a hint that the stomach has been surgically transposed into the mediastinum. The thick-walled structure with the irregular lumen is a part of the stomach (**129**), not an esophageal tumor. At the moment of data acquisition the stomach was contracting and is therefore not as easily identified as in Figure 91.2.

4 Points

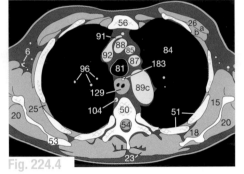

Fig. 224.4

Solution to exercise 26 (p. 101):

You are already familiar with this tragic case of bronchial carcinoma in a young pregnant woman (thus no CM enhancement, see Fig. 98.2). The anterior locule of the malignant effusion (3 points) had caused the right lung to collapse (2 points) and was therefore drained. After the fibrin clot had been removed from the catheter the lung was reinflated and the mother's life was prolonged until the birth of her healthy child. Did you notice the metastatic LN in the right axilla? (1 point)

6 Points

Solution to exercise 27 (p. 101):

6 Points

Perhaps the first thing you noticed was the irregular contour of the diaphragm (**30**) (1 point), but this is a normal finding. The patient was a smoker and had complained of weight loss. You should first ask for lung windows in order to check for meta-

stases (**7**) or primary bronchial carcinoma (5 points). When a chest is examined, it should become your standard procedure to use both soft-tissue and lung windows (Fig. 224.5 a).

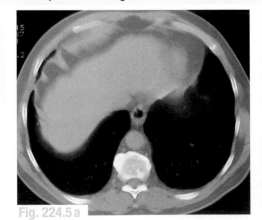

Fig. 224.5 a   Fig. 224.5 b

Solution to exercise 28 (p. 101):

6 Points

These two images show an aberrant branch of the aortic arch: The subclavian artery passes posterior to the trachea and the esophagus toward the right side of the body. You may remember that this anatomic variation was mentioned, but not shown, on page 120.

In addition to the air–fluid levels in the dilated bowel (2 points) associated with an ileus, you should have seen the dilated right ureter anterior to the psoas muscle (2 points). The correct diagnosis is therefore ileus and hydronephrosis. You may recognize this particular case as the same one shown in Figure 127.2, at a slightly more cranial level.

This is a case of left inguinal hernia (**177**) (1 point). There are normal LN bilaterally (**6**) (1 point). Did you identify the femoral artery (**119**), the profunda femoris artery (**199a**), the femoral vein (**120**), the deep femoral vein, and the gluteal vessels (**162**) (1 point each)?

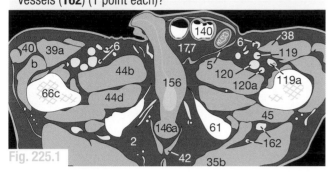

Fig. 225.1

You should have seen the adenoma (**134**) in the right adrenal gland (2 points). For $1/2$ point each you should be able to name ten other organs. Consult the number legends if you are uncertain.

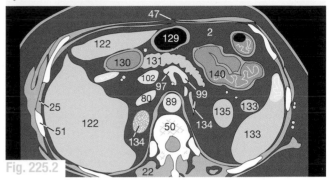

Fig. 225.2

This is indeed a case of situs inversus (2 points). You will also have noticed that the attenuation of the liver (**122**) is abnormally low: fatty liver (2 points).

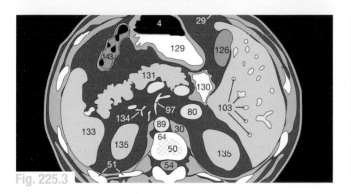

Fig. 225.3

The question itself will have drawn your attention to the atherosclerotic plaques (**174**) in the common iliac arteries (**113**) (1 point). The left one is part of an aortic aneurysm (2 points).

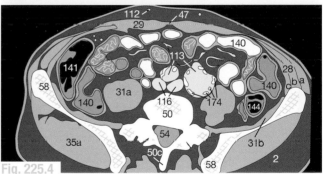

Fig. 225.4

Hopefully you saw the fairly large, irregular metastasis (**7**) in the posterior segment of the liver (**122**) (1 point). Did you also see the smaller, more anterior metastasis? (3 points). The DD may have included an atypical hepatic cyst (1 point) or, for the anterior lesion, partial volume averaging of the falciform ligament (1 point).

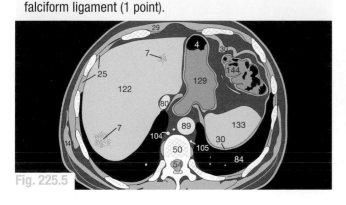

Fig. 225.5

The two cysts (**169**) in the right kidney (**135**) are impossible to miss (1 point). But there are also multiple, hypodense lesions in the spleen (**133**), due to splenic candidiasis (3 points). You may also have considered a rare case of nodular lymphoma or melanoma metastases in the spleen ($1/2$ point each).

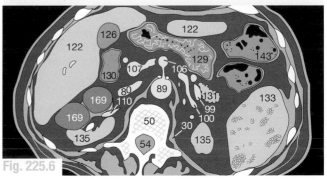

Fig. 225.6

Solution to exercise 36 (p. 150): **6 Points**

Figure 226.1 is the section next to the one in Figure 150.1 and shows that the hypodense area in the liver is the gallbladder. If you suggested doing anything else, for example aspiration or biopsy, before seeing adjacent sections, take 3 points away.

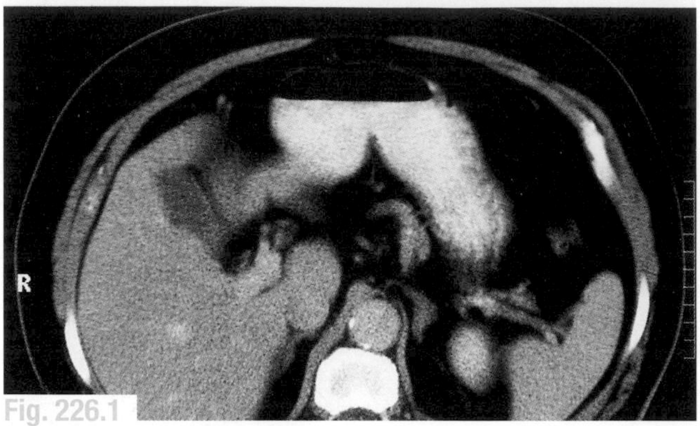

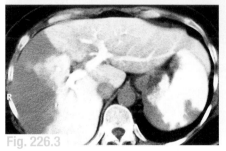

Fig. 226.1

Solution to exercise 37 (p. 150): **5 Points**

You may have thought that the hyperdense foci next to the rectum (**146**) represent calcified LN (**6**) (1 point). However, the lymphatics are so well demarcated because they are still opacified after lymphography (3 points). Did you also notice the atherosclerotic plaques (**174**) in the femoral arteries (**119**) (1 point)?

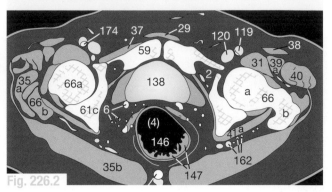

Fig. 226.2

Solution to exercise 38 (p. 150): **3 Points**

You will achieve the most accurate densitometry of a cyst if you select a section without any partial volume effects from renal parenchyma as in Figure 150.3b (1 point). Results of measurements in Figure 150.3a would be too high (2 points). Since this very case was discussed on page 133, take away 2 points for the incorrect answer.

Solution to exercise 39 (p. 150): **7 Points**

The illustration showed only one metastasis in the right lobe of the liver (1 point) in a case of hepatomegaly (1 point). By using triphasic SCT, additional metastases become visible (2 points). CT arterial portography (3 points) is more invasive than SCT alone, but it demonstrated that the spleen also has metastases.

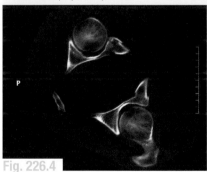

Fig. 226.3

Solution to exercise 40 (p. 150): **6 Points**

For further documentation you should ask to see bone windows (2 points) and of course the adjacent sections (2 points) in order to assess the pelvic fracture. It is also important to determine whether the acetabular fossa was involved (2 points). The fractures of the pubic bones were already visible on soft-tissue windows (Fig. 150.5) because the fragments were slightly displaced.

Fig. 226.4

Solution to exercise 41 (p. 151): **10 Points**

If you detected the fresh thrombosis (**173**) in the right femoral vein (**118**), you get 3 points. Did you also see the synovial cyst (**175**) on the left (3 points)? Your DD may have included a lymphoma, a femoral or inguinal hernia, or a metastasis (1 point each). If you mistook the cyst for thrombosis of the left femoral vein as well, take away 3 points! The vein (**118**) lies next to the cyst.

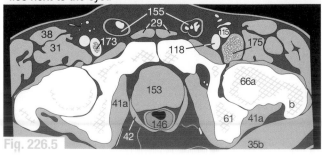

Fig. 226.5

Solution to exercise 42 (p. 151): **7 Points**

Another example of a partial volume effect: the sigmoid colon was only apparently "within" the urinary bladder (4 points). The first thing you should have asked to see was adjacent sections (2 points). You may remember that this case was discussed on page 116 (see Fig. 116.5a). There's also pararectal ascites (1 point).

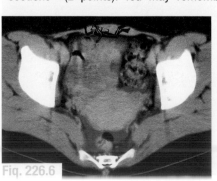

Fig. 226.6

Solution to exercise 43 (p. 151): **11 Points**

The beam-hardening artifacts (**3**) due to drainage tubes (**182**) were a hint that this image was taken shortly after surgery (2 points). The abnormal structures containing gases (**4**) are surgical packs (5 points) placed to control bleeding after multiple trauma. When the patient's condition had stabilized they would be removed in a second operation. Your DD may have included fecal impaction in Chilaiditi's syndrome (2 points) or an abscess with gas-forming bacteria (2 points).

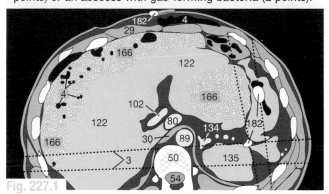
Fig. 227.1

Solution to exercise 44 (p. 151): **8 Points**

You may have thought that Figure 151.4 shows a gastric pullthrough for esophageal carcinoma (1 point) or that the esophageal walls are thickened due to metastases (2 points). However, this was a case of a paraesophageal sliding hiatus hernia (3 points). If you forgot to ask for lung windows, you will not have seen the large right paramediastinal emphysematous bulla (→) (2 points).

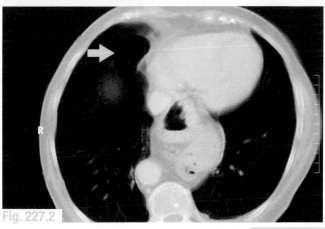
Fig. 227.2

Solution to exercise 45 (p. 151): **11 Points**

In Figure 151.5 a poorly defined tangential section of a diverticulum of the urinary bladder can be seen next to the rectum on the right side (✳) (5 points). Your DD may have included a pararectal LN (2 points). The irregularities in the attenuation values of the urine are due to CM and the 'jet phenomenon' (2 points each). Figures 227.3 and 227.4 are adjacent to Figure 151.5.

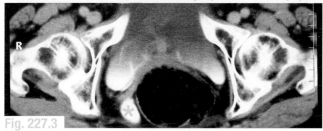
Fig. 227.3

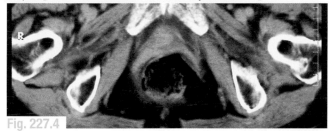
Fig. 227.4

Solution to exercise 46 (p. 151): **4 Points**

The same old problem! The hyperdense (enhanced) C-shaped structure in the pancreas (**131**) in Figures 151.6 or 227.5 is a loop of the splenic artery (**99**) (4 points). The adjacent sections (Fig. 227.5 c, d, and e) show that the splenic artery can be very tortuous.

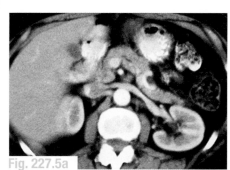
Fig. 227.5a

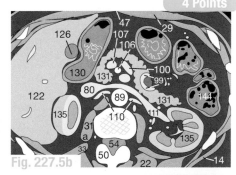
Fig. 227.5b

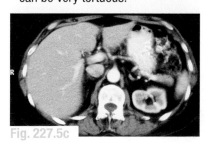
Fig. 227.5c

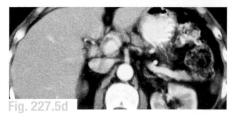
Fig. 227.5d

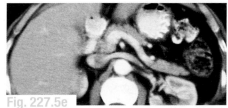
Fig. 227.5e

Solution to exercise 47–49 (p. 190): **6 Points**

A stenosis of the thoracic aorta is clearly identified (Fig. 190.1), as well as a thrombus in the right pulmonary vessels (Fig. 190.2) and an inflow effect of contrast medim into the superior vena cava as differential diagnosis of a genuine cava thrombosis (Fig. 190.3).

[1]   **Prokop M, Galanski M:** Spiral and Multislice Computed Tomography of the Body. Stuttgart, New York: Thieme, 2003.

[2]   **Lanfermann H, Raab P, Kretschmann HJ, et al:** Cranial Neuroimaging and Clinical Neuroanatomy. 4th ed. Stuttgart, New York: Thieme; 2019

[3]   **Burgener FA, Herzog C, Meyers S et al:** Differential Diagnosis in Computed Tomography. 2nd ed. Stuttgart, New York; Thieme; 2011

[4]   **Hosten N, Liebig T, Kirsch M et al:** Computertomographie von Kopf und Wirbelsäule. 2nd ed. Thieme, Stuttgart 2006

[5]   **Stäbler A, Ertl-Wagner B, Hartmann M:** Radiologie-Trainer Kopf und Hals. 3rd ed. Thieme, Stuttgart 2019

[6]   **Duerck JL, Pattany PM:** Analysis of imaging axes significance in flow and motion. Magn. Reson Med 7 (1989): 251

[7]   **Laub G:** Displays for MR angiography. Magn Reson Med 14 (1990): 222-229

[8]   **Boehm I, Lombardo P: Letter to the Editor:** How to document adverse reactions induced by gadolinium based contrast agents? A plea for type A and type B reactions. Eur Radiol. (2020);30: 1755-1756

[9a]   **Thumma S, Manchala V, Mattana J:** Radiocontrast-Induced Thyroid Storm. Am J Ther. (2019);26: e644-e645

[9b]   **Woeber KA:** Iodine and thyroid disease. Med Clin North Am. (1991);75:169-78

[9c]   **Kornelius E, Chiou JY, Yang YS et al:** Iodinated Contrast Media-Induced Thyroid Dysfunction in Euthyroid Nodular Goiter Patients. Thyroid. (2016);26: 1030-8

[10a]   **Brundridge W, Perkins J:** Iodinated Contrast Administration Resulting in Cardiogenic Shock in Patient with Uncontrolled Graves' Disease. J Emerg Med. (2017);53: e125-e128

[10b]   **Brabant G:** Clinical relevance of new normative data for TSH. MMW Fortschr Med 2010, 152: 37-39

[10c]   **Barbesino G:** Drugs affecting thyroid function. Thyroid 2010, 20: 763-770

[11]   **European Society of Urogenital Radiology:** ESUR Guidelines on Contrast Agents. Version 10.0. http://www.esur.org/esur-guidelines/ Accessed Nov, 2020

[12a]   **Kornelius E, Chiou JY, Yang YS et al:** Iodinated Contrast Media Increased the Risk of Thyroid Dysfunction: A 6-Year Retrospective Cohort Study. J Clin Endocrinol Metab. (2015);100: 3372-9

[12b]   **Hsieh MS, Chiu CS, Chen WC et al:** Iodinated Contrast Medium Exposure During Computed Tomography Increase the Risk of Subsequent Development of Thyroid Disorders in Patients Without Known Thyroid Disease: A Nationwide Population-Based, Propensity Score-Matched, Longitudinal Follow-Up Study. Medicine (Baltimore), (2015);94: e2279

[13a]   **Kusirisin P, Chattipakorn SC, Chattipakorn N:** Contrast-induced nephropathy and oxidative stress: mechanistic insights for better interventional approaches. J Transl Med. (2020);18: 400

[13b]   **Oloko A, Talreja H, Davis A et al:** Does Iodinated Contrast Affect Residual Renal Function in Dialysis Patients? A Systematic Review and Meta-Analysis. Nephron. (2020);144: 176-184

[13c]   **Levey AS et al.:** For the Chronic Kidney Disease Epidemiology Collaboration (CKD-EPI). A New Equation to Estimate Glomerular Filtration Rate. Ann Intern Med. 2009; 150: 604-612

[13d]   **Mosteller RD.** Simplified calculation of body-surface area. NEJM 1987; 317: 1098-9

[14a]   **Jung J, Cho YY, Jung JH et al:** Are patients with mild to moderate renal impairment on metformin or other oral anti-hyperglycaemic agents at increased risk of contrast-induced nephropathy and metabolic acidosis after radiocontrast exposure? Clin Radiol. (2019);74: 651.e1-651.e6

[14b]   **Boehm I, Morelli J, Nairz K et al:** Beta blockers and intravenous roentgen contrast materials: Which risks do exist? Eur J Intern Med. (2016);35: e17-e18

[14c]   **Böhm I, Morelli J, Nairz K et al:** Myths and misconceptions concerning contrast media-induced anaphylaxis: a narrative review. Postgrad Med. (2017);129: 259-66

[15a]   **Katayama H, Yamaguchi K, Kozuka T et al.:** Adverse reactions to ionic and nonionic contrast media. A report from the Japanese Committee on the Safety of Contrast Media. Radiology (1990);175: 621–8

[15b]   **Böhm I, Heverhagen JT, Klose KJ:** Classification of acute and delayed contrast media-induced reactions: proposal of a three-step system. Contrast Media Mol Imaging. (2012);7:537-41

[15c]   **Böhm I:** Three Important Points on the Documentation of Contrast Hypersensitivity Reactions to Improve Contrast Medium Safety. J Am Coll Radiol. (2020);17:207

[15d]   **Böhm I:** Limited duration of hypersensitivity reactions to contrast and exact documentation of such adverse events. Reg Anesth Pain Med. (2020);45: 246

[15e]   **Böhm I, Nairz K, Morelli JN et al:** Iodinated Contrast Media and the Alleged „Iodine Allergy": An Inexact Diagnosis Leading to Inferior Radiologic Management and Adverse Drug Reactions. Röfo. (2017);189: 326-32

[15f]   **Böhm I, Hasembank Keller PS, Heverhagen JT.** „Iodine Allergy" - The Neverending Story. Röfo. (2016);188: 733-4

[15g]   **Böhm I, Alfke H, Klose KJ.** Hypersensitivity reactions and contrast medium injection: are they always related? Eur J Radiol. (2011);80: 368-72

[16a]   **Tramer MR, von Elm E, Loubeyre P et al:** Pharmacological prevention of serious anaphylactic reactions due to iodinated contrast media: systematic review. BMJ. (2006); 333:675

[16b]   **Böhm IB:** Lower dose and lower injection speed of iodinated contrast media: a new strategy to reduce the incidence rate of immediate hypersensitivity reactions. Quant Imaging Med Surg. (2020);10: 883-5

[17]   **Van Leeuwen MS, Noordzij J, Feldberg MA et al:** Focal liver lesions: characterization with triphasic spiral CT. Radiology. (1996); 201: 327-36

[18a]   **Boehm I, Morelli J, Nairz K et al:** Risks of contrast media applied via the gastrointestinal route. Eur J Intern Med. (2017);42: e19-e21

[18b]   **Meindl TM, Hagl E, Reiser MF et al:** Comparison of 2 different protocols for ingestion of low-attenuating oral contrast agent for multidetector computed tomography of the abdomen. J Comput Assist Tomogr. (2007);31: 218-22

[18c]   **Mazzeo S, Caramella D, Belcari A et al:** Multidetector CT of the small bowel: evaluation after oral hyperhydration with isotonic solution. Radiol Med. (2005);109: 516-26

For further references [19] – [37] , please see back cover flap.